D0321849

ONDON HOSPIT
COLLEGE

OPPENHEIMER'S
DIAGNOSTIC NEUROPATHOLOGY

Oppenheimer's
Diagnostic Neuropathology
A PRACTICAL MANUAL

MARGARET M. ESIRI MA, DM, FRCPath
Clinical Reader in Neuropathology, The Radcliffe Infirmary, and
Professional Fellow, St Hugh's College, Oxford

FOREWORD BY
L.J. RUBINSTEIN

SECOND EDITION

**Blackwell
Science**

© 1989, 1996 by
Blackwell Science Ltd
Editorial Offices:
Osney Mead, Oxford OX2 0EL
25 John Street, London WC1N 2BL
23 Ainslie Place, Edinburgh EH3 6AJ
238 Main Street, Cambridge
    Massachusetts 02142, USA
54 University Street, Carlton
    Victoria 3053, Australia

Other Editorial Offices:
Arnette Blackwell SA
    224, Boulevard Saint Germain
    75007 Paris, France

Blackwell Wissenschafts-Verlag GmbH
    Kurfürstendamm 57
    10707 Berlin, Germany

    Zehetnergasse 6
    A-1140 Wien
    Austria

First published 1989
Second edition 1996

Set by Excel Typesetters, Hong Kong
Printed and bound in Italy
by Rotolito Lombarda SpA, Milan

The Blackwell Science logo is a
trade mark of Blackwell Science Ltd,
registered at the United Kingdom
Trade Marks Registry

DISTRIBUTORS

Marston Book Services Ltd
PO Box 269
Abingdon
Oxon OX14 4YN
(*Orders:* Tel: 01235 465500
          Fax: 01235 465555)

USA
Blackwell Science, Inc.
238 Main Street
Cambridge, MA 02142
(*Orders:* Tel: 800 215-1000
          617 876-7000
          Fax: 617 492-5263)

Canada
Copp Clark, Ltd
2775 Matheson Blvd East
Mississauga, Ontario
Canada, L4W 4P7
(*Orders:* Tel: 800 263-4374
          905 238-6074)

Australia
Blackwell Science Pty Ltd
54 University Street
Carlton, Victoria 3053
(*Orders:* Tel: 03 9347 0300
          Fax: 03 9349 3016)

A catalogue record for this title
is available from the British Library

ISBN 0-86542-915-4

Library of Congress
Cataloging-in-Publication Data

Esiri, Margaret M.
    Oppenheimer's diagnostic neuropathology :
    a practical manual/
    Margaret M. Esiri ;
    foreword by L. J. Rubinstein. — 2nd ed.
        p.   cm.
    Rev. ed. of: Diagnostic
    neuropathology. 1989.
    Includes bibliographical references
    and index.
    ISBN 0-86542-915-4
    1. Nervous system—Pathophysiology.
    2. Nervous system—Diseases—Diagnosis.
    I. Oppenheimer, D. R. (David Richard)
    II. Esiri, Margaret M.
    Diagnostic neuropathology.   III. Title.
    [DNLM: 1. Nervous System Diseases—
    pathology.   WL 100 E75o   1996]
    RC347.E84 1996
    616.8'047—dc20
    DNLM/DLC
    for Library of Congress   95–18625
                                              CIP

Contents

Foreword to the First Edition

Textbooks of neuropathology, like people and microglia, generally appear in one of two forms: thin and lean; or fat and crammed. The former are designed to sketch the bare bones of the subject for the otherwise overburdened medical student. The latter, replete with minutiae, are addressed to the practitioner already experienced in the field.

Rarer are those books which fall between these extremes and in which the balance between the skeletal outline and a profusion of details has been carefully adjusted, and the mixture blended with art. The present manual, authored by Drs Esiri and Oppenheimer, fits the description. The writers, whose experience is based on the extensive neuropathological material examined at the Radcliffe Infirmary at Oxford, have combined forces to share their considerable, and complementary, skills. The product of this labour of love is an exemplary model of what a specialized textbook should be.

What does this book supply, and to whom is it addressed? Obviously it is too detailed for the medical student. The authors state that it is chiefly aimed at the apprentice in neuropathology and at the general pathologist with, as they say, 'an interest'. They view its purpose as largely practical rather than systematic. They are too modest by half; I should predict that by reason of its unusual features and because of the manner in which it has been conceived and executed it will find its place on the shelves of even the most seasoned neuropathologist.

This work, understatingly labelled 'a practical manual', but in which so much reflection and wisdom has gone into the making of it, has, first, all the requirements that make it a reliable guide. It is abundantly and clearly illustrated, contains many apposite diagrams and tables, furnishes selected references at the end of each chapter and provides a wealth of useful recommendations. These include the types of neural tissue to be secured and reserved after consultation of the clinical notes; discussions on the problems of brain biopsies and on the brain smear technique; a timely review of the immunoreactivities of brain tumours based on a wide panel of antibodies; precautions to be taken in slow virus diseases; and of course the expected tabulated lists of metabolic central and peripheral nervous system disorders. The clinical neurological correlations that can be established with the sites and the nature of the neuropathological changes, both gross and microscopic, or with the localization of selective cell losses are succinctly, but comprehensively presented. But perhaps the most innovative aspects are the special features that cannot usually be found in comparable texts: not only an emphasis on an interpretative approach that closely correlates the clinical neurological picture and the pathological findings but separate chapters on the aetiology of epilepsy, on the diverse neuropathology of the very young, on a large number of different malfunctions that may involve the central and the peripheral nervous systems and on which neuropathological data are often scanty or incomplete, even on sundry but relevant matters such as the ceremony of brain cutting, advice on how to avoid reporting delays, suggestions on the manner of reporting, and counselling on the relationships to be maintained with one's colleagues and one's laboratory staff. The candour with which the advice is given, and these points made, should endear both neuropathology and the authors to even the least sympathetic reader.

Thus the contents, spirit and tone of this manual belie the austerity of its title. The writing is cheerful, alert and graceful, not devoid of its wry touches—even where it examines some of the causes of head injury, when the reader will momentarily muse on the dangers attending the fall of coconuts in the groves of Papua. The authors persistently ask questions, often leaving them unanswered, but always pointing the way to further questions and, sometimes, to possible solutions. Bearing the fruits of personal experience, this book counsels a modesty which is becoming to a relatively esoteric specialty. But it exudes the pleasure of problem-solving and breathes the joy of neuropathology.

L.J. Rubinstein
University of Virginia

Preface to the Second Edition

It must be a source of pleasure to most authors, as it was to me, to be invited to prepare a second edition of a book. It suggests that the original aims have at least approximately been met, to the extent that sufficient copies of the original have been sold to hold out a prospect of a further edition being worth the time and effort to prepare.

In the case of *Diagnostic Neuropathology* the invitation to prepare a second edition came after its senior author, David Oppenheimer, had died. The publishers and I have decided to alter the title of the book to *Oppenheimer's Diagnostic Neuropathology* in affectionate recognition that his hand and mind are indelibly stamped on the book, both through his own contributions to it and through his influence as mentor and guide on me.

In preparing this edition I have retained almost all the original text, altering it only to incorporate new information or to attempt to make points clearer. The main alterations to the book lie in the illustrations. Some of those I have tried to improve on and many of them now appear in colour. I hope readers will agree that this enhances the impact of the photographs and aids interpretation as well as giving a more telling hint of the aesthetic pleasures of neurohistology.

Another major addition in this new edition is the many magnetic resonance imaging (MRI) illustrations corresponding to the pathological specimens. This serves to provide the neuropathologist with an introduction to MRI and emphasizes the excellent anatomical information that is achieved by this imaging technique. MRI is sensitive and optimally delineates disease extent in the central nervous system. Additionally, MRI is capable of imaging in any plane and the coronal and axial scans correlate well with the actual brain slices obtained in the pathology laboratory.

The book is offered as a guide to those pathologists, neurologists, neurosurgeons and neuroradiologists sufficiently intrigued by neuropathology to want to understand it better and to those who wish to practice it themselves.

In addition to the works of reference listed in the preface to the first edition, the following books are recommended.

Adams JH, Duchen LW (Eds). 1992. *Greenfield's Neuropathology*, 5th edn. Edward Arnold, London.

Brodal P. 1992. *The Central Nervous System: Structure and Formation*. Oxford University Press, Oxford.

Carpenter MB. 1991. *Core Text of Neuroanatomy*, 4th edn. Williams and Wilkins Ltd.

Williams PL, Warwick R, Dyson M *et al.* (Eds). 1989. *Gray's Anatomy*, 37th edn. Churchill Livingstone, Edinburgh.

Paxinos G (Ed). 1990. *Human Neuroanatomy*. Academic Press, New York, 859–1244.

Okazaki H, Scheithauer BW. 1988. *Atlas of Neuropathology*. Gower Medical Publishing, New York.

Schochet SS, Nelson J. 1989. *Atlas of Clinical Neuropathology*. Appleton and Large, Connecticut.

M.M. Esiri
Department of Neuropathology
Radcliffe Infirmary
Oxford, UK

Preface to the First Edition

Some years ago one of the authors of this book, as a junior neuropathologist, was accustomed to receiving from outside sources a succession of more or less damaged and distorted brains and spinal cords. Some of these had been sliced and diced into unrecognizable fragments in the post mortem room. Some were accompanied by an inch-square section of an unidentified part of the brain stained with haematoxylin and eosin. Sometimes an undistorted, well-fixed brain arrived, accompanied by a good set of clinical notes which made it clear that the main site of the patient's disorder lay in the spinal cord or peripheral nerves.

The recipient of these tantalizing specimens spoke of his frustrations to a fatherly, much respected, senior colleague, who was duly sympathetic. But when the young man spoke of his intention of writing a little pamphlet giving guidance to general pathologists on the handling of material from neurological cases, he was met with an alarming display of mock rage. 'You must do no such thing!' the old man thundered. 'If the priests reveal the mysteries of their craft to the multitude, what will become of them? If we allow the general pathologists to discover how simple our work is and how lacking in mystery, they will start doing it themselves, and we shall be out of a job.'

On reflection, we think the old man's fears were exaggerated. Many pathologists, we know, regard the nervous system and its diseases with distaste, or even fear, and are only too happy to unload the neurological material that comes their way, leaving more time to pursue the subjects that interest them. Others—especially those facing specialist examinations—are not averse to rounding off their general competence with a course of simple neuropathology. Yet others—and it is from these that the priesthood is mainly recruited—positively enjoy the subject; and it would be both selfish and impolitic to erect barriers to their initiation.

Of the two authors of this book, one underwent a preliminary indoctrination in general pathology, the other in clinical neurology and neuro-anatomy. In the course of 15 years or so of collaboration, often in different areas of the neuropathological field, each of us has profited from the effects of the other's apprenticeship, to the extent of acquiring at least a rough grasp of what the other was doing and thinking, and even, on occasion, offering useful criticism. In this, we think we have been more fortunate than many others.

With these and similar considerations in mind, we are presenting this book as a guide to neuropathological methods, aimed principally at apprentices in neuropathology and at general pathologists with, as they say, an interest. It consists partly of advice on how to avoid the embarrassment of being shown to have destroyed or thrown away the evidence which should have led to a diagnosis. It contains a certain amount of descriptive matter, which overlaps with the conventional textbooks of neuropathology; but it is not, and is not intended to be, comprehensive. On the other hand, there are places where we have included theoretical, or speculative, remarks, based on our own observations, on matters which tend to be neglected in standard textbooks of neuropathology. Nor is it systematic in the sense of being arranged in separate categories of disease—inflammatory, degenerative, neoplastic and so forth. The chapter headings correspond for the most part to the immediate questions facing the neuropathologist in the post mortem room, such as 'what had caused this patient's epilepsy?', 'why was he so weak?', or 'why, after what seemed to be a successful neurosurgical procedure, did he suddenly die?'

The title *Diagnostic Neuropathology* entails a brief explanation of what we mean by 'diagnosis'. In our view, to write 'multiple sclerosis' at the end of a post mortem report is not an adequate diagnosis, unless the report has expressed an opinion on how the patient's history, signs and symptoms are related to the lesions and to their distribution, severity and chronicity. Similarly, 'chromophobe adenoma of the pituitary' is an inadequate diagnosis unless the report gives an idea of the size, manner of growth and hormonal activity of the tumour, with a view of how it affected the patient's state, and why he is now dead.

We realize that our criteria for the adequacy of a diagnosis may seem too demanding of effort to some readers and too easily satisfied to others. If a line is to be drawn between 'routine diagnosis' and 'research', there is no agreed principle deciding where it should be drawn. In this book, we have proposed what seem to us reasonable standards for routine diagnosis, but make no claim to have arrived at a generally acceptable system. We would like to think that in areas of neuropathology in which the dividing line between routine diagnosis and research is particularly ill-defined, our comments may encourage our readers to contribute to further knowledge by systematic study of their own material. Regarding research, we have worked on the assumption that the user of this book will have some research interests, which will be based on material acquired in the course of his diagnostic work. He will also probably be called on to do some teaching at graduate or undergraduate level. We would ask our readers to bear these points in mind if at times they feel that our recommendations are unduly fussy and demanding of time and effort.

This book will inevitably contain some errors in presenting the facts, and some questionable recommendations. We, the perpetrators, would be very grateful for the help of readers who take the trouble to point out our shortcomings. Magnifications accompanying illustrations in the book are, we believe, accurate to within 10%.

A working knowledge of the basic anatomy of the nervous system, including its wrappings, is assumed throughout. For those in doubt, the following works of reference may be recommended:

Brodal A. 1981. *Neurological Anatomy in Relation to Clinical Medicine*, 3rd edn. Oxford University Press, Oxford.

Carpenter MD, Sutin J. 1983. *Human Neuroanatomy* (8th edn. of Strong OS, Elwyn A. *Human Neuroanatomy*). Williams and Wilkins, Baltimore and London.

For detailed descriptions of neuropathological states, we recommend:

Adams JH, Corsellis JAN, Duchen LW (Eds). 1984. *Greenfield's Neuropathology*, 4th edn. Edward Arnold, London.

Russell DS, Rubinstein LJ. 1989. *Pathology of Tumours of the Nervous System*, 5th edn. Edward Arnold, London.

Burger PC, Vogel FS. 1976. *Surgical Pathology of the Nervous System and its Coverings*. John Wiley, New York.

For more summary textbooks, we recommend:

Escourolle R, Poirier J. 1978. *Manual of Basic Neuropathology* (translated from the French by LJ Rubinstein). WB Saunders, Philadelphia.

Okazaki H. 1983. *Fundamentals of Neuropathology*, Igaku-Shoin, New York and Tokyo.

And for illustrated guides, the following:

Adams JH, Murray M. 1982. *Atlas of Post Mortem Techniques in Neuropathology*. Cambridge University Press, Cambridge.

Weller RO. 1984. *Colour Atlas of Neuropathology*. Oxford University Press, Oxford.

Barnard RO, Logue V, Reaves PS. 1976. *An Atlas of Tumours involving the Central Nervous System*. Baillière Tindall, London.

More specialized chapters, monographs and articles are referred to at the ends of the relevant chapters. In general, we have cited individual papers only when the information in them is not readily available in textbooks.

M.M. Esiri
D.R. Oppenheimer
Department of Neuropathology,
Radcliffe Infirmary,
Oxford, UK

Acknowledgements

I am particularly indebted to Dr Shelley Renowden and the radiographers of the Oxford MRI unit for the provision of the MRI scans that appear in the second edition.

For reading parts of the text in the first edition, and in many cases providing illustrations, I express my thanks to Drs M Al-Izzi, RO Barnard, JV Clark, F Cruz-Sanchez, P Da Costa, L Horton, JT Hughes, J Keeling, D McCormick, B McDonald, CS Morris, JH Morris, TH Moss, R Menai-Williams, M Rossi, A Sheehan and M Squier; and to Professors JB Cavanagh and B Lake.

For invaluable assistance in the preparation of figures, I thank Miss P Deacon, Miss J Dyer, Mr D Gardner, Mr J Haywood, Mr G Richardson and Mr D Webster.

For preparation of most of the material used for photomicrography I am deeply indebted to the late Mr R Beesley, Mr R Cross, Miss P Deacon, Miss H Kidd and Miss M Reading. Dr F Sheriff, Mr R Cross and Miss N Sullivan kindly assisted with the preparation of Appendix A.

For permission to reproduce figures or tables originally published in other books or journals, I wish to thank the editors and/or publishers of the following:

Books

Autonomic Failure, Ed. R Bannister, 2nd edn (1988), Oxford University Press, Oxford. (Figs 15.3, 15.5 and 15.6.)

Developmental Neuropathology, by R Friede (1975), Springer, Berlin. (Table 21.1.)

Development of the Human Brain by F Gilles, A Leviton and E Dooling (1983), PSG Publishing Company, Inc., Littleton, MA. (Table 21.2.)

Fetal and Neonatal Pathology, Ed. J Keeling (1987), Springer, Berlin. (Fig. 23.22.)

Gray's Anatomy, 36th edn (1980) Eds P Williams and R Warwick, Churchill Livingstone, Edinburgh. (Fig. 21.1.)

Greenfield's Neuropathology, 3rd edn (1976; Eds W Blackwood and JAN Corsellis) and 4th edn (1984; Eds JH Adams, JAN Corsellis and LW Duchen), Edward Arnold, London. (Figs 14.1, 15.1, 15.2, 15.12, 15.13, 15.14 and 15.18.)

Handbook of Clinical Neurology, vol. 37 (1979). Eds PJ Vinken and GW Bruyn. Elsevier/North-Holland, Amsterdam. (Figs 20.2–20.4.)

Muscle Biopsy: a Practical Approach, by V Dubowitz (1985), Baillière Tindall, London. (Tables 23.1 and 23.2.)

Pathology of Peripheral Nerve, by A Asbury and P Johnson (1978), WB Saunders, Philadelphia. (Fig. 22.2.)

Viral Encephalitis, by J Booss and M Esiri (1986), Blackwell Scientific Publications, Oxford. (Fig. 10.26.)

Journals

Acta Neuropathologica, Berlin (Figs 13.34 and 13.39). *AIDS* (Fig. 10.36). *Brain* (Figs 3.9, 15.8a).

International Journal of Leprosy (Fig. 22.17).

Journal of Neurology, Neurosurgery and Psychiatry (Figs 3.46, 15.1a and 22.5).

Journal of the Neurological Sciences (Figs 10.17, 10.18, 10.29, 15.19, 20.7 and 23.31).

Neuropathology and Applied Neurobiology (Fig. 2.21).

Quarterly Journal of Medicine (Figs 10.30, 10.32 and 10.34).

1   The Post Mortem

This chapter is concerned only with points where the recommended procedures for neurological cases differ from routine methods.

Removal of the brain

The usual procedure is to reflect the scalp, and remove a cap of bone by a circumferential saw-cut. If this is carefully done, the dura will not be damaged, and will remain covering the brain. At this stage the superior longitudinal sinus is tested for patency either by opening it or more simply by running a fingertip along it and observing any movement of the contained blood.

If the brain is to be fixed by suspension from the basilar artery (see p.7), the dura is incised on each side and reflected medially, cutting through the bridging veins with scissors or knife (if they are torn, they may give rise to a false appearance of subdural or subarachnoid bleeding). The anterior attachment of the falx is divided, and the dura is reflected backwards. If fixation is to be by suspension from the dura of the vertex, the bridging veins are left intact, and the falx is divided with scissors both in front and behind, i.e. it is separated from the crista galli in front and from the tentorium behind.

The frontal lobes are gently lifted away from the floor of the anterior cranial fossa, leaving the olfactory bulbs attached to the brain if possible. The optic nerves, internal carotid arteries, pituitary stalk and oculomotor nerves are cut cleanly across close to the base, as they come into view. The tentorium is exposed, first on one side then on the other, by gently lifting the temporal lobes; and the attachments of the tentorium to the petrous temporal bones are cut with a sharp knife. The same cut will sever the roots of the trigeminal, facial and auditory nerves as they pierce the dura. It is important at this stage to retract the cerebral hemispheres as little as possible, as overstretching very easily results in tearing the midbrain (Fig. 1.1).

In the gap which appears between the pons and the clivus, the abducent nerves are seen and cut. Not so clearly seen are the lower cranial nerves and the vertebral arteries, which are still holding the brain stem down. These must be cut, either with a knife or with long-bladed scissors, without damaging the lower brain stem. This can usually be carried out blind, but cutting as far as possible to each side. After the vertebral arteries have been cut the lower brain stem and upper cervical cord rise into view, and are cut across with the knife. All that remains to be cut after this is

Fig. 1.1 Appearance, after formalin fixation, of a midbrain which has been torn during removal of the brain. (This happened to be a case of Parkinson's disease, in which the histology of the substantia nigra of the midbrain is of prime interest.)

a number of bridging veins, including the great vein of Galen, which drains blood from the deeper cerebral grey matter into the straight sinus. During the whole performance, if the operator is holding the knife in his right hand, the brain should be supported by the left hand, and tension and distortion kept to a minimum. When the brain is free it should be placed, base upwards, in a suitably sized bowl rather than being laid on a flat surface.

There are many circumstances in which this routine has to be modified — too many, in fact, to be enumerated here. The most obvious ones are when the patient has undergone a neurosurgical operation. Often, of course, the neurosurgeon will welcome an invitation to come to the post mortem room and explore the outcome of his operation in person. In any case, it is important that the pathologist should have a clear grasp of what the surgeon has done, as well as of the clinical state before and after the operation. In cases where a ventriculo-atrial shunt has been carried out for the relief of obstructive hydrocephalus, it is best to explore the shunt mechanism before the cranium is opened. This entails finding the tube as it lies in the internal jugular vein (usually on the right side), cutting it, and testing the patency of the proximal and distal parts of the tube. Where there is a flushing device lying beneath the scalp overlying the burr-hole, a few squeezes should result in the escape of ventricular fluid from the proximal cut end.

In cases where high pressure in the posterior fossa has resulted in herniation of the lower medulla oblongata and cerebellar tonsils into the foramen magnum, the final severance of the brain from the spinal cord is hard to achieve without making an ugly oblique cut through the medulla itself; this, however, can usually be avoided by cautious manipulation. In any case, this cut, if it is performed from within the cranial cavity, will be an oblique one, reaching a lower level at the back of the cord than in front. If for some reason it is desirable to make a detailed anatomical study of structures near the junction of cord and medulla, it is best to make a *transverse* cut through the cord at the desired level before removing the brain.

Special care is needed in taking out *infants' brains*. Not only is the brain tissue itself softer and more friable but the leptomeninges are also very delicate; it is only too easy to drive an injudicious thumb through the cerebral cortex, or even to wipe a considerable area of cortex away from the rest of the brain. In some centres, the dangers of manipulation are reduced by removing the brain under water.

Preliminary inspection of the brain

If any serious anatomical study is contemplated, the brain should not be sliced before fixation. Because of the soft, soufflé-like consistency of the unfixed brain, it is impossible to make clean parallel cuts through it; when fresh-cut slices are fixed their surfaces are found to be irregular, wavy and pitted (Fig. 1.2). Unless a diagnosis is urgently needed, the examination of the brain at post mortem should be confined to significant surface features — in particular, features associated with brain swelling, such as flattening of cerebral convolutions and marks of tentorial or foraminal herniation (see p.9). Cautious palpation may disclose softenings due to infarction or tumour, or less often hardenings due to tumours, or to scarring, or to oddities such as tuberous sclerosis. Such hardenings are much more difficult to detect after fixation.

A firm diagnosis of *multiple sclerosis* (MS) can often be made without cutting into the brain, from the presence of clearly-defined grey patches on the surface of the pons, or on the cut surfaces of the optic nerves (Fig. 14.1).

The presence of frank pus in the subarachnoid space clearly calls for swabs and specimens for bacteriology. In cases of subacute or chronic meningitis the changes are generally far less striking, and to the naked eye may be identical with those of diffuse malignant spread. In case of doubt, a couple of wet films stained with, say, methylene blue and Gram's stain, will quickly make the distinction (for method, see p.80).

Blood in the subarachnoid space is best cleared away before fixation (see p.114), after noting where it seems to be coming from — a contused surface, or a ruptured aneurysm, or the exit foramina of the fourth ventricle. Aneurysms, in particular, should be dissected free of their surroundings while the vessels from which they arise are still supple.

In cases of proven or suspected *meningitis* or *encephalitis*, and in various other conditions, one may wish to collect samples of cerebrospinal fluid (CSF), preferably uncontaminated by blood. Clear CSF may be obtained, before removal of the brain, by aspiration with a hollow needle from an anterior or posterior horn of a lateral ventricle. However, if the hemispheres are swollen, this may be both ineffectual and disruptive. Ventricular fluid may be obtained from the fourth ventricle by gentle compression of the brain, and subarachnoid fluid from the pre-pontine space when the lower cranial nerves are being cut across, or from the spinal subarachnoid space by tilting the lower spinal column upward after the brain is removed.

Dissection of the skull

After removing the brain, and noting any abnormalities in the dura at the base of the cranial cavity, the principal venous sinuses (straight, lateral, sigmoid, superior longitudinal) are checked for patency. In cases of head injury the dura is stripped to reveal fractures at the base of the skull. For examining the internal carotid arteries, and at the same time the ear-drums and middle ears, a hammer and a 2 cm chisel are used. The chisel is applied to the floor of the middle cranial fossa at the point shown in Fig. 1.3; a sharp

(a)

(b)

Fig. 1.2 Appearance, after fixation, of brain which has been sliced fresh.

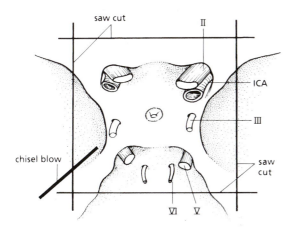

Fig. 1.3 Removal of sphenoid block, using the vibrating saw. For the anterior cut, the saw is directed downward and backward; for the lateral cuts, downward and medially; and for the posterior cut, forward through the clivus. If the cuts are deep enough, the block is easily detached. The thicker line on the left of the picture indicates the site where a chisel blow will expose the carotid canal and the middle ear, displacing the ridge of the petrous temporal bone backward. ICA = internal carotid artery; II = optic nerve; III = oculomotor nerve; V = trigeminal nerve; VI = abducent nerve. The block includes the pituitary gland, the cavernous sinus and the gasserian (trigeminal) ganglia.

blow with the hammer will then display the middle ear and ear-drum, and the internal carotid artery lying within the carotid canal, whence it can be followed into the wall of the cavernous sinus. The frontal and ethmoidal sinuses (and after removal of the pituitary, the sphenoid sinus) are similarly opened and displayed.

A specimen containing the *pituitary* and portions of the second to sixth *cranial nerves*, including the gasserian ganglia, can be obtained with a de Soutter vibrating saw, applied in the planes indicated in Fig. 1.3. The block can be fixed and dissected at leisure, with the anatomical relations perfectly preserved. A more thorough examination of the *optic nerves* is desirable in cases with a suspected diagnosis of MS. For this, the simplest procedure is to remove the thin bony roofs of the orbits with bone forceps and nibblers, incise the soft tissues anteriorly, and cut carefully down until the eyeball is reached. The optic nerve is severed just behind the globe, and the remaining orbital contents are dissected away from the globe and from the bone of the orbit, back to the optic foramen. The specimen containing optic nerve, external ocular muscles, oculomotor nerve and ciliary ganglion, all embedded in fat, can be fixed for later dissection, with very little distortion.

Removal of the spinal cord

If this is to be performed in the post mortem room, the cord can be approached either from behind or from the front.

For the *posterior approach*, the sacrospinal muscle mass is cleared away from neck to sacrum and the exposed vertebral laminae are sawn through, using either an electric vibrating saw, which is quicker, or a hand-saw, which is very much safer if the cord is not to be damaged. Directions for the saw-cuts are shown in Fig. 1.4. The cuts are directed forward and slightly inward, starting about 2 cm from the midline on each side. A rather narrower margin is adequate for the thoracic region. Provided that the spine is straight and symmetrical, the result will be that a bony strip, consisting of the vertebral spines and the medial halves of the laminae, will lift backward, leaving the spinal dura (theca) exposed. If the saw-cuts are too lateral, the bone will need to be cut away with bone shears—a safe but laborious procedure. If the saw-cuts are too medial, the

saw will make its embarrassing way into the substance of the cord. If, as often happens, there is some degree of scoliosis, there is a danger of entering the cord on one side while failing to enter the spinal canal on the other. If X-rays are available, they may help in avoiding this mishap.

When the theca is exposed, a decision must be made as to whether any *sensory ganglia* need to be examined (for instance, particular ganglia require to be looked at in cases of herpes zoster). These can be found in the intervertebral foramina by exploration with knife and nibbler, and left attached to the cord by their nerve roots. In a case of tabes dorsalis or of Friedreich's ataxia, several lumbar and cervical ganglia should be preserved. In extracting the cord, the main concern should be to avoid undue kinking, which alone can cause considerable damage. The lower end of the theca can be secured with artery forceps, and the cord lifted gently backwards, cutting nerve roots on each side from below upward. After extraction the cord must not be curled up or subjected to pressure. If its length makes fixation difficult, it should be divided into two or even three sections by clean transverse knife-cuts made after opening the dura; cutting the cord within the dura will cause damage by compression.

The other standard method of removing the cord is *from in front*, after clearing away the thoracic and abdominal viscera. If it is desired to examine the sympathetic chains, this is the moment to remove them. They come into view after stripping away the pleura and peritoneum, running up and down at the level of the exit foramina of the spinal nerves. Saw-cuts are made immediately in front of these, in a coronal plane. These cuts, if well placed, will expose the anterior surface of the dura as well as numerous nerve-roots and ganglia. This anterior approach is preferable if multiple spinal ganglia are wanted. It also entails less risk of damage to the cord than the posterior approach.

An alternative to both these methods is to *remove the entire vertebral column* and extract the spinal cord after fixation. The approach is from the front. Oblique saw-cuts are made, separating the sacrum from the iliac bones, and through the vertebral ends of the ribs. The vertebral column is lifted forward, and separated from the skin of the back with a long knife. Finally, it is detached from the skull with knife-cuts through the atlanto-occipital joints. This involves inserting the sharp tip of a stout knife into these joints at just the right point and just the right angle. The manoeuvre requires skill and practice. The young pathologist, if in a hurry, is well advised to leave the joints in peace and saw blithely through the atlas vertebra. Little if any damage will result, except to the vertebral arteries. A broom handle, or similar piece of wood, is cut to an appropriate length and the upper end is tapered to fit tightly into the foramen magnum. The advantages of this method are that the time consumed in the post mortem room is much shortened, and the final dissection can be performed at

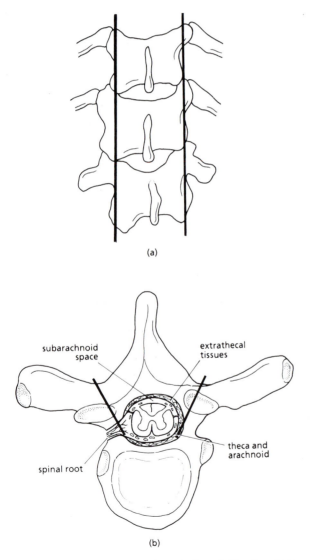

(a)

subarachnoid space

extrathecal tissues

spinal root

theca and arachnoid

(b)

Fig. 1.4 Posterior approach to the spinal cord. The drawings indicate the position and angulation of the saw-cuts.

leisure; the cord is kept safe from damage and distortion during fixation; and the resulting specimen includes all the spinal ganglia and both sympathetic chains, as far upward as the stellate ganglia, and the intravertebral parts of the vertebral arteries. The disadvantage, in some quarters, may lie in the need for a competent and cooperative post mortem room attendant.

Dissection of the neck

It is often desirable to study nerves, ganglia, muscles and blood vessels from deep in the neck. This is difficult if the skin incision is the one most commonly used in Britain—that is, in the midline from the larynx downwards. The alternative is a V- or U-shaped incision, running from the mastoid processes down to the upper end of the sternum. The skin flap is reflected upward, giving easy access to the anterior and posterior triangles of the neck. We recommend this approach for all cases of cerebral vascular disease, as it affords access to the *internal carotid arteries* up to their entry into the skull; also for cases with suspected peripheral neuropathy, in which the lower cranial nerves may be involved. A suggested procedure to follow is shown below.

1 Expose the *sterno-mastoid* muscle, from which samples may be taken for transverse and longitudinal sections from the middle of its length, where the spinal accessory nerve penetrates its deep surface; then reflect the cut ends upward and downward.

2 Identify the intermediate tendon of the *digastric muscle*, which runs through a fibrous pulley attached to the hyoid bone (Fig. 1.5). The pulley is slit open, and the muscle is retracted by an artery forceps applied to the tendon. The anterior belly, going to the chin, and the posterior belly, going to the mastoid process in company with the stylohyoid, can be cleaned without damage to muscle tissue, and detached from their bony attachments and kept for histology if required.

3 Expose and explore the *carotid sheath*, which contains the common and internal carotid arteries, the *internal jugular vein* and the *vagus* nerve. Follow the vagus upward to the skull, and expose its *inferior ganglion*, which is a fairly conspicuous swelling. The glossopharyngeal and accessory nerves emerge close to the vagus; just behind these, lying ensheathed in loose connective tissue on the surface of the prevertebral muscles, is the *superior cervical ganglion*—the topmost, and much the largest, element in the sympathetic chain (Fig. 1.6). Following the chain downward, one comes to the middle cervical ganglion, and below this, just below the point where the *vertebral artery* disappears into the

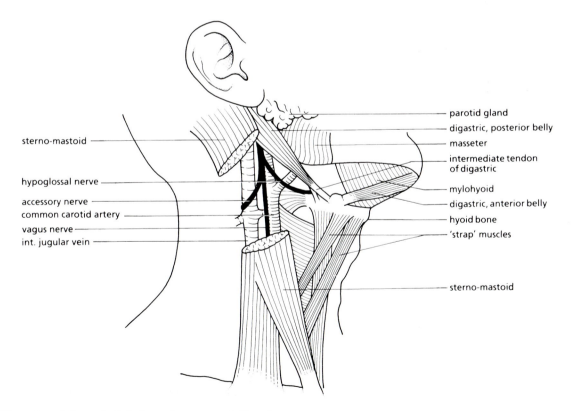

Fig. 1.5 Dissection of the neck. Relations of sterno-mastoid and digastric muscles with deeper structures. The submandibular gland and lymph nodes have been removed.

inferior ganglion of vagus

transverse process of atlas

transverse process of axis

C3 root

C4 root

phrenic nerve

C5 root

scalenus medius

C6 root

C7 root

C8 root

lower trunk of
brachial plexus

subclavian artery

scalenus anterior

clavicle

superior cervical ganglion

glossopharyngeal nerve

internal carotid artery

external carotid artery

middle cervical ganglion

common carotid artery

vertebral artery

inferior cervical ganglion

stellate ganglion

vagus

vertebral artery

subclavian artery

innominate artery

recurrent laryngeal nerve

Fig. 1.6 Deeper dissection of the neck showing relations of the lower cranial nerves with the sympathetic chain and ganglia.

spinal column, is the *inferior cervical ganglion*, which is often fused with the *stellate ganglion*. In any case of autonomic failure, a portion of the vagus, including its inferior ganglion, and the superior cervical and stellate ganglia, should be examined histologically; if facilities for histochemistry are available, specimens of these may be deep-frozen. Since some cases of progressive autonomic failure suffer from laryngeal palsy, the *larynx* should also be taken for later dissection. Of the remaining cranial nerves, the *glossopharyngeal* is found running between the internal carotid artery and the internal jugular vein on its way to the pharynx, and the *hypoglossal* follows a similar course on its way to the tongue, looping around the internal carotid close to the inferior ganglion of the vagus.

4 Examine the *carotids*. In general, the common carotids are found to be free of atheroma; the trouble begins at the bifurcation, in particular at the bulbous lower end of the internal carotid, where turbulence is presumably at its greatest.

Muscles and nerves

In cases suspected of neuropathy or neuromuscular dis-

ease, the minimum requirements are the spinal cord, with anterior and posterior nerve roots, and samples of nerve and muscle from the neck and from proximal and distal parts of upper and lower limbs. For muscles innervated from the brain stem we recommend the *digastric* (anterior belly supplied by the trigeminal, posterior belly by the facial nerve), the *sterno-mastoid* (accessory nerve) and the *tongue* (hypoglossal nerve). In the choice of *nerves*, it is better to avoid those that are apt to be traumatized during life, such as the median nerve at the wrist and the sciatic nerve in the buttock. The main nerves of the *upper arm*—median, ulnar and radial—are better protected, and easy of access. For the *lower limb*, the femoral nerve is readily accessible in the abdomen as it emerges from the psoas muscle, and the medial and lateral popliteal nerves are easy to find in the popliteal fossa (Fig. 1.7). More distally, the *sural nerve* lies beneath the skin just behind the lateral malleolus (Fig. 1.8). This slender nerve, which is almost purely sensory, provides control material for sural biopsies.

For the *hand*, an incision such as that shown in Fig. 1.9 gives access to the muscles of the thenar and hypothenar eminences, lumbricals and interossei, as well as to the

Fig. 1.7 Dissection of popliteal fossa.

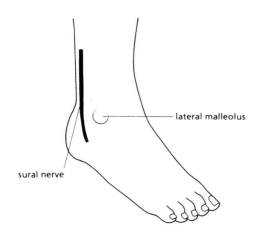

Fig. 1.8 Position of sural nerve.

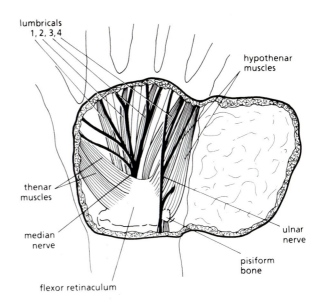

Fig. 1.9 Dissection of the palm of the hand.

distal branches of the median and ulnar nerves. The short hand muscles supply useful material for the study of motor end-plates, and of muscle spindles, with which they are richly supplied.

In taking specimens of muscle it is important to take an adequate (3 cm or more) length, and to avoid trauma and distortion, so that accurately oriented transverse and longitudinal sections can be examined histologically. If part of a long muscle is taken, this should be from somewhere near the motor point, which is generally near the middle of the muscle belly.

Fixation of specimens

If the *brain* is to be fixed entire, it must on no account be left resting on the bottom of a hard container. Not only does

this cause distortion, it also prevents the fixative from reaching the tissue where it is in contact with the floor. The most usual procedure is to *suspend* the brain in a plastic bucket, where it remains for at least two weeks. A hook or a loop of string is passed between the pons and the basilar artery, which is normally strong enough to support the weight of the brain *in water*, though not in air. If the basilar artery is diseased or damaged, pieces of string may be passed around two or more other basal arteries. An alternative, causing less distortion of the brain stem, is to suspend the brain topside upwards, by means of a few stitches passing through the dura of the vertex, which is left attached when the brain is removed. Whatever the method, suspension is from a loop of string running between the ends of the bucket handle. Plastic curtain hooks are preferable to pieces of wire or safety pins, which deposit rust, and are more apt to tear through the basilar artery. Once in its bucket, the brain should be left there, and not carried about, as minor accelerations may cause tearing of the artery.

If *biochemical* or *enzyme studies* are planned, selected portions of the brain can be excised at post mortem and put without delay into a low-temperature freezer. If cryostat sections are required the small blocks of tissue can be placed on cork discs, labelled with the case number and site of origin of the tissue, on their undersides. A dab of Tissue Tek or similar mountant-material serves as glue and the disc with its attached tissue block is plunged into liquid nitrogen for a minute or so before being taken out and stored, wrapped in foil to prevent drying out, in a deep freezer or liquid nitrogen container. In some cases multiple sites in the brain may undergo biochemical investigation, and the results tabulated alongside the histological findings in the corresponding areas on the other side. The brain is cautiously bisected, passing a long, sharp knife through the corpus callosum and other cerebral commissures and splitting the hindbrain as near as possible to the midline. One-half of the brain is then frozen; the other half is either suspended in formalin or placed, resting on its medial cut surface, on a thick layer of cotton wool in a container, and periodically lifted and replaced over the next few days.

Diffusion of fixing fluid into normal brain tissue is rapid enough to ensure good fixation throughout; but this is not so when there are areas of *oedema*. Unless special precautions are taken, a swollen brain, when it is sliced, may contain areas (in particular the lentiform nucleus and centrum ovale) which are almost liquid, look like toothpaste and have a sour smell due to post mortem bacterial growth. The most effective precaution is to make a slit in the corpus callosum, to ensure that the fixative reaches the interior of the hemispheres from the lateral ventricles. If one suspects blockages at the interventricular foramina, the insertion of a scalpel blade for a few millimetres in the midline between the mamillary bodies ensures access of fixative to the third ventricle. Another fixation artefact is attributable to leaving the brain unfixed at room temperature for many hours. The inner parts are invaded by gas-forming anaerobic bacteria, giving rise to the so-called Swiss cheese artefact (Fig. 2.18).

If the *spinal cord* is taken out at post mortem, it should be suspended in, for instance, a tall measuring cylinder filled with formalin, preferably with a weight attached to the theca at the lower end. This is because the theca tends to shrink longitudinally in the fixative, while the cord does not. As a result, the cord may buckle in many places and in the end look like a giant caterpillar. If the tall jar is not available no harm is done if the cord is divided by a clean transverse cut.

For reliable fixation of the whole *vertebral column*, there must be access of fixative to all parts of the subarachnoid space. This is hindered by tumours in the cord or elsewhere in the vertebral canal, and also by inflammatory exudates in the subarachnoid space. One precaution is to make a clean transverse cut through the whole specimen. This may be a necessary procedure if a fixing tank of sufficient length is not available. An alternative is to nibble away one of the thoracic spines and adjacent laminae, expose and incise the theca, and slit the underlying arachnoid before plunging the specimen into the tank.

Specimens of *muscle* and *nerve* should be laid, as soon as they are taken, on pieces of stiff card, on which their provenance is written with a grease pencil. They are left undisturbed for a few minutes, during which their natural juices congeal and act as a glue, thus preserving the orientation of the specimens. It is very difficult to obtain true transverse and longitudinal sections from specimens which have lain free in fixative. Pinning the specimens to a cork mat guards against later drift. This can be achieved using hedgehog quills, which, although not easy to obtain, do not rust.

Method for hydrocephalic children

Before examining the viscera, the skin is incised in the midline down the back. The incision is carried to the mastoid process on one side, then continued over the vertex to the opposite mastoid process. The anterior part of the scalp is reflected forward as far as the eyebrows and zygomatic processes. This entails cutting through the external auditory meatuses. The posterior part of the scalp is reflected sideways and the suboccipital muscles removed. Now the vertebral column is mobilized, cutting or sawing through the sacro-iliac joints and rib attachments. The column is dissected away from the soft tissues and displaced backward until the occipital bone immediately in front of the foramen magnum is exposed.

The orbital contents are dissected free from the roofs of the orbits and displaced downward. A saw-cut is then made in a plane passing from the orbital roofs to the angle between the occipital bone and the body of the atlas vertebra (Fig. 1.10). After this, the cranium and vertebral column, with their contents, come away as a single specimen, leaving the face and eyes behind. If the saw-cut is accurately performed, it may graze but will not seriously damage the lower surfaces of the temporal lobes. The subsequent reconstruction involves sewing up the scalp and stuffing it with some kind of wadding. If this is carefully done, the appearance of the child's head is often less horri-

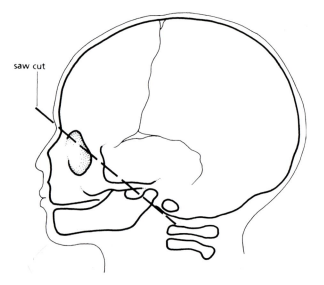

Fig. 1.10 Diagram showing direction of the saw-cut separating the vault of the skull from the bones of the face. Care must be taken to avoid damage to the eyeballs. The cut should barely graze the undersurfaces of the temporal lobes.

fying than it was during life. Finally, the viscera are extracted backward and examined. The vertebral column is replaced with a length of wood.

The object of this manoeuvre is to avoid the usual combination of distortion and disruption attendant on the attempt to extract a hydrocephalic brain. For fixation, the vertebral column may be cut transversely below the level of a Chiari malformation (see p.287) of the cerebellar tonsils. If there is a meningomyelocele, i.e. a backward protrusion of cord, nerve roots and meninges through a defect in the bony column (spina bifida), this will be included in the specimen. For good fixation, formalin should be introduced into the ventricular system. This can be done with a large syringe and hollow needle, either through a fontanelle or through the exposed temporal lobes. Some caution in needed here as the blown-out cerebral hemispheres have a tendency to fall inward away from the skull.

Causes of death

The pathologist who has just completed a post mortem may be faced with two questions, (i) what was the patient's underlying disease? and (ii) what was the immediate cause of death? The answer to the first may have been clear from the start; or it may take a couple of months to decide; or it may never be found. To the second question—why did the patient die when he did?—an immediate answer may be required, for a coroner's report, or for a cremation certificate. The finding of a blocked coronary artery, or of bronchopneumonia, or of an intracranial haemorrhage, may supply a ready answer, but the pathologist is well aware that all these are compatible with continued life. On occasion, after reading the clinical notes, one may conclude that the principal cause of death was the patient's lack of desire to go on living. In such cases the answer to the coroner will be determined by common sense rather than by physiological expertise.

Sometimes the immediate cause of death is obvious from an inspection of the brain—in particular of the brain stem, in which the so-called vital centres are lodged. There may be a fresh pontine haemorrhage, or a thrombosed basilar artery. Commoner than either of these is some form of *internal herniation* causing distortion, haemorrhage or ischaemia in the upper or lower brain stem.

Tentorial herniation

This is the commonest type of herniation. It occurs at the tentorial opening, usually as a result of swelling of one or both cerebral hemispheres. The swelling may be caused by haemorrhage, or oedema, or tumour. Other causes of transtentorial herniation are compression from massive blood clots in the epidural or subdural compartments, and acute or subacute hydrocephalus from blocking of the flow of

CSF through the ventricular system. The effects differ according to whether the space-occupying lesion is on one side or both, and whether it is in front or behind. When both hemispheres are affected the diencephalon—thalamus and subthalamic region—is thrust downward into the posterior fossa (see Fig. 2.8); at the same time the medial parts of the temporal lobes—unci and parahippocampal gyri—are thrust medially and downward over the tentorial edge, causing a mixture of downthrust and side-to-side compression of the midbrain and upper pons (see Fig. 2.9). At post mortem the visible effects of this sequence are (i) flattening of the cerebral convolutions, with diminution of the subarachnoid spaces, and (ii) deep grooving of the under surfaces of the *parahippocampal gyri* (see Figs 2.8–2.10). (Note that a shallow groove is normally present about 4 mm from the tip of each uncus (see Fig. 2.8a): it is caused by the edge of the tentorium, but does not indicate raised pressure.)

When cerebral swelling or compression is predominantly one-sided, grooving of the parahippocampal gyrus is deeper, and involves a greater area of the gyrus, on that side. The *mamillary bodies* are visibly displaced towards the opposite side. Not uncommonly, the midbrain is displaced strongly enough to cause bruising of the opposite cerebral peduncle from pressure against the free edge of the tentorium (see Fig. 2.10). During this process, branches of the posterior cerebral artery may be pinched on *either* side, causing infarction (usually haemorrhagic) of a large area on the inferior surface of the temporal lobe and of the visual cortex.

Bilateral swelling in the anterior part of the cerebrum results in backward displacement of the diencephalon, and herniation of the *unci*, which pinch the cerebral peduncles between them (see Fig. 2.9b). When the swelling is more posterior, the herniated parahippocampal gyri similarly pinch the tegmentum of the midbrain. A further effect of posterior swelling is that pressure is exerted on the upper surface of the tentorium. This reduces the amount of transtentorial herniation, but increases congestion in the posterior fossa. A common result is that a *foraminal* hernia is added to the tentorial one.

Foraminal herniation

The foramen magnum is approached from above by way of a conical basin, in which the lower medulla, flanked by the cerebellar tonsils, normally lies in a capacious bath of CSF, the *cisterna magna*. When increased congestion in the posterior fossa drives these structures downward, the bath empties, and unless the pressure is relieved herniation ensues. Medulla and tonsils are impacted in the foramen, and are moulded by the surrounding bone into a conical shape, which has given rise to the popular term 'coning' for the whole pathological process (see Fig. 2.15).

Clinical concomitants

The clinical concomitants of these two types of herniation are different. The cardinal signs of impending death from tentorial herniation are a lowering level of consciousness, rising blood pressure, stertorous or Cheyne–Stokes breathing, and loss of pupillary reflexes, leading to a fixed, dilated pupil, first on one side, later on both sides. This last feature has been attributed by some to compression of the oculomotor nerves by herniated unci; however, in most cases a more plausible explanation is that as the midbrain is forced downward, the oculomotor nerves become *kinked* as they cross the posterior cerebral arteries which, being tethered, cannot move downward. Such kinking can sometimes be observed at post mortem; but if the brain is fixed by suspension from the basilar artery, kinking occurs as a normal post mortem artefact.

Acute foraminal herniation, such as can occur from an injudicious lumbar puncture in the presence of raised pressure in the posterior fossa, can be horrifyingly sudden

in its effects. Breathing and heart-beat stop, and the patient is lifeless within seconds. When the process is more gradual, a common effect is the onset of pulmonary oedema, probably attributable to vagal irritation. This may give rise to a form of positive feedback, since impaired gas exchange causes hypercapnia and hypoxaemia, which in turn give rise to brain swelling.

Reverting to the coroner's question regarding the cause of death, we wish to record that the coroners with whom we have had dealings have been reasonable and kindly people, who wish to conclude their enquiries as quickly and painlessly as possible. In a case where poisoning is one of the possibilities, they will wait for the necessary investigations to be carried out. In a case of fatal road traffic accident, they will want a quick, easily intelligible report, rather than a detailed account of anatomical and physiological events following the injury. They may even be satisfied with the statement that the cause of death was a fracture of the skull.

We do not wish to moralize on these matters, but we

Table 1.1 Recommended selection of specimens to be taken at post mortem, after consulting the clinical notes.

Type of disease	What to take away	Type of disease	What to take away
Primary brain tumours (most cases)	Brain	Peripheral neuropathies	Brain, cord, nerves, ganglia and muscles
Dementia and psychosis (if no suspicion of CJD)	Brain‡	Myasthenia gravis	Brain, cord, nerves, ganglia and muscles
Epilepsy	Brain	Motor neuron diseases	Brain, cord, nerves, ganglia and muscles
Malformation of brain	Brain		
Perinatal brain damage	Brain	Head trauma	Brain, cervical spine
Parkinsonism	Brain‡	Cervical spondylosis	Brain, cervical spine
Brain tumours with clinical evidence of spread via CSF pathways	Brain and spinal cord	Cerebral vascular disease	Brain, heart, neck arteries
		Vascular disease of cord	Spinal column, aorta
		Friedreich's ataxia	Brain, cord, heart, sensory ganglia and nerves
Medulloblastoma	Brain and spinal cord		
Meningitis	Brain and spinal cord*, serum, CSF	Tuberous sclerosis	Brain, heart, kidney
Encephalitis	Brain and spinal cord*, serum, CSF		
CNS degenerations not affecting PNS	Brain and spinal cord	Intoxications, including Reye's syndrome	Brain, cord, nerves, liver, kidneys‡
Myelopathies, all types	Brain and spinal cord		
Multiple sclerosis	Brain and spinal cord†	Congenital hydrocephalus	Brain and spinal column (see also p.287)
Metabolic disorders	Brain, cord, peripheral nerves and ganglia‡	Hypopituitarism	Sphenoid block (see p.3)
Degenerations involving PNS and CNS	Brain, cord, peripheral nerves and ganglia‡	Pituitary and parapituitary tumours	Sphenoid block
Autonomic failure	Brain, cord, peripheral nerves and ganglia‡	Ataxia–telangiectasia	Brain, spleen, lymph nodes, gonad, pituitary, sensory ganglia

CSF, cerebrospinal fluid; CJD, Creutzfeldt–Jakob disease; PNS, peripheral nervous system.
*include specimens for microbiology.
†take optic nerves.
‡consider keeping tissue for freezing.

would suggest that in such cases it would serve the cause of veracity, without causing unnecessary confusion, if the immediate cause of death was given as compression and distortion of the brain stem, with supplementary information on the causes of such fatal distortions. These causes may not be clear until the brain has been dissected, preferably after fixation; but fatal herniations at the tentorial opening and the foramen magnum are generally obvious if they are looked for as soon as the brain is taken out of the cranium. These are discussed in more detail in the next chapter.

Use of clinical information

Most pathology departments have a standard form on which the main post mortem findings and the final diagnoses are entered. Such forms usually have a space—sometimes regrettably small—for a summary of the patient's clinical history, along with details of relevant investigations. There is no need to dwell here on the general usefulness of such clinical summaries, or on the advantages of conveying as much relevant information in as few words as possible. It is worth pointing out, however, that the neuropathologist, unlike the general pathologist, is often faced with a delay of weeks or months between the post mortem and the cut-up, and may need to be reminded of the points on which he is expected to find an answer. Once the clinical notes have been returned to the Records Department it may be a little difficult to retrieve them. When cutting the brain from a case of MS it is irritating if one does not know whether the patient could walk or see, or hold an intelligible conversation. In short, the clinical summary should give clear indications of the problems to be solved (see Table 1.1).

In neurosurgical cases, it is usually prudent to keep hold of the relevant X-rays and computerized axial tomography (CT) or magnetic resonance imaging (MRI) scans up to the time of cutting-up. In this and in many other respects, friendly relations with the neurosurgeons and neuroradiologists are of great importance.

Safety in the post mortem room

Neuropathologists are called on from time to time to undertake post mortem examinations on cases where there is a risk of infection. The reader is referred to Appendix C for advice about precautions to take when dealing with such cases. It should be pointed out here that this risk will not have been invariably uncovered by clinicians before death. Therefore, when reading the clinical information available before a post mortem examination is performed pathologists should always come to their own judgment of whether such a risk exists and take appropriate steps accordingly.

2 The Cut-up

Dissection of the fixed brain

A brain should be left soaking in formalin for 3 weeks or more. If it is sliced after a fortnight, no harm will be done, but the uneven colours seen on the cut surfaces usually betray incomplete fixation, and the inner tissues will not be ready for histological examination. Photography, too, will give unsatisfactory pictures. As it is advisable to have one's camera ready before starting on the dissection, a word on *equipment* will be inserted here.

We use a single-lens reflex 35 mm camera, with a 5 cm lens and extension rings for close-up photography. Using two camera backs, one can alternate readily between monochrome and colour film. The camera is mounted on a copying stand, with movable lamps on each side (Fig. 2.1), and kept close to the cutting-up bench.

Before examination, the brain should be washed in running water for at least 2 hours, and left soaking overnight. Many pathologists have lived to regret the casual attitude to formalin vapour of their earlier days. It is probably advisable to give the brain an extra wash after making the first cut into the ventricular system, especially if the specimen is hydrocephalic and contains a large reservoir of formalin. Formalin also affects the skin, and rubber gloves should always be worn when handling fixed tissues.

Superficial features

Features which may call for photography before slicing include such things as tumours, old infarcts, aneurysms, signs of tentorial or foraminal herniation, cerebral cortical atrophy (either generalized or localized, as in Pick's disease, Fig. 17.5), relative atrophy of the brain stem, as in pontocerebellar atrophy (Fig. 15.7), or hypertrophy, as in

diffuse astrocytomatous infiltration (Fig. 12.3). Some dissection is needed before slicing in order to expose aneurysms of the middle cerebral artery, lying in the lateral fissure, or of the anterior communicating artery, between the two gyri recti. This involves a little disruption of cortical tissue, of no great consequence, but one should watch

copying stand　　reflex camera

lamp

brain slice

Fig. 2.1 A simple set-up for photography of specimens.

Key to Figs 2.2 to 2.5

Cerebral gyri

ang	angular
cing	cingulate
cun	cuneus
fus	fusiform (occipito-temporal)
gr	g. rectus
if	inferior (third) frontal
ilo	inf. lateral occipital
ins	insula
ip	inf. parietal lobule
it	inf. (third) temporal
lin	lingual
lo	lateral orbital
mf	middle (second) frontal
mo	medial orbital
mt	middle (second) temporal
occ	occipital gyri
ph	parahippocampal
post	postcentral (sensory)
pre	precentral (motor)
precun	precuneus
sf	superior (first) frontal
slo	sup. lateral occipital
sm	supramarginal
sp	sup. parietal lobule
st	sup. (first) temporal
trans	transverse (Heschl's)

Central grey matter

am	amygdaloid nucleus
c	caudate nucleus
cl	claustrum
gp	globus pallidus
hip	hippocampus
hyp	hypothalamus
lgb	lat. geniculate body
mam	mamillary body
p	putamen
rn	red nucleus
sn	substantia nigra
sub	subthalamic nucleus
t	thalamus

Central white matter

ac	anterior commissure
cc	corpus callosum
f	fornix
ic	internal capsule

Other features

aq	aqueduct
CALC	calcarine sulcus
CENT	central (Rolandic) sulcus
cereb	cerebellum
ch pl	choroid plexus
LAT	lateral (sylvian) fissure
lat vent	lateral ventricle
n	cranial nerve
olf	olfactory tract
ot	optic tract
ox	optic chiasm
PO	parieto-occipital sulcus
vent 3	third ventricle

Fig. 2.2 Lateral view of the brain. The line indicates the plane of the initial cut for horizontal slicing.

out for local brown staining by blood pigments, i.e. evidence of earlier haemorrhages. Such superficial staining should also be looked for in the brains of epileptics, especially in the anterior temporal, orbital and frontal regions (Fig. 18.2).

The main *arteries* of the brain should be examined at an early stage. The *circle of Willis* is inspected before or after fixation, and its pattern noted (for normal pattern see Fig. 7.15). In cases of stroke, emboli may be found, the commonest sites being the bifurcation of an internal carotid artery, and the origin of a branch of a middle cerebral artery. Sites of atheromatous narrowing should be noted, and transverse scalpel cuts made in identified vessels to test for occlusion. If old or recent softenings are revealed in slicing the brain, an attempt should be made to relate these either to occluded arteries or to the border zones between arterial territories (see Chapter 7; Figs 7.14–7.22).

A special case calling for preliminary dissection is when there is a history of speech disturbance or hearing loss attributable to a cerebral vascular accident. The auditory cortex, consisting mainly of Heschl's gyri, and Wernicke's speech area, centred on the posterior third of the left first temporal gyrus, can be exposed by cutting the arachnoid covering the lateral fissure, and cleanly amputating the temporal lobe. After photography the temporal lobe may be replaced and sliced along with the rest of the cerebrum.

Slicing

The *first incision* is normally the one separating the hindbrain (brain stem and cerebellum) from the cerebral hemispheres. This should be made by a clean transverse cut across the midbrain, at right angles to the long axis of the brain stem (Fig. 2.9a). It is easier to see what one is doing after cutting the arachnoid overlying the cerebral peduncles. It is bad practice to make two separate oblique cuts through the cerebral peduncles, as this makes it almost impossible to examine the anatomy of the midbrain, tegmentum and subthalamic region.

It is customary to *weigh* the brain before slicing. If one wants to compare the weights of the two hemispheres – for instance, when one hemisphere is relatively swollen by tumour or oedema, or relatively shrunken from old trauma or infarction – they can be separated without damage by gently cutting through arachnoid attachments and making a midline incision in the corpus callosum from above, followed by midline cuts through the optic chiasm, hypothalamus, anterior and posterior commissures, and interthalamic connexus. The hemispheres can then be sliced together or separately.

For slicing, we use a long (40 cm or so), not too flexible, knife, a resin-covered cutting board, and pairs of L-shaped stainless steel guides, 1 cm, 0.7 cm and 0.5 cm thick respectively. In Oxford, two alternative planes of slicing are used: coronal and horizontal. For *coronal slicing* we make the first cut through the mamillary bodies (Fig. 2.3), passing through the anterior margin of the thalamus. The anterior part of the cerebrum is then placed, cut surface down, between a pair of centimetre guides, and successive slices taken at centimetre intervals or less and laid out, posterior surface upward, with the right side on the right. The procedure is repeated with the posterior part. For convenience in description, the slices are numbered; slices in front of the initial cut are A1, A2, A3, etc., progressing forward, and those behind it are P1, P2, P3, etc., progressing backward. Because of variations in size and proportions between one brain and another, the structures seen in slices A1 and P1 will be almost the same in all brains, the correspondence becoming progressively less in subsequent slices. When giving an anteroposterior *level*, the posterior aspect of the slice is referred to; thus the mamillary bodies are always level A1 (Fig. 2.4).

To produce accurate centimetre-thick slices, a little

Fig. 2.3 Base of the brain.

practice is needed. Assuming that the knife is held in the right hand, the blade is directed to the left and slightly downward, and the left palm holds the left side of the specimen down. If the blade is directed upward the knife will ride upward, and the slice will be too thick on the left. If the pressure exerted by the left hand is inadequate, the brain will ride upward, and the slice will be too thin on the left.

The alternative—horizontal—plane of slicing may be preferred, especially in cases which have undergone CT scans during life, making possible a comparison between the actual and the radiographic slices. The usual initial cut is indicated in Fig. 2.2. From then on the procedure is as with coronal slices, except that rather longer cutting guides are required: 22 × 18 cm, say, as against 19 × 16 cm. The slices are laid out, upper surface upward, with the right side on the right. Figures 2.4 and 2.5 show the structures normally displayed in coronal and horizontal slices respectively.

Comparison of brain slices with magnetic resonance imaging (MRI) scans

Remarkably accurate comparisons can now be made between lesions seen in fixed brain slices and in MRI scans (Figs 2.4–2.6). If no MRI scans were obtained during life but are thought desirable they can be taken after washing the well-fixed brain very thoroughly in water (about a week's soaking with daily changes in the water) (Boyko *et al.* 1994). The thoroughly washed brain can then be scanned in its container of water.

Nomenclature

Here we propose to digress on the subject of neuro-anatomy. Normal people forget, in the course of a few years or months, information which has been acquired purely for the purpose of an examination. This commonly includes the topology of the brain. Luckily relearning, when the need arises, is far easier than the initial learning. Apprentices in neuropathology need feel no shame if they have forgotten the difference between, say, the dentate nuclei and the dentate fascia; but it is incumbent on them, if their post mortem reports are to be of any value whatever, to relearn much of what they have forgotten. This will involve spending a lot of time over their first few brain-slicings, simply reminding themselves of the relations of parts, and of their names.

The facts of neuro-anatomy are one thing; nomenclature is another. Professional anatomists enjoy meeting each other from time to time in order to change the terminology in current use. In this they resemble experts in tumour pathology, taxonomic botanists, and the promoters of new translations of the Bible. Although the new terminology is naturally superior to the old, this may create problems for outsiders using obsolete textbooks. In some cases, glossaries of old and new terms may help. A somewhat different problem arises with terms in common use which have no precisely defined application. An example is the word *brain*, which some people use as a synonym for *cerebrum*, while others (more correctly, we think) apply it to the whole of the intracranial part of the central nervous system. Another is *basal ganglia*, which is sometimes an alternative to *corpus striatum*, and at other times includes not only the caudate and lentiform nuclei but also the thalamus, hypothalamus, amygdala and subthalamic grey matter. We prefer the wider application. Even the terms *grey matter* and *white matter*, familiar as they are to laymen, are rather hard to define. Grey matter, of course, is central nervous tissue containing nerve cell bodies, whereas white matter is composed almost exclusively of axons, myelin and neuroglia. In the cerebral and cerebellar hemispheres and the spinal cord, the distinction is clear; but what of the brain stem? There is an analogy here with pork butchery. In a conventional joint, there is a clear separation of lean meat from fat; but what of streaky bacon? This is not mere pedantry. It is well known that what makes white matter white is myelin; but it is sometimes forgotten that there is plentiful myelin in grey matter. Hence the utterly false statement, seen in old textbooks of neurology, that MS is a disease of white matter. In fact, demyelination may occur throughout the CNS.

Regarding the terminology in this book, we have tried to remember, when two or more synonymous terms are in common use, to mention the synonyms (e.g. dorsal (Clarke's) nuclei; sensorimotor (Rolandic) cortex; pyramidal (corticospinal) tracts). For the terminology of the central cerebral grey matter, we use the conventions shown below:

Corpus striatum—caudate and lentiform nuclei, claustrum, internal and external capsules.

Lentiform nucleus—putamen and pallidum (globus pallidus).

Striatum—caudate nucleus and putamen.

Hippocampus we regard as interchangeable with *Ammon's horn*.

Subthalamic nucleus we regard as interchangeable with *corpus Luysii*.

Tegmentum and *subthalamic grey matter* can be used interchangeably; in practice, one or other is used according to whether the brain stem or cerebrum is being discussed.

Dissection of the hindbrain

After severing the midbrain, one can observe whether transtentorial herniation has taken place. The main visible signs of this are (i) grooving of the parahippocampal gyrus,

Fig. 2.4 Coronal slices of the cerebral hemispheres, cut at 1 cm intervals, from before backward and the same slices in coronal SPGR (spoiled GRASS) MR images of the normal brain. Compare corresponding A (anterior) and P (posterior) numbered slices. In MR images CSF is of a very low signal and grey matter is of a much lower signal than white matter, reflecting the different water content.

Fig. 2.4 *continued.*

Fig. 2.4 *continued.*

Fig. 2.4 *continued.*

Fig. 2.4 *continued.*

Fig. 2.5 Normal T1 sagittal midline MRI.

on one side or both, and (ii) lateral compression of the upper brain stem (Fig. 2.9). For slicing the hindbrain, there are two commonly practised routines. The first (the one we normally follow) is to cut through the upper medulla at the level of the *lateral apertures* (foramina of Luschka) in a plane vertical to the long axis of the medulla, and continue the cut through the cerebellum. This displays the *fourth ventricle* at its broadest extent, the *dentate nuclei*, and the flocculi, uvula and nodulus of the cerebellum. Further cuts are made through the lower part of the specimen, using 5 mm guides, until it comes to an end. If the anatomy of the brain stem nuclei is of interest (as it very often is), wedge-shaped slices may give rise to later confusion. Figure 2.27 shows a series of hindbrain sections, stained for myelin.

In the upper part of the specimen, it is often the case that the upper and lower cut surfaces are not parallel, and the specimen is somewhat wedge-shaped, being thicker in the ventral than in the dorsal part. It should then be cut free-hand, after taking 5 mm slices from the upper (midbrain) and lower (caudal pons) ends, making sure that each slice shows a complete transverse section of the pons.

The alternative routine may be preferred if interest is directed to regional differences between areas of the cere-bellum. The cerebellum is separated from the brain stem by oblique cuts through the cerebellar peduncles into the fourth ventricle. Oblique cuts can then be made at right angles to the folia on the upper surface, and a midline cut will display the whole of the cerebellar vermis (Fig. 2.28). The brain stem is sliced at 5 mm intervals as before.

In slicing the brain, the knife may come across areas of gritty resistance. These may be due to calcification in the pineal gland and/or choroid plexus. Larger foci of calcification, up to the size of a date (so-called brain stones) occur, mainly in cases with endocrine disturbances, and have characteristic sites—in particular, the lentiform nuclei, thalami, and dentate nuclei. They are described and discussed on p.346.

Until the normal appearances of the slices are so familiar that any abnormality leaps to the eye, it is well to conduct one's inspection in a routine order. Apart from gross haemorrhages, large infarcts, tumours and malformations, it is important to note signs of brain swelling and herniation.

Signs of brain swelling and herniation

Some of these—convolutional flattening, grooving of the

Fig. 2.6(a) (See p. 25 for legend)

C

B

D

Fig. 2.6(b)

Fig. 2.6(a) *continued.*

E

G

F

Fig. 2.6 (a)(A) Vertex of the brain. (B–G) Horizontal slices of the cerebral hemispheres, cut at 1 cm intervals, from above downward. (b) Series of spin echo T2W axial MR images of the normal brain (horizontal). Compare the corresponding images. In the MR images CSF is of very high signal (white) and white matter is of lower signal than grey matter and is darker. The difference in signal reflects the water content. Blood vessels are seen as areas of signal void (black). The red nuclei and substantia nigra are of lower signal than the remainder of the midbrain because of their iron content. Most pathological processes are hyperintense (of higher signal: whiter) to brain on T2W.

Fig. 2.6(b) *continued.*

parahippocampal gyri, and 'coning' of the medulla and cerebellar tonsils—will have been observed before slicing (see above, pp.2–9). Others are best seen at a later stage. One of these is an increased concavity on each side of the upper surface of the cerebellum. This is caused by downward pressure on the tentorium from the temporal lobes. In cases of tentorial herniation—even of mild extent—it is important to assess the degree of *diencephalic downthrust*. This can be done with a fair amount of accuracy by noting the position of the mamillary bodies (level A1) in relation to a line joining the lateral angles of the inferior horns of the lateral ventricles (Figs 2.7 and 2.8). Normally the mamillary

(a)

(b)

Fig. 2.7 The Greenhall line. At coronal level A1 a line between the inferior horns of the lateral ventricles normally lies above the mamillary bodies (arrowed). In the presence of cerebral swelling, the diencephalon, including the mamillary bodies, descends below this line. (a) Normal, (b) diencephalic downthrust.

bodies lie 1 or 2 mm above this line (Greenhall 1977). A severe downthrust brings them 5 mm or more below it.

Unilateral cerebral swelling or compression causes a shift of midline structures to the opposite side (Figs 2.9 and 2.10). At levels including the septum lucidum, this shift is easily measured by halving the distance between the lateral surfaces of the hemispheres, and noting the difference from the actual position of the septum. Other signs of a sideways shift are a grooving or indentation of the cingulate gyrus (Fig. 2.10) where it has come against the free edge of the falx cerebri. (Incidentally, there is no known clinical correlate of this type of subfalcine herniation.) Posteriorly, the falx comes close to the splenium of the corpus callosum: in front, the free edge of the falx lies a centimetre or more above the callosum.

Another type of herniation which is not often referred to, but which can be a very real threat to life, is an *upward* hernia through the tentorial opening. This occurs in the presence of tumours or haemorrhages in the posterior fossa, and can be precipitated by the sudden withdrawal of fluid from the lateral ventricles, or even, on occasion, by the turning of an osteoplastic flap, increasing the differential pressures above and below the tentorium. When the brain is cut, it will be found that the upper surfaces of the cerebellum, instead of being slightly concave, are convex, and display a distinct groove, caused by pressure on the free edge of the tentorium (Fig. 2.11).

The most important, i.e. the deadliest, effects of herniation are seen in slices of the brain stem. After a fatal tentorial hernia, the midbrain is distorted—mainly by lateral compression—and frequently haemorrhagic. The haemorrhages are usually symmetrical, mainly in the midline of the tegmentum, and may extend downward into the upper half of the pons (Fig. 2.12). This pattern differs somewhat from that seen in traumatic haemorrhage, which tends to affect one or both superior cerebellar peduncles (Fig. 2.13), or in primary spontaneous pontine haemorrhage, which is more disruptive but tends to spare the upper brain stem (Fig. 2.14). Lesions due to coning look rather different. The herniated tissue is softened and diffusely haemorrhagic (Fig. 2.15), apparently as a result of mechanical compression of veins and capillaries, whereas the upper brain stem haemorrhages are attributed to stretching and tearing of intrinsic arteries. Various causes of herniation are discussed in Chapter 11.

Appearance of the ventricles

The lateral ventricles may be larger or smaller than normal, or unequal. When they are larger than normal this may be due to loss of cerebral tissue, or to increased intraventricular pressure, which in turn is often due to an obstruction to the normal circulation of CSF. An account of the normal CSF pathways, and of the sites at which ob-

(a)

(b)

(c)

Fig. 2.8 Coronal level A1. (a) Normal. The mamillary bodies lie well above the Greenhall line. (b) Diencephalic downthrust in a case with bilateral cerebral swelling. (c) Downthrust in a case with right-sided haemorrhagic infarction due to phlebo-thrombosis. Note the midline shift to the left, herniation of the right cingulate gyrus, and bruising and grooving of the right parahippocampal gyrus (arrowed).

struction may occur, is given on pp.142−4. Briefly, in a brain with enlarged ventricles there are various points to note.

1 Whether the ventricles contain *blood*. Intraventricular bleeding can cause obstruction of the CSF pathway (for instance, in the aqueduct) by blood clots. Arterial bleeding will immediately expand the lateral ventricles, and may cause transtentorial herniation, resulting in compression of the aqueduct.

2 Whether the subarachnoid spaces between the cerebral sulci and in the basal cisterns are more or less capacious than normal. If more, there is a presumption of cerebral atrophy; if less, a block in the CSF pathway must be looked for.

3 Whether the ventricular dilatation affects the whole or only a part of the ventricular system; if only a part is affected, whether the difference can be accounted for by local atrophy or tissue destruction.

4 Whether the narrow places in the CSF pathway−the interventricular foramina, aqueduct, apertures of the fourth ventricle and cisterna ambiens (the subarachnoid space surrounding the midbrain)−are fully patent. Some of the causes of obstruction at these levels are mentioned in Chapter 8. The special case of the Chiari type 2 (Arnold–Chiari) malformation is discussed on pp.287−8; and some of the sequelae of perinatal injuries in Chapter 21, on pp.366−8.

The common causes of unduly *small* ventricles are external

(a)

(b)

Fig. 2.9 Base of cerebrum after severing the midbrain. (a) Normal. (b) Showing effects of one-sided cerebral swelling. Same case as in Fig. 2.8c. The midbrain is laterally compressed and shifted to the left (right side of picture). The right parahippocampal gyrus is deeply grooved by the free edge of the tentorium (arrowed).

compression (e.g. by a blood clot or a meningioma), infiltrating or expanding tumours, and oedema. The last two may be combined, since some gliomas and some carcinoma deposits evoke an inflammatory type of response (Fig. 11.4). In this context, it is worth noting that adhesions often occur between apposed ependymal surfaces. Such adhesions are presumably congenital, and perfectly innocent. The *interthalamic connexus* is one such: and the tips of the posterior horns of the lateral ventricles are normally obliterated to some extent, often asymmetrically. The same process often produces adhesions between the corpus callosum and the head of a caudate nucleus (Fig. 2.16).

Scanning for lesions

No cut-and-dried instructions can be given here. As would be expected, the more practice one has the easier it becomes to identify significant changes, and to ignore insignificant ones. Even practised neuropathologists, however, tend to refer to photographs and diagrams of normal structures and often need to settle doubts on naked-eye pathology by resorting to microscopy.

In scanning for lesions, the first guidance comes from the clinical notes. If MS has been suspected, one searches for plaques (see Chapter 14). If there was a parkinsonian syndrome, one looks for pigment loss in the substantia nigra and locus ceruleus (Fig. 2.17). If the patient was ataxic or dysarthric, special attention is paid to the pons, medulla and cerebellum. If he was blind, from other than ocular disease, the visual pathway, from optic nerves to visual cortex, should be looked at; and so forth.

It is important to learn—as soon as possible, in order to avoid wasting one's own and the technician's time—to recognize common *artefacts*. A few of these, such as

Fig. 2.10 Coronal slice, showing effects of a haemorrhagic tumour in the left cerebral hemisphere. Midline structures are shifted to the right, and there is a subfalcine herniation of the left cingulate gyrus, and bruising of the left parahippocampal gyrus (arrowed), as in Fig. 2.8c. The midbrain (on the right) shows lateral compression and a midline haemorrhage caused by distortion. The right crus (on the left) shows bruising from lateral pressure on the free edge of the tentorium.

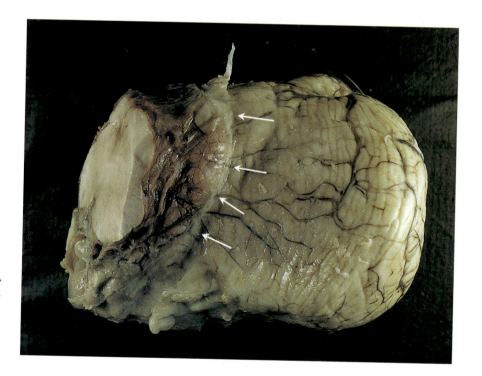

Fig. 2.11 Upward transtentorial hernia. A cerebellar tumour has displaced the brain stem upward, and the upper surface of the cerebellum has been grooved (arrowed) by the free edge of the tentorium.

'Swiss cheese' artefact (Fig. 2.18) and toothpaste softening, have been mentioned above (p.8). Common minor artefacts include pink haloes, a few millimetres or more in diameter, around small blood vessels (Fig. 2.19). These are found, on microscopy, to contain bacteria, which have presumably left the bloodstream and proliferated at some time between death and diffusion of the fixative. They may be mistaken for small perivenous plaques of MS. Some doubts concerning the significance of colour changes may be settled by putting the cut slices back into formalin for a few days.

A change commonly seen in the cerebellum is a bluish discoloration of the cortex, often referred to as *état glacé*. It is believed to be due to post mortem autolysis, and is said to be commoner when there has been a delay between death and necropsy. Histological examination of the affected tissue shows dissolution of the cells of the granular layer, though the neighbouring Purkinje cells are unaffected (Fig. 2.20).

Patches of grey discoloration are commonly seen on cut surfaces in slices of the brain stem. These may even mimic

Fig. 2.12 Haemorrhages in the upper brain stem caused by distortion, with over-stretching of vessels, in the course of a tentorial hernia. Such haemorrhages are characteristically in or near the midline.

Fig. 2.13 Haemorrhages in the upper brain stem following an acceleration injury to the head, with 6 days' survival. The upper pons contains haemorrhages which were probably due to sudden stretching at the time of injury.

Fig. 2.14 'Spontaneous' pontine haemorrhage, ploughing into the upper and lower brain stem and erupting into the fourth ventricle. The causes of such haemorrhages are not always clear, but some undoubtedly arise from vascular malformations.

plaques of MS. Histology shows no abnormality. We are at a loss to explain this phenomenon. Another form of discoloration is seen in slicing brain tissue which has been kept for many months in formalin. Here, the tissue has a dirty yellow hue for a distance of several millimetres inward from the exposed surfaces. Contact with blood clot in the storage jar inevitably causes dark discoloration of the tissue.

Fingertip palpation is a useful supplement to visual inspection. An area of fresh infarction may look almost nor-

mal, though the softening and the demarcation from the adjoining arterial territory is immediately apparent on palpation. Oedematous white matter and diffuse astrocytoma may look alike, but the former is soft and slimy, the latter firm and dry. Owing to the hardening effect of formalin, the altered consistency of plaques of MS is hard to appreciate in fixed tissue; but in some conditions, such as globoid-cell and sulphatide leucodystrophies, fibrous gliosis of the affected tissue confers an almost wood-like hardness. In tuberous sclerosis the firm consistency of the tubers in the

Fig. 2.15 'Coning' in a case of acute brain swelling due to pneumococcal meningitis. The herniated cerebellar tonsils, and the ventral part of the lower medulla, are disrupted and haemorrhagic.

Fig. 2.16 'Coarctation' of a lateral ventricle. Adhesions between the corpus callosum and the caudate nucleus, although of no pathological significance, sometimes gave rise to diagnostic errors. Note that the midline is not displaced.

cerebral cortex, easily felt in the unfixed brain, is still just appreciable after fixation.

Dissection of the fixed spinal column

In cases of peripheral neuroathy, particularly if this is complicated by autonomic disturbances, one may wish to examine parts of the *sympathetic chains*. These are easily identified after stripping off the remains of pleura and peritoneum overlying the sides of the vertebral bodies, up to the level of the stellate ganglia. They should be removed before beginning the dissection of the backbone.

The *tools* needed for the dissection are a metre of solid bench, a pair of strong vices, a stout knife, scissors and forceps, bone shears and nibblers, and a short handsaw and/or electric vibrating saw. The spinal column, fixed and well washed, is held dorsum upward in the vices, and the erector spinae musculature cut away. The laminae are sawn through and removed with the spinous processes as described on p.8, with the same precautions against inflicting damage to the spinal cord. Spinal roots and ganglia are exposed at the desired levels, and dissected away from the bone of the intervertebral foramina. An artery forceps is placed on the lowest part of the theca, in the sacral part of the spinal canal, and the cord, enclosed in the theca, is gradually eased backward, cutting nerve roots with a sharp knife. During this procedure, there should be as little sideways or backward bending of the cord as possible. Although the cord is much firmer than before fixation, it is also more liable to crumble if it is bent, giving very unsatisfactory histological sections. Longitudinal stretching of the theca, on the other hand, is harmless.

For most of the distance (unless there is extrathecal tumour tissue) the theca will come away from the anterior wall of the spinal canal with only slight encouragement from the knife. In elderly subjects, however, dense fibrous

Fig. 2.17 Slices of midbrain. On the right, normal pigmentation of the substantia nigra; on the left, loss of pigment in an advanced case of paralysis agitans (Parkinson's disease).

Fig. 2.19 Slices through cerebrum and hind-brain showing areas of pink discoloration caused by post mortem bacterial contamination.

Fig. 2.18 'Swiss cheese' artefacts in cerebrum and cerebellum, due to invasion by gas-forming organisms during the interval between death and fixation.

Fig. 2.20 'Etat glacé'. The cells of the granular layer of the cerebellum show post mortem digestion. Purkinje cells (arrowed), though showing signs of agonal hypoxia, are preserved. ×220.

adhesions are often encountered in the lower cervical region, the usual cause being *osteoarthritic and spondylotic changes*, with osteophytosis of the vertebral bodies and discs.

Cranial and spinal meninges

In the cranial cavity the dura mater consists of two layers, of which the outer layer is in effect the periosteum of the bone, and is continuous, via the various bony foramina, with the pericranium. Over the vault, the dura is relatively easily detached from the bone, as occurs in the formation of an epidural haematoma simply from the force of arterial pressure. The inner layer is closely bound to the outer layer over most of its extent, but leaves it at certain points to

form infoldings such as the falx and tentorium. It is along these lines of infolding that venous sinuses occur. At the base, the dura is more firmly stuck down—densely so at and just below the foramen magnum. Below this the two layers separate, the outer layer becoming the periosteum of the spinal canal. The inner layer becomes the spinal *theca*, which is separated from the periosteum by a layer of loose connective tissue, containing fat and blood vessels. Until adhesions form, there is free movement between the theca and the bony canal, unrestrained by the spinal nerve roots, which lie loosely in the extrathecal space, and are covered with an epineurium derived from the theca.

The *arachnoid* membrane, though it is attached to the pial covering of the entire brain and cord, is everywhere in direct contact with the inner surface of the dura. Over the cerebral hemispheres, there is free gliding movement, checked only by dural folds and by bridging veins running between brain and dura. This presumably affords the brain some protection against the effects of accelerations. At the base, however, such a slipping plane would be useless because of the numerous nerves and blood vessels traversing the subdural space. Here, such movement as occurs is mainly in the subarachnoid space, and is checked by the excellent packing of the hindbrain within the posterior fossa.

In the spinal canal, as in the posterior fossa, the presence of numerous nerve roots would render a subdural slipplane useless. The arachnoid, though easily stripped from the theca, only loses contact in peculiar circumstances, for instance, when a lumbar puncture is performed with a blunt or hooked needle. The subarachnoid space, however, is capacious, and the arachnoid is only loosely and intermittently attached to the pia of the cord, by the denticulate ligaments and the spinal nerve roots.

Movement of the cord relative to the bony canal—shown at its most impressive by gymnasts, acrobats and some dancers—is made possible by the elasticity of the cord tissue, and by the existence of two planes of movement, the epidural and the subarachnoid. In the presence of cervical osteoarthritis and spondylosis, the former is reduced or abolished. It has been suggested that this may have a bearing on the predominant patterns of cord lesions in MS.

In dissecting the spine, a note should be made of any dense fibrous adhesions met with during removal of the cord, and of any excrescences, tumorous or otherwise, projecting into the spinal canal. After the cord has been removed, the walls of the canal should be inspected and herniated discs identified. It is also worth making a midline saw-cut through at least the cervical part of the bony column, to reveal the ravages, if any, of cervical spondylosis—the degenerate discs and osteophytes, the obliteration or exaggeration of the normal cervical lordosis, and so forth (Fig. 2.21).

(a)

(b)

Fig. 2.21 Cervical spondylosis. The spinal cords have been removed after laminectomy, and midline saw-cuts made through the bodies of the cervical vertebrae. The specimens are displayed with the anterior longitudinal ligaments in the middle and the interior of the spinal canal at the sides. (a) From a man aged 80, with a sensory level at C6. The cervical spine has lost its normal lordosis. The C2–3 and T1–2 discs appear normal, but all the intervening discs are either narrowed or grossly

degenerate. Detachment of the anterior and posterior longitudinal ligaments from the bone has resulted in the formation of osteophytic projections. Anterior osteophytes are relatively harmless, whereas posterior osteophytes become adherent to the theca, and narrow the spinal cord from before back. (b) From a woman of 83, with a long history of MS. Here the cervial lordosis is exaggerated. Discs C3–4 and C4–5 are narrowed. C4–5 is disrupted, and shows anterior and posterior osteophytes.

Examination of the spinal cord

If it is clear, from palpation, that there is more inside the theca than is accounted for by the cord and nerve roots, a transverse cut should be made before opening the theca. This may reveal pus, clear fluid, subarachnoid tumour, or a swollen cord. Otherwise, the theca can be slit open longitudinally, back and front, and peeled away from the arachnoid. The arachnoid itself should be delicate and transparent. It becomes somewhat thicker and more opaque in later life, and may develop a number of so-called *arachnoid plaques*. These are white, opaque, less than 0.5 mm thick, and often over 1 cm long (Fig. 2.22). Being composed of cholesterol they disappear completely in fat solvents. They are of no known pathological significance.

After the theca and arachnoid have been slit open, the front and back of the cord are easily distinguished by the pattern of surface vessels; behind, there are many small venous tributaries to the posterior spinal veins, whereas in front there is a prominent midline vein, accompanied by the anterior spinal artery. *Segmental levels* are most easily

worked out by counting upward and downward from the first thoracic root, which is the lowest *large* root of the cervical enlargement.

Some yellow–brown staining may be seen in the leptomeninges (arachnoid and pia) at the lower end of the cord, and on the roots of the cauda equina. The pigment is *haemosiderin*, and the intensity of the staining is usually an indication of the number of lumbar punctures that the patient has undergone. More widespread brown staining (*superficial siderosis*) involving the brain, at least at the base, is due to intermittent small haemorrhages from a variety of sources. Blackish-brown discoloration of the pia covering the upper cervical cord and lower medulla is normal. The pigment here is melanin.

Acute and chronic meningitis

Purulent meningitis (i.e. pus in the subarachnoid space) is readily recognized. The more chronic forms, such as tuberculous or syphilitic meningitis or the mysterious non-infective chronic arachnoiditis, show less exudate,

Fig. 2.22 Arachnoid plaques. These are thin white scales, embedded in the spinal arachnoid, especially in the lower regions. They are common in elderly subjects, and have no known clinical or pathological significance.

more discoloration, and conspicuous thickening of the leptomeninges (Fig. 9.17). This appearance may be mimicked in cases of diffuse spread of tumour through the CSF pathways.

Such spread is very characteristic of medulloblastomas, but rare with gliomas. It occurs with some carcinomas (especially of the breast and stomach), and is commonly referred to as 'carcinomatous meningitis' rather than the more correct *meningeal carcinomatosis* (Fig. 13.54).

'Angioma' of the spinal cord

In elderly patients with a history of progressive paraplegia, one may find a dilated, grossly tortuous vein overlying the back of the lower part of the cord (Fig. 2.23). This condition, sometimes referred to as 'angioma of the cord', is in fact the result of an *arteriovenous fistula* arising in or close to the vertebral column. Subjection to arterial pressure causes the posterior spinal vein to dilate, elongate, and develop a thick wall. This leads to changes in the substance of the cord, where venules undergo fibrous thickening and hyaline change, with eventual obliteration of the lumen. The cord tissue becomes ischaemic and undergoes patchy necrosis.

Spinal nerve roots

The proximal, intrathecal parts of the spinal nerve roots should be examined at an early stage, and histological blocks taken in cases with a history of neuropathy and/or diabetes. Samples of anterior and posterior roots can be taken from the cauda equina for transverse and longitudinal cutting; likewise, *sensory ganglia*, which are easily accessible in the sacral region. Anterior nerve roots are visibly wasted in motor neuron disease (amyotrophic lateral sclerosis) and after severe *poliomyelitis* (Fig. 2.24). Posterior roots are wasted, more in the lumbosacral region than higher up, in *tabes dorsalis* (Fig. 2.25) and *Friedreich's ataxia*. The spinal cord itself is wasted in Friedreich's ataxia, and in some long-standing cases of MS.

Swelling of the cord

Local swellings of the spinal cord (other than the cervical and lumbar enlargements) are attributable to *intrinsic tumour* (Figs 11.10 and 11.13), *syringomyelia* (Fig. 8.14) or inflammation. The commonest tumours are *gliomas*—ependymomas, subependymomas, and astrocytomas (see Chapter 12). Deposits of secondary carcinoma are rare. The division of fluid-filled cavities, or syrinxes, into those lined with ependyma (hydromyelia) and those not so lined (syringomyelia) is probably somewhat artificial. The subject of the origin and pathology of these lesions is still an area of dispute (see p.150).

Examples of *inflammatory* lesions causing swelling of the cord are poliomyelitis (p.171), perivenous encephalomyelitis (p.179) and acute MS (Fig. 11.11). As the pia mater is somewhat inelastic there is a tendency for the lesion to extend itself upward and downward, producing the clinical state of 'ascending myelitis' (see p.196).

Segmental levels

The cords of paraplegic patients (other than those with MS) will generally show a sharply defined locus of thinning or destruction, due to compression or to trauma. The segmental level of such a lesion should be determined (see below), and compared with the assessed sensory level recorded in the clinical notes. If the vertebral column is still available, the vertebral level of the lesion, which is numerically higher than the segmental level in the cord, should be ascertained.

In assessing segmental levels by reference to the vertebral column, it must be remembered that the first cervical nerve roots emerge below the occipital bone, *above* the first cervical vertebra; similarly, the seventh cervical roots emerge *above* the seventh cervical vertebra, the eight cervical roots appear between the seventh cervical and first

(a)

(b)

Fig. 2.23 (a) 'Angioma' of the spinal cord. The posterior surface of the lower part of the cord is covered by an exceedingly tortuous, dilated, and thick-walled vein, clothed in thickened pia and arachnoid. (Courtesy of Dr JT Hughes.) (b) Venous angioma of the cord after dissection.

thoracic vertebrae, and from there downward, each pair of roots emerges *below* the similarly numbered vertebra.

Close to the cord, the entering and emerging roots are split into a number of rootlets which form an almost uninterrupted series in front and behind. The cord segment is defined as the portion receiving and emitting the rootlets of a particular root – a rather imprecise definition, as the division between one set of rootlets and the next may be at different points on the cord in front and behind. In an adult, each cervical and thoracic cord segment measures a little over 1 cm from above down. Below this the segments are progressively shorter so that the lower sacral segments are no more than 2 or 3 mm long.

If the vertebral column is not available, segmental levels may be worked out by counting upward and downward from the first thoracic segment. T1 is normally the lowest segment in the cervical enlargement, and the T1 roots are the lowest *large* nerve roots in that region. In case of doubt, two transverse cuts may settle the matter. The upper half of T1 cord segment has a typical 'cervical' appearance, with massive anterior grey horns; the lower half has a typical 'thoracic' shape, with slender anterior horns and well-defined lateral horns.

Transverse slicing

Transverse slicing of the cord may reveal certain features.
1 Areas of *softening* or even disruption. If these are not the immediate effect of trauma, they are probably due to infarction. Causes of infarction include: atheroma of the aorta, with occlusion of one of the major radicular arteries supplying the anterior spinal artery; surgical procedures in the posterior abdominal wall, with damage to an important radicular artery; compression of a nerve root carrying

(a)　　　　　　　　(b)　　　　　　　　(c)

Fig. 2.24 Anterior roots of the cervical enlargement. (a) The roots are normal, but there is a shrunken, discoloured plaque of MS at the lower end. (b) Atrophic roots from a case of motor neuron disease. (c) Even more wasted roots from an old case of severe poliomyelitis.

such an artery by tumours, especially neuroblastomas, lymphomas, myelomas and secondary carcinomas (one of the commoner causes of '*malignant paraplegia*'); and fat or air *embolism*. In cases with inflammatory cord swelling, a common finding is a *plug of necrotic tissue* which has been forced upward or downward into the posterior white columns by pressure within a tightly stretched pia mater.

2 Well-defined *patches of grey discoloration*, unrelated to grey–white boundaries or to tracts in the white columns, or to areas of vascular supply. These can be confidently diagnosed as plaques of MS. They are more frequent in the cervical cord than elsewhere, and tend to affect the lateral columns more than the rest of the cord. In long-standing cases of MS, the outlines of the plaques may be blurred as a result of wallerian degeneration in long tracts.

3 *Grey discoloration* of such long tracts as are large and compact enough to be distinguished by the naked eye. It should be remembered that in wallerian (anterograde) degeneration loss of myelin from the affected tracts is a slow

(a)　　　　　　　　(b)

Fig. 2.25 Posterior lumbosacral roots. (a) Normal; (b) from a case of tabes dorsalis. The roots are wasted, and there is some meningeal fibrosis. The discoloration is probably due to traumatic lumbar punctures.

process; thus it may be several weeks before the effects of a hemiplegic stroke are reflected in naked-eye changes in the relevant corticospinal tract.

Bilateral degeneration of the crossed and uncrossed corticospinal (pyramidal) tracts is seen *below* the lesion after cord transection (p.109); in Friedreich's ataxia (p.278), and in most cases of motor neuron disease (p.271). Bilateral degeneration of upgoing pathways (posterior columns and spinocerebellar tracts) is seen *above* a cord transection and in Friedreich's ataxia, and of the posterior columns alone in tabes dorsalis. In Strümpell's *familial spastic paraplegia*, where it appears that the cells of origin are unable to maintain the vitality of very long axons, one finds pyramidal tract degeneration in the lower part of the cord, and posterior column and spinocerebellar tract degeneration in the upper part (see p.285).

Choice of blocks for histology

In some neuropathological departments a standard number of blocks, taken from standard sites, are embedded, sectioned and stained from every brain examined. We feel that this practice is unnecessarily wasteful of time, technical skill, materials and storage space. Ideally, in our view, each block, and each stain, should serve the purpose of answering one or more questions; thus, if the technician were to ask 'why did you take that block?' or 'why did you ask for that stain?' the pathologist should be ready with a satisfying answer.

Neuropathologists have been laughed at by general pathologists for demanding sections of extravagantly large size, requiring very expensive glass slides and coverslips. In return, general pathologists are mocked for examining sections no bigger than postage stamps, stained with haematoxylin and eosin, and labelled simply 'brain'. We do not wish to argue these points, apart from maintaining that there are situations demanding large sections, and that there should be technicians able to prepare them.

Freezing and embedding

In selecting blocks for histology there is an initial choice to be made between *frozen sections* and *paraffin* or *celloidin embedding*. If fat stains are required, frozen or cryostat sections are obligatory, since fat is dissolved away during the embedding process. Some of the most used metallic impregnations—for instance, Cajal's gold sublimate method for astrocytes, or the Weil–Davenport method for microglia—require frozen sections. For most other purposes, blocks are embedded, and the choice lies between paraffin and celloidin embedding.

The advantages of celloidin embedding are listed below:

1 large sections are easier to handle than paraffin sections of comparable size;
2 Nissl-type stains for neurons, and haematoxylin stains for myelin, are generally clearer, more vivid, and thus more suited for photography than in paraffin sections.

The main disadvantages are:

1 it is sometimes difficult to achieve perfect flatness of the section. This can be a drawback in high-power photography;
2 the process of embedding is slow, and the pathologist may have to wait several months for his/her sections;
3 the blocks, which are stored in dilute alcohol, deteriorate over the years, becoming very hard, and difficult to stain effectively when cut, whereas paraffin-embedded blocks last indefinitely;
4 nitrocellulose (celloidin) is an explosive substance, and the solvent is ether. The handling and storage of these materials entails certain hazards.

By and large, the disadvantages of celloidin outweigh the advantages, especially if the technician has acquired the skill needed for handling large paraffin sections. We currently use paraffin almost exclusively.

No rigid rules can be laid down regarding choice of blocks for embedding, except that some at least should be relevant to the probable diagnoses. For instance, blocks from the brain of a patient with parkinsonism must include the *putamen* (Fig. 2.26), *substantia nigra* (Fig. 2.27A) and *locus ceruleus* (Fig. 2.27D). In the case of an elderly patient with progressive dementia, in the absence of naked-eye lesions, samples of *cerebral cortex*, including a temporal lobe, must be looked at, as recommended on p.311. In a case of heart failure, or if there is reason to think there was cerebral ischaemia or hypoxaemia shortly before death, elements known to be particularly sensitive to hypoxia should be examined. These include the *thalamus, hippocampus*, and *Purkinje cells* of the cerebellum.

More often than not, the clinical notes and the naked-eye appearances provide one with a firm, or at least a provisional, diagnosis. When this is not the case, one may be reduced to scanning for lesions with the microscope. For this purpose there are certain useful blocks which include a number of different structures in a single section. For example, a block can be taken at level A1 (Figs 2.4 and 2.26D) which includes third ventricle, hypothalamus, mamillary body, striatum, pallidum, amygdala and insula. Similar blocks from P1 and P2 show anterior and posterior thalamic levels, medial and lateral geniculate bodies, and hippocampus (Figs 2.4 and 2.26E–G). A section taken at or just below the lateral apertures of the fourth ventricle shows the medullary pyramids, inferior olives, medial lemnisci, descending trigeminal tracts and nuclei, dorsal vagal nuclei, inferior cerebellar peduncles, cerebellar cortex and dentate nuclei (Fig. 2.27G and H). If interest is focused on cerebellar topography, the cerebellum should

Fig. 2.26

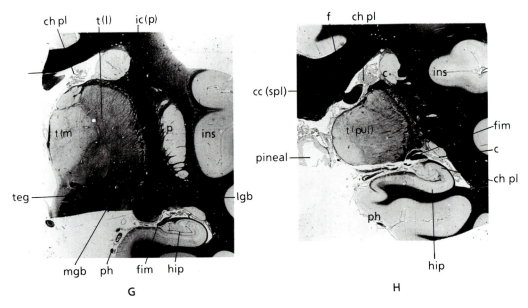

Key

	Basal ganglia				
		gp (i)	globus pallidus (internal segment)	olf	olfactory tract
		gr	gyrus rectus	ot	optic tract
ax	anterior commissure	hip	hippocampus	p	putamen
am	amygdaloid nucleus	hyp	hypothalamus	ph	parahippocampal gyrus
aps	ant. perforated substance	ic (a)	internal capsule, anterior limb	rn	red nucleus
c	caudate nucleus	ic (g)	internal capsule, genu	sn	substantia nigra
cc	corpus callosum	ic (p)	internal capsule, posterior limb	spl	splenium of corpus callosum
ch pl	choroid plexus	ins	insula	sub	subthalamic nucleus (Luys)
cing	cingulate gyrus	lgb	lateral geniculate body	t (a)	thalamus, anterior nucleus
cl	claustrum	mam	mamillary body	teg	tegmentum
f	fornix	mgb	medial geniculate body	t (l)	thalamus, lateral area
fim	fimbria	mo	medial orbital gyrus	t (m)	thalamus, medial area
gp (e)	globus pallidus (external segment)	n bas	nucleus basalis (subst innominata)	t(pul)	pulvinar of thalamus

Fig. 2.26 (*above and previous page*) Myelin-stained sections, taken at roughly 7 mm intervals, of the central part of the right cerebral hemisphere. The levels correspond with levels A3–P3 in coronal slices (Fig. 2.4).

be severed from the brain stem (p.21), and sections taken of the midline and of one or both hemispheres, with a cut at right angles to the folia on the upper surface, passing through the dentate nucleus (Fig. 2.28a and b).

Routines for brain and cord

Routine histology on the spinal cord is carried out on transverse slices at various levels—for instance, one from the cervical enlargement (C5 to T1), two from upper and lower thoracic levels, and one from the lumbosacral enlargement (Fig. 2.29). The lowest block should include anterior and posterior nerve roots. These are liable to fall away from the cord during processing, but can be kept in place until the last moment by tying a piece of thread around the specimen. In cases of peripheral neuropathy, a bundle of roots, with the tip of the conus medullaris to distinguish between anterior and posterior aspects, is simi-

larly wrapped. All specimens of cord and cauda equina should be clearly labelled with at least approximate levels, and inked on the surface opposite the one from which sections are to be cut.

In cases of MS, longitudinal sections may be desirable, in order to distinguish between normal, degenerate and demyelinated tracts. Either coronal or paramedian planes may be used; but the former, passing through both left and right sides of the cord, are somewhat easier to interpret.

Examination of long tracts

An important part of the examination of a diseased nervous system consists of tracing degeneration through the *long myelinated tracts* of the brain and spinal cord. For this, the most usual approach is to look for unnatural localized pallor in low-power views of myelin-stained sections. This negative, so to speak, impression of tract degeneration can be reinforced by stains which give positive evidence of myelin breakdown (for methods, see below). To avoid confusion, we propose to define 'tract' as a bundle of myelinated fibres of similar origin and destination, sufficiently large and homogeneous to be identified by low-power microscopy. In this sense, the optic radiation

Key

Brain stem

acc cun	accessory cuneate nucleus
ambig	nucleus ambiguus
ant	anterior horn (C.1)
aq	aqueduct
ch pl	choroid plexus
c teg	central tegmental tract
cun fun	cuneate funiculus (column of Burdach)
cun nuc	cuneate nucleus
dent	dentate nucleus
dors coch	dorsal cochlear nucleus
dors vag	dorsal vagal nucleus
fr pont	frontopontine tract
grac fun	gracile funiculus (column of Goll)
grac nuc	gracile nucleus
icp	inferior cerebellar peduncle (restiform body)
inf col	inferior colliculus (inf. corpus quadrigeminum)
inf ol	inferior olive
lat ap	lateral aperture (foramen of Luschka)
lat lem	lateral lemniscus (lateral fillet)
lat vest	lateral vestibular nucleus
loc cer	locus ceruleus (locus pigmentosus pontis)
mcp	middle cerebellar peduncle (brachium pontis)
med lem	medial lemniscus (medial fillet)
mgb	medial geniculate body
mlf	medial longitudinal fasciculus
mo nuc 5	motor nucleus of trigeminal nerve
m vest	medial vestibular nucleus
n3	oculomotor nerve
n4	trochlear nerve
n5	trigeminal nerve
n6	abducent nerve
n7	facial nerve
n8	cochleo-vestibular (acoustic) nerve
n9	glossopharyngeal nerve
n10	vagus nerve
n12	hypoglossal nerve
nuc 3	oculomotor nucleus
nuc 4	trochlear nucleus
nuc 6	abducent nucleus
nuc 7	facial nucleus
nuc 12	hypoglossal nucleus
par pont	parieto-pontine tract
pyr	pyramid
pyr tr	pyramidal (corticospinal) tract
pyr x	decussation of pyramidal tract
retic	reticular formation
rn	red nucleus
scp	superior cerebellar peduncle (brachium conjunctivum)
sn	substantia nigra
sp nuc 5	spinal nucleus of trigeminal nerve
sp tr 5	spinal (descending) tract of trigeminal nerve
sp vest	spinal (inferior) vestibular nucleus
sup col	superior colliculus (sup. corpus quadrigeminum)
sup ol	superior olive
sup vest	superior vestibular nucleus
tr sol	tractus solitarius
vent coch	ventral cochlear nucleus
vent 4	fourth ventricle

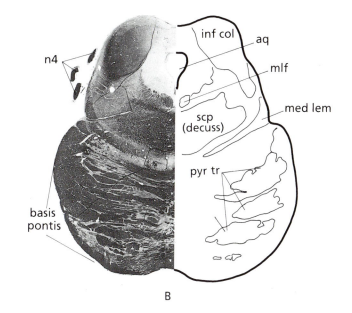

Fig. 2.27 Myelin-stained transverse sections of the brain stem. Intervals between sections are unequal, being larger in the pons and smaller in the medulla.

Fig. 2.27 *continued.*

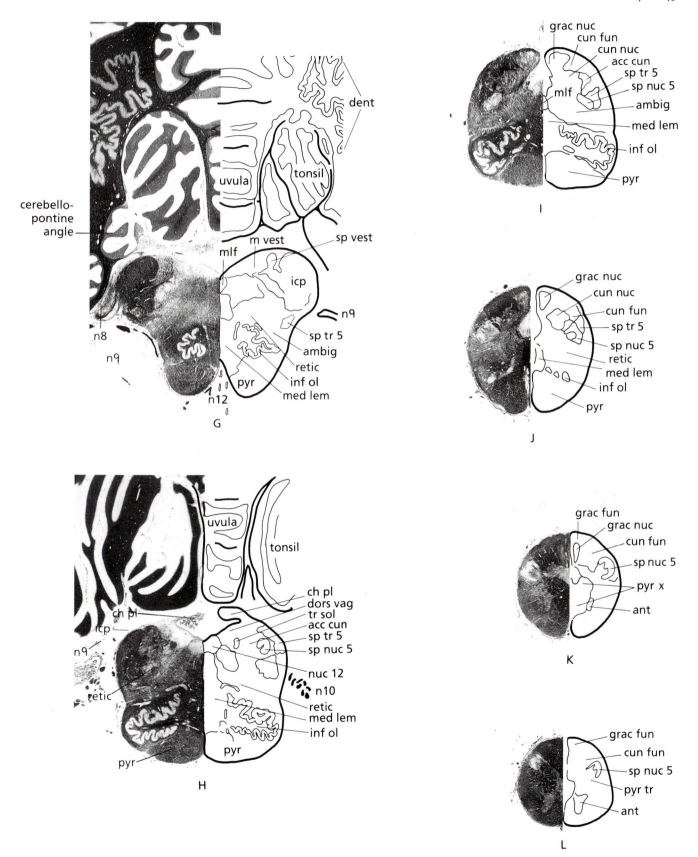

Fig. 2.27 *continued.*

Key

ant	anterior lobe
D	dentate nucleus
l	lingula
mb	midbrain
med	medulla
n	nodulus
p	pyramis
post	posterior lobe
t	tonsil
u	uvula
1	primary fissure
4	fourth ventricle

(a)   (b)

Fig. 2.28 Sections through the cerebellum: (a) in the midline, showing divisions of cerebellar vermis; (b) oblique, passing through the dentate nucleus.

(running from the lateral geniculate body to the visual cortex), the medial lemniscus (running from the gracile and cuneate nuclei to the thalamus), the superior cerebellar peduncle (running from the dentate nucleus to the red nucleus and thalamus on the opposite side) and the middle cerebellar peduncle (running from the pontine nuclei to the opposite cerebellar cortex) are *tracts*; whereas the spinothalamic pathway, running in the anterior quadrant of the spinal cord, being mixed with many other pathways, is not a tract in this sense.

The longest, and most famous, tract in the CNS is the *pyramidal* (corticospinal) tract. Its course is indicated in Figs 2.27, 2.29 and 2.30. This tract originates in the cerebral cortex on both sides of the central sulcus (not merely in the motor cortex, as is sometimes stated) and courses downward through the posterior limb of the internal capsule to the brain stem and beyond. In the internal capsule, it lies well behind the position ascribed to it in older anatomy textbooks. It occupies the middle third of the crus of the cerebral peduncle, the medial and lateral thirds of which terminate among the pontine nuclei. In the pons it is broken up into several bundles, which come together as the *pyramid*, from which the tract takes its name, in the medulla oblongata. At the junction of the medulla and spinal cord, most of the pyramidal fibres decussate (i.e. cross to the opposite side), and run downward in the lateral columns of the cord. A variable proportion, on one side or both, continues downward, as the uncrossed pyramidal tracts, and decussates at lower levels. The fibres terminate in the grey matter of the spinal cord, and exert an influence on the motor cells of the anterior horns. The more rostral fibres (the corticobulbar tracts) exert a similar influence on cells in the motor nuclei of the brain stem.

The pyramidal tract has traditionally been regarded as the essential pathway for 'willed' movements. Since cases have been described in which interruption of the tract has not been followed by permanent hemiplegia, this view can no longer be treated as dogma; but it remains true that in

most cases of hemiplegic 'stroke' the relevant pyramidal tract is found to have degenerated a few months later.

The positions of other important tracts are indicated in Figs 2.27 and 2.29. Some of the commoner degenerative conditions, in which individual tracts undergo progressive decay, are discussed in Chapter 15. Table 2.1 is intended to show the origins and destination of some of these tracts, along with some of the common conditions in which tract degeneration can be observed by low-power light microscopy. It is probably the case that not one of these tracts is 'pure', i.e. homogeneous in its origin and destination. The table merely indicates the *predominant* fibre composition.

In addition to those listed in the table, there are a number of conspicuous bundles of myelinated fibres, of mixed origin and destination, in which it is often possible to detect degenerative changes. These include: the *corpus callosum*, which is mainly composed of fibres connecting corresponding areas of cerebral cortex in the right and left hemispheres; the *anterior commissure* (Fig. 2.26C), similarly connecting the right and left temporal lobes; the *internal capsule*, which comprises not only the corticobulbar and corticospinal pathways but the many projections running from thalamus to cortex and cortex to thalamus; the *fornix*, which consists largely of fibres running from the hippocampus to the mamillary body and septal nuclei of the same side; the *lateral lemniscus* (lateral fillet), which contains auditory fibres on their way to the inferior colliculus and sensory fibres running to the thalamus; the *central tegmental tract*, with mainly descending fibres from the thalamus and other basal nuclei to the olives and other brain stem structures; the *medial longitudinal fasciculus*, which connects the nuclei of the third, fourth and sixth cranial nerves with each other and with the various vestibular nuclei; and the *inferior cerebellar peduncle* (restiform body), which carries the fibres of the dorsal spinocerebellar tract and its cranial equivalent, arising in the accessory cuneate (lateral cuneate) nucleus to the cerebellum, as well as fibres from the opposite inferior olive, and fibres run-

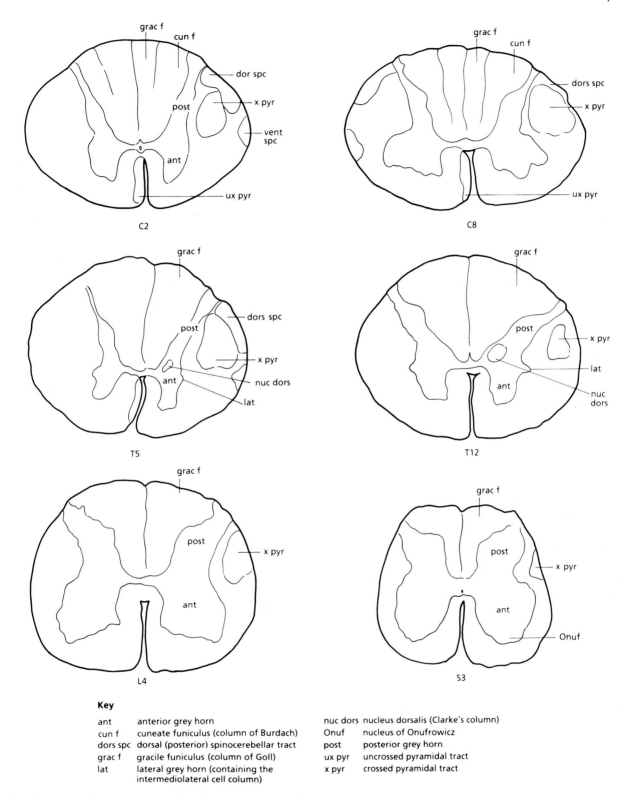

Key

ant	anterior grey horn	nuc dors	nucleus dorsalis (Clarke's column)
cun f	cuneate funiculus (column of Burdach)	Onuf	nucleus of Onufrowicz
dors spc	dorsal (posterior) spinocerebellar tract	post	posterior grey horn
grac f	gracile funiculus (column of Goll)	ux pyr	uncrossed pyramidal tract
lat	lateral grey horn (containing the intermediolateral cell column)	x pyr	crossed pyramidal tract

Fig. 2.29 Drawings of sections of spinal cord at levels C2, C8, T5, T12, L4 and S3.

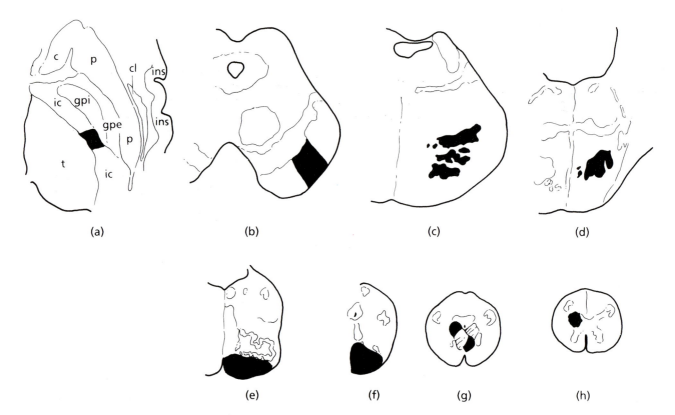

Fig. 2.30 Position of pyramidal (corticospinal) tracts in the brain. (a) Basal ganglia in horizontal section. See key to Fig. 2.26.

ning in both directions between the vestibular nuclei and the emboliform, fastigial and globose nuclei in the roof of the fourth ventricle.

In the spinal cord, the *posterior columns* (gracile and cuneate funiculi) are relatively pure, consisting of the central processes of primary sensory ganglion cells. The crossed and uncrossed pyramidal tracts, the dorsal spinocerebellar tracts, and less conspicuously the ventral spinocerebellar tracts, are tracts in the sense given above. The rest of the lateral and anterior white columns consists of a mixture of ascending and descending fibres, having various origins and destinations. The neatly defined 'tracts', so commonly illustrated in textbooks of neurology, are mainly the product of the passion for systematization of an older generation of German anatomists.

Loss of nerve cells

The other major preoccupation in the exploration of a sick brain or cord is the search for loss of, or pathological changes in, *nerve cells* in relevant areas. In general, the detection of cell loss is more troublesome than scanning for tract degeneration. It may involve careful (but often inconclusive) comparison with 'control' materials, or even cell counting in selected sites. It hardly needs saying that

familiarity with the normal appearances is conducive to speed. In addition, there are two well-tried ways of making the task less formidable. One is the use of glial stains, which draw attention to foci of tissue loss or damage (see below). The other is to examine the efferent pathways serving the cells in question. For instance, loss of fibres in anterior nerve roots is a reliable indication of anterior horn cell loss; and loss of cells in a dentate nucleus is reflected in the superior cerebellar peduncle (Fig. 15.14).

Visual pathways

When there is a clinical history of *visual disturbances*, the reason for which is not readily apparent, it may be helpful to remind oneself of the anatomy of the visual pathways, the main points of which are shown in Fig. 2.31. It should be clear from this that a defect in the sight of *one* eye will result from a lesion in that eye or in its optic nerve. A defect in the temporal fields of *both* eyes points to a lesion affecting the fibres from the medial halves of both retinae. This may happen with a tumour such as an olfactory groove meningioma, lying just in front of the chiasm, or from one lying just behind the chiasm such as pituitary adenoma. A defect in corresponding areas of the visual fields of *both* eyes (homonymous hemianopia) indicates a lesion in the optic tract on the side opposite the field defect, or in the related lateral geniculate body, optic radiation or calcarine,

Table 2.1 Some myelinated tracts in the CNS.

Tract	Origin	Principal destination	Conditions (other than MS) causing degeneration
Olfactory	Olfactory bulb	Pyriform cortex (uncus and parahippocampal gyrus)	Head injury, with avulsion of olfactory bulb (see p.109) Neurosurgery, with retraction of frontal lobe
Optic nerves and tracts	Retinae, with hemidecussation at chiasm	Lateral geniculate bodies	Retinal disease. Glaucoma. Ocular trauma. Orbital tumours Optic neuritis. Pituitary and parapituitary tumours (see Chapter 13) Methyl alcohol or clioquinol poisoning (pp.358, 353). Tobacco/alcohol amblyopia (p.354)
Geniculostriate (optic radiation)	Lateral geniculate body	Striate (visual) cortex	Cerebral tumours and vascular accidents Leucodystrophies (see Chapter 19)
Fimbria and fornix	Hippocampus	Septal nuclei and mamillary body	Mesial temporal sclerosis (see p.326). Cerebral tumours (see Chapter 12). Neurosurgery
Pyramidal (corticobulbar and corticospinal)	Pre- and postcentral cortex	(Via interneurons) contralateral motor nuclei of brain stem and cord.	(Unilateral) cerebral trauma, tumour or vascular accident (Bilateral) cord compression. Motor neuron disease (p.271) Friedreich's ataxia (p.278). Strümpell's paraplegia (p.285) B_{12} deficiency (p.361). Toxins, including organophosphorus and clioquinol (Chapter 20)
Medial lemniscus (medial fillet)	Contralateral gracile and cuneate nuclei	Thalamus (nuc. ventralis lateralis)	Acceleration injuries (see p.106). Brain stem tumours (see Chapter 12)
Superior cerebellar peduncle (brachium conjunctivum)	Dentate nucleus	Contralateral red nucleus and thalamus	Acceleration injuries (p.106). Friedreich's ataxia (p.278) Progressive supranuclear palsy (p.282). DRPLA (p.283)
Middle cerebellar peduncle (brachium pontis)	Pontine nuclei	Contralateral cerebellar cortex	Pontocerebellar degeneration (see p.276)
Inferior cerebellar peduncle (restiform body)	Dorsal, accessory cuneate and vestibular nuclei: contralateral inferior olive	Cerebellar cortex	Cerebellar and spinocerebellar degenerations (p.275) Syringobulbia (p.151)
Solitary	Ganglia of facial, glossopharyngeal and vagus nerves	Nucleus of solitary tract	Peripheral neuropathies (Chapter 22) Multiple system atrophy
Cuneate funiculus (column of Burdach)	Cervical and thoracic sensory ganglia	Cuneate nucleus; accessory cuneate nucleus	Ascending, from lower spinal trauma or tumour Friedreich's ataxia and other system degenerations (Chapter 15)
Gracile funiculus (column of Goll)	Lumbar and sacral sensory ganglia	Gracile nucleus Thoracic nucleus	Peripheral neuropathies (Chapter 22). B_{12} deficiency (p.361) Carcinomatous radiculopathy (p.184). Tabes dorsalis. Toxins, including organophosphorus, clioquinol and vincristine (Chapter 20)
Dorsal spinocerebellar	Dorsal nucleus (Clarke's column)	Cerebellar cortex	Ascending, from lesions of lower spinal cord Friedreich's ataxia and other system degenerations (Chapter 15) Chronic meningitis and other causes of marginal degeneration of the spinal cord (p.155)

DRPLA, dentato-rubro-pallido-luysian atrophy; MS, multiple sclerosis.

Fig. 3.10 Ferrugination. In an area of old infarction, the bodies of dead neurons in the cerebral cortex, instead of undergoing phagocytosis, have been mummified and impregnated with iron and calcium salts. In an H&E preparation they appear densely basophilic. H&E, ×350. (The resemblance to silver-impregnated neurofibrillary tangles (Fig. 3.14) is fortuitous.)

Fig. 3.11 Chromatolytic motor cell from the anterior horn of the spinal cord. The cells are large, with widely spreading dendrites. H&E, ×600. Compare with Fig. 3.3.

Fig. 3.12 Cerebellar Purkinje cells (arrowed) in a case of multiple system atrophy (p.273). The axon of one cell is expanded by a so-called 'torpedo'—a sign that the distal part of the axon is damaged. Holmes silver, ×1400.

Fig. 3.13 Cerebellar cortex from which Purkinje cells have been lost. The molecular layer occupies much of the field with the granule-cell layer at top right and lower left. Between them can be seen basket cell processes that terminate in the 'baskets' which normally envelop the bodies of the Purkinje cells. Here, the Purkinje cells have died, leaving empty baskets (arrowed). Holmes silver, ×160.

have so far revealed nothing to suggest a connection with virus infections. It is otherwise with the eosinophilic cytoplasmic inclusions of rabies, and nuclear inclusions of herpes simplex encephalitis and subacute sclerosing panencephalitis. These are described and discussed in Chapter 10.

Fig. 3.14 (a) Neurofibrillary tangles in the subiculum (Fig. 2.32) in a case of progressive supranuclear palsy (p.282). von Braunmühl silver impregnation, ×270. (b) Neurofibrillary tangles can also be seen with routine H&E stain, ×500.

(a)   (b)

Fig. 3.15 Pigmented cell from the locus ceruleus in the pons, in a patient with Parkinson's disease. The nucleus is seen on the right; on the left there is a typical laminated Lewy inclusion body. Lendrum's phloxine-tartrazine, ×1600.

Fig. 3.16 'Senile' plaques in the cortex of a patient with Alzheimer's disease. Methenamine silver, ×300.

Neuroglia

Neuroglial cells—astrocytes, oligodendrocytes and ependymal cells—originate, like central neurons, from the embryonic neural tube, the common ancestral cell being the spongioblast. The secretory epithelium of the choroid plexus consists of modified ependymal cells.

Astrocytes

Astrocytes are distributed throughout the central (but not the peripheral) nervous system. They have two (perhaps three) known functions (others which have been ascribed to them have not yet been generally accepted). The first of these is based mainly on electron-microscopical studies, which show that while nerve cells have no direct contact with capillary blood vessels, the processes of astrocytes make intimate contact both with nerve cell bodies and with capillaries. It is inferred that certain astrocytes perform the duties of wet-nurses to neurons. The second function is that of reacting to various kinds of local damage—cell death, axonal degeneration, demyelination, etc.—by proliferating, enlarging and putting out long processes

Striking changes are seen, mainly in the larger cells of the central and peripheral nervous system, in the *lipidoses*. These are for the most part familial disorders, with autosomal recessive inheritance, in which deficiency of an enzyme results in abnormal accumulations of a normal or abnormal lipid substance in the cytoplasm of nerve cells (Fig. 19.2). The histological appearances tend to be similar in different types of lipidosis. These conditions are discussed in Chapter 19. A number of antibodies to cytoskeletal components can be used to demonstrate nerve cells and their processes. For example, neurofilament antibodies demonstrate axons well and antibodies to the lysosomal enzyme cathepsin D clearly demonstrate pyramidal neurons (Fig. 3.42).

which in due course become glial fibres, forming a glial scar (Figs 3.17–3.20). The term *gliosis* is commonly (and confusingly) used to denote both hypertrophy and hyperplasia of astrocytes on the one hand, and glial scarring on the other. We think the term is best reserved for the latter. The third function plausibly ascribed to these cells is the maintenance of the *blood–brain barrier* by means of their 'end-feet', which surround the walls of small vessels (Fig. 3.18a) and the similar terminal expansions applied to the pial and ependymal linings of the brain.

In conventional cell stains, and even in metallic impregnations, normal resting astrocytes are unimpressive. The cytoplasm is scanty and the cell outline indistinct. The nucleus is ellipsoid rather than globular, and smaller than that of most nerve cells, rather pale, with a stippling of chromatin. In a reactive astrocyte, the cytoplasm enlarges and becomes more eosinophilic, and the nucleus is displaced to the side (Fig. 3.17). Binucleate forms are not uncommon, and should not be regarded as evidence of neoplasia. In a Holzer preparation (see p.65) one can see cell processes extending in all directions; there are fibrils, presumably the precursors of glial fibres, running from one such process through the cytoplasm, ending in another process, and criss-crossing with other similar fibrils. In metallic impregnations, of which Cajal's gold chloride method is the general favourite, less is seen of intracellular details, but more of the cell processes (Fig. 3.18a and b). Some of these processes, thicker than the rest, terminate as 'end-feet' on the walls of capillaries and venules (Fig. 3.18a). Others, on the surface of the brain and cord, end in intimate contact with the pia mater. Astrocytes, with their

processes, may also be demonstrated by treatment with an anti-GFAP (glial fibrillary acidic protein) antiserum or monoclonal antibody (Fig. 3.40; see p.70).

Following Cajal, a distinction is often drawn between 'fibrillary' and 'protoplasmic' astrocytes (Fig. 3.18a and b), and these terms have been applied to the cells in astrocytic tumours. The physiological significance of this distinction is not known. The change referred to as 'clasmatodendrosis'—i.e. fragmentation of astrocytic processes—is seen in metallic impregnations of what are thought to be moribund astrocytes. Of the few recognized pathological cell changes, two were first described in cases of Wilson's disease (hepatolenticular degeneration; see p.335). The cells referred to as 'Alzheimer glia, type 1' appear to be grossly enlarged astrocytes, with bizarre polyploid nuclei (Fig. 19.4). Similar cells are seen, not only in glial tumours, but also in *Richardson's disease* (progressive multifocal leucoencephalophathy; see p.173). Alzheimer type-2 glia is more commonly met with, and appears to be pathognomonic of hyperammonaemia due to liver failure (see p.345). The cells appear in conventional cell stains as naked nuclei within almost empty spaces. These nuclei are pale, globular or lobulated, larger than those of normal astrocytes, with a diffuse stipple of chromatin, and a conspicuous nucleolus (Fig. 19.3). They occur mainly in grey matter, in any region of the brain.

Oligodendrocytes

Apart from vascular endothelium, oligodendrocytes are the most numerous cells in the CNS. The 'few dendritic

(a)

(b)

Fig. 3.17 Reactive astrocyte in an active plaque of MS.
(a) GFAP, ×800; (b) H&E, ×250.

(a)

(b)

(c)

Fig. 3.18 Reactive astrocytes. (a) In the cerebral cortex in a case of Creutzfeldt–Jakob disease. Astrocytes are increased in numbers and in size. Some of the thicker cell processes can be seen terminating in 'end-feet' (arrowed) on the walls of a small blood vessel. Cajal's gold sublimate, ×180. (b) So-called protoplasmic astrocytes in the neighbourhood of a malignant tumour. The cell bodies are smaller than those of the fibrillary astrocytes shown in Fig. 3.18a; the processes are more numerous and more finely divided. Cajal's gold sublimate, ×180. (c) In a plaque of acute MS. The cells are pleomorphic, and in some instances multinucleate. In biopsy specimens of lesions of this kind there is a temptation to rush into a diagnosis of astrocytoma. Holzer, ×420.

Fig. 3.19 Gliosis of the cerebellar cortex in a case of Creutzfeldt–Jakob disease. There has been a massive loss of neurons in the granular layer (lower half of picture), and almost all the cells seen in this area are reactive astrocytes. Above this, there are Purkinje cells in normal numbers. The molecular layer (above) is crammed with the fibrillar processes of astrocytes (the so-called Bergmann glia) situated in the Purkinje cell layer. The glial fibrils lie parallel with each other (so-called 'isomorphous gliosis') because they are replacing the axons of dead granule cells, which themselves lie at right angles to the surface. Holzer, ×60.

will increase understanding of many nervous system diseases, and that they will eventually find a use in diagnosis. The extent to which immunohistological techniques are used at present depends to a great extent on local expertise and preference; also on expense, since some commercially available antibodies are very expensive, (though to set against this is the high cost of silver stains). For the present, probably the most widely used antibodies in routine diagnostic use are those directed against glial fibrillary acidic protein (GFAP), which identify normal, reactive and neoplastic astrocytes (Fig. 3.40). Other immunological cell markers are also of use, particularly for identifying cells that are hard to stain by routine techniques. In our hands, oligodendrocytes can best be demonstrated in paraffin sections with antibodies to carbonic anhydrase isoenzyme II (Morris *et al.* 1993). Oligodendrocytes also react with antibodies to galactocerebroside, and with the monoclonal antibody, anti-Leu 7, which detects myelin-associated glycoprotein, some neural crest-derived cells, and natural 'killer' cells of haemopoietic origin. Neurons can be identified by use of neurofilament antibodies and of antibodies to neuron-specific enolase, or better, synaptophysin or cathepsin D (Fig. 3.42). Neurofibrillary tangles, abnormal neuronal inclusions, can be demonstrated with antibodies to hyperphosphorylated tau protein. The abnormal argyrophilic plaques seen in cerebral cortex in many old people and in greater number in Alzheimer's disease (Chapter 18) are well shown with antibody to β-amyloid as well as with silver (Fig. 3.44). There are some macrophage monoclonal antibodies that react with microglial cells (e.g., HAM 56 and binding of the lectin

Fig. 3.41 Increased numbers of oligodendrocytes with cytoplasm reactive for carbonic anhydrase isoenzyme II (red) at the edge of a subacute multiple sclerosis plaque. Counterstained with Mayer's haemalum, ×150.

(a)

Fig. 3.42 Hippocampus showing a strong reaction for the lysosomal enzyme cathepsin D in the cytoplasm of CA4 and dentate gyrus neurons. Counterstained with Mayer's haemalum, ×100.

(b)

Fig. 3.40 Immunohistochemical staining of astrocytes. (a) Resting. (b) Reactive. GFAP method, ×420.

Fig. 3.43 Neurofibrillary tangles in the entorhinal region revealed with an antibody to hyperphosphorylated tau protein. ×200. (Compare with Fig. 3.14.)

(a)

Fig. 3.44 Argyrophilic plaques in cerebral cortex of an elderly person revealed with an antibody to β-A4 protein. ×100. (Compare with Fig. 3.16.)

(b)

Fig. 3.45 Immunohistochemical staining of microglial cells using *Ricinus Communis* agglutinin 1 lectin binding (a) mildly reactive microglial cells in white matter (b) 'rod' cells in the hippocampus in encephalitis associated with HTLV-1 infection. Note close relationship of microglial cell processes to pyramidal neurons. Both counterstained with haematoxylin (a) ×250, (b) ×400. (This lectin also binds to endothelial cells.) (Slides prepared by Dr CS Morris.)

Ricinus communis agglutinin 1 also shows microglial cells well) (Fig. 3.45). The use to which some of these and other antibodies can be put in tumour diagnosis is discussed in Chapter 4 and in encephalitis in Chapter 10.

Warnings

Teachers of histopathology are familiar with the tendency of students to turn to the high powers of the microscope before they have scanned the specimen by the low power, and with the need to combat this tendency. The principle that one should survey the wood before examining the trees applies to the exploration of the nervous tissue even more than to the examination of the lungs or liver. Apart from sharply localized lesions, one sample of a liver will look much like another, whereas sections of the lower brain stem may yield quite different information from that derived from the upper brain stem or cervical cord. What is more, the most important bits of information will usually be revealed by the use of the naked eye, hand lens, or dissecting microscope.

In this, as in other activities, it is of some importance to avoid wasting one's time in vain pursuits. In biopsy work, for instance, there is no profit in trying to decide on the exact nature of cells which have been crushed by forceps or frizzled by diathermy. It is therefore important to learn, as soon as possible, to recognize features in histological preparations which are of no pathological significance, or which are actually misleading. Such features are of two main kinds: (i) genuine, but non-specific, tissue changes, and (ii) so-called artefacts. Some of these are listed below.

Non-specific changes in nervous tissue

By 'non-specific' we mean merely that we do not know what the changes signify, and do not associate them with any well-recognized disease. Some of them may one day turn out to be of great diagnostic importance. It is worth remembering that the great TH Huxley spoke of the pituitary gland as a vestigial structure of no physiological importance.

Aberrant nerve fibres

Disputes continue concerning the capacity for sprouting and regeneration of nerve fibres within the CNS, but there is no doubt about the sprouting ability of peripheral nerve fibres. These include the axons of motor neurons, and the central processes of sensory ganglion cells. If for any reason a small or large chunk of spinal cord dies, the necrotic tissue is liable to be invaded by nerve fibres, with Schwann cells in attendance, derived from either anterior or (more commonly) posterior spinal nerve roots. The invading fibres acquire sheaths of myelin of peripheral type (Fig. 11.12). Lacking any orientating influence, they do not form parallel bundles, but get twisted into dense tangles, resembling the neuromas arising from the cut ends of peripheral nerves (Fig. 3.46). The same process may occur on a small scale, and it is not at all uncommon to see tiny neuromas in the substance of the cord or brain stem, with no evidence as to the original lesion.

Calcification

Calcified pineal glands and choroid plexus are normal in later life, and may be visible in straight X-rays of the head. Massive calcification in brain tissue ('brain stones') has been mentioned earlier (p.26). Minor degrees of calcification, unassociated with symptoms, or with any recognized disease, are commonly met with in stained sections. They occur for the most part in elderly people, and are

Fig. 3.46 Central neuromas in the spinal cord. Fourteen years before death the patient had suffered a very severe acute polyneuritis, with very slow and incomplete recovery. Although there was little, if any, loss of sensory ganglion cells, there was severe loss of their central processes. Regeneration from sensory ganglia resulted in invasion of the cord by regenerated axons, accompanied by Schwann cells. Within the cord, these fibres formed neuromas, i.e. dense tangles of myelinated axons. In this longitudinal section, stained with silver, surviving CNS tracts contain fine, straight axons, whereas the regenerated fibres are coarse and darkly stained. Holmes silver, ×85.

commonest in the lentiform nucleus. They occur either as rows of tiny calcospherites along the course of capillary vessels, or as tubular deposits in the medial wall of larger vessels (Fig. 19.22). They stain positively for iron as well as for calcium.

Corpora amylacea

These are globular basophilic bodies, 10–50 μm in diameter, most commonly seen in the subpial tissue of the brain and cord in elderly subjects (Fig. 3.47). Favourite locations are the lips of the lateral fissures and the white columns of the spinal cord. They stain positively with PAS and

Fig. 3.47 Accumulation of corpora amylacea in the subpial tissue at the base of the cerebrum. The appearance, though striking, is non-specific. It must not be confused with the picture of cryptococcal meningitis. PAS, ×250.

iodine. They are currently believed to develop within astrocyte processes, and to indicate some form of neural decay. They must not be confused with yeasts, such as *Cryptococcus*.

Lipofuscin

This yellowish fatty material accumulates in the cytoplasm of nerve cells with advancing age. It is seen in many sites, but is often most abundant in the large neurons of the thalamus (Fig. 3.48).

Fig. 3.48 Lipofuscin in thalamic nerve cells. Buff-coloured lipid may occupy over half the volume of the cell. As with corpora amylacea, the appearance is non-specific, becoming more prominent with increasing age. H&E, ×420.

Subependymal and subpial astrocytes

These normally form sheets of fibroglia, which grow denser with age. Here, too, the change is not regarded as pathological until it is deemed to be excessive. How much is too much is a question individual neuropathologists must decide for themselves, on the basis of their experience. Truly pathological causes include acute and chronic meningitis, and subarachnoid blood from burst aneurysms, head trauma, etc.; and subpial and subependymal gliosis is said to result from repeated epileptic fits.

Myelin pallor

One of the most familiar problems in the histopathology of the CNS lies in deciding whether failure of the myelin in a particular area to take up the stain is due to disease, or to non-specific causes, or to an artefact. 'True' myelin pallor can be caused by oedema (see Chapter 11), demyelination (see Chapter 14), leucodystrophy (see Chapter 19) or by wallerian tract degeneration. Most of the lesions of MS are easily recognized as such, but 'shadow plaques' often give rise to doubts. Doubts of this kind can often be disposed of by the use of a Holzer or similar stain, which reveals a glial reaction to the lesion.

In the spinal cords of elderly people there is sometimes a marginal rim, a millimetre or so wide, of poorly staining, or even absent, myelin. This is often combined with fibrous thickening of the pia mater and subpial gliosis. The cause is generally uncertain. It is important not to mistake this appearance for specific tract degeneration—in particular, of the dorsal and ventral spinocerebellar tracts.

Artefactual causes of myelin pallor are discussed below (p.75).

'Slight cell loss'

This phrase is only too familiar from published neuropathological reports. It may occasionally be taken on trust, but more often it represents an attempt by authors to hedge their bets. They are unsure of their observations, they do not want to be thought to have been neglectful, or to have failed to examine the relevant part; also, they do not wish to commit themselves to a positive statement that the tissue is diseased. In a few places, such as the Purkinje layer of the cerebellum, a mild degree of cell loss may actually be detectable without recourse to cell counting. Elsewhere, it is usually exceedingly difficult. Admitting that even we may not be free of sin, we strongly deplore the tendency to report on 'slight cell loss'. Honesty, we maintain, is still the best policy.

Fig. 3.49 The wavy pattern commonly seen in longitudinal sections of peripheral nerve may be partly due to differential shrinkage of the connective tissue during fixation. ×150.

'Wavy pattern' in peripheral nerves

A common observation in longitudinal sections of peripheral *nerves* is a more or less regular pattern of waves, as in Fig. 3.49. This is merely the expression of the nerve's elasticity. If the specimen is fixed under moderate longitudinal tension, the waves are not seen. Another common appearance is the apparent disruption of myelin sheaths by a series of so-called Schmidt–Lanterman clefts (Fig. 3.50). There has been some dispute as to whether these clefts are natural or artefactual, or a bit of each. At any rate, they do not have a pathological significance. They are discussed by Thomas, Landon & King (1984).

Peri-tendinous muscle

Sections of *muscle* taken from near a tendinous insertion may show features which would be regarded as pathological if they occurred in the belly of the muscle. These include increased perimysial collagen, splitting of muscle fibres, and internal nuclei (see Chapter 23).

Artefacts

In archaeology, the word 'artefact' means an object thought to be the product of human artifice: a stone wall, for instance, or a potsherd, or a flint showing signs of pressure-flaking. In histology, the word means an unintended by-product of a technical procedure, or merely the result of bad technique. Artefacts of these kinds occur at all stages in the processing of pathological material. Tissues decompose if the cadaver is not adequately chilled. If the delay between death and fixation of tissues is excessive, bacteria

Fig. 3.50 Schmidt–Lantermann clefts. These are very commonly seen in longitudinal sections of myelinated peripheral nerve fibres. Their origin is still disputed. Myelin stain, ×300.

which entered the bloodstream in the agonal phase may escape into the tissues and proliferate there. When the organisms are of a gas-forming persuasion, this results in the 'Swiss cheese' artefacts illustrated in Fig. 2.18. More commonly, the organisms are non-gas-forming anaerobes. Their presence in the fixed brain tissue is signalled by

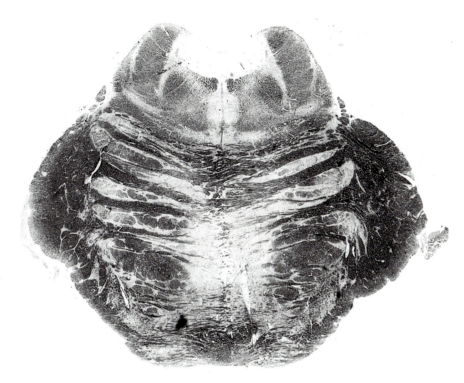

Fig. 3.51 Myelin pallor in the centre of the pons, in the absence of disease, may be due to poor fixation. When the brain is suspended in the formalin bucket from the basilar artery, the pons lies close to the surface of the fluid, resulting in poor penetration of fixative.

the appearance of tiny red rings around venules on the cut surfaces (Fig. 2.19). This can be confirmed by Gram stains.

Inadequate or delayed fixation

The effect of inadequate, or delayed, fixation of oedematous brain tissue has already been described (pp.7–8). Apart from oedema, access of formalin may be delayed mechanically—for instance, if the brain is improperly suspended, and parts of the surface are resting on the bottom of the bucket. Hydrostatic pressure may also play a part in fixation. When the brain is slung from the basilar artery, the part nearest the surface of the fluid, where the hydrostatic pressure is lowest, is the pons. It is not unusual to find that the centre of the pons stains poorly for myelin, as in Fig. 3.51. It is important not to mistake this artefact for the genuine pathological condition of central pontine myelinolysis (p.347).

An artefact most commonly seen in sections from biopsy specimens of cerebral cortex is the so-called *'dark cell'*. Near the edge of the specimen one sees shrunken, deformed pyramidal cells, sometimes with prominent, corkscrew-like apical dendrites (Fig. 3.52). It is now generally agreed that this is an effect of mechanical trauma (Duchen 1992).

An artefact which we have encountered in brains removed and fixed in departments other than ours is a wide-

Fig. 3.52 'Dark cells'. In biopsies of cerebral cortex, the pyramidal cells of layers 3 and 5 appear in stained sections as plump, rounded shapes, with globular nuclei and prominent nucleoli (slender arrows), as compared with the isosceles triangles seen in post mortem material. Near the margins of the specimen, one commonly sees shrunken, dark-staining neurons, often with dark, corkscrew-like apical dendrites (thick arrows). This is a mechanical artefact, without pathological significance. Nissl, ×200.

Fig. 3.53 A narrow band of haematoxyphil staining close to, and parallel with, the pial surface, was known locally as the St Elsewhere's artefact but now occurs in our department too since we started using buffered formalin. H&E, ×50.

Fig. 3.55 Weird patterns may also be seen in tissues which have been subjected to diathermy. Artefacts from this cause can usually be recognized in an H&E section by a disagreeable purplish discoloration. ×90.

Fig. 3.54 Firm application of the forceps to biopsied tissues often gives rise to bizarre deformations of the affected structures. On occasion, these may mimic pathological changes. ×200.

spread deposition of haematoxyphil material in a narrow band deep to the pia covering the cerebral cortex (Fig. 3.53). We were unable to account for it until the recent introduction of the use of buffered formalin into our own department brought this artefact with it.

In biopsy material, the commonest artefacts are either mechanical or thermal. Good surgeons are more concerned with the patient's interests than with the pathologist's; they will therefore tend to include damaged tissues in the specimen pot rather than leave them inside the patient. If the specimen is a piece of peripheral nerve, they will make it as short as possible, and apply the jaws of the forceps to the specimen rather than to the remaining cut ends. Thus pathologists learn to confine their attention to the middle of the specimen. Figure 3.54 shows some artefacts caused by the application of forceps; Fig. 3.55 shows the effects of diathermy on sensitive tissues.

Muscle preparations

Artefacts in histological preparations of muscle include zones of contraction affecting segments of muscle fibres, which then appear abnormally eosinophilic and homogeneous (Fig. 4.47). In frozen sections, ice crystals may leave empty spaces in the centres of fibres.

Artefacts in general constitute a nuisance and, on occasion, a serious trap for the unwary. It is important to recognize them and, as far as possible, avoid their creation. In biopsy work, this may involve a little frank discussion with the surgeons.

Further reading and references

Cajal S. Ramón y 1928. *Degeneration and Regeneration in the Nervous System.* Oxford University Press, Oxford.

Cross RB. 1982. Demonstration of neurofibrillary tangles in paraffin sections—a quick and simple method using a modification of Palmgren's method. *Med Lab Sci* **39**, 67–9.

Duchen LW. 1992. General pathology of neurons and neuroglia. In Adams JH, Duchen LW (Eds) *Greenfield's Neuropathology,* 5th edn. Edward Arnold, London, Chapter 1.

Harriman DGF. 1992. Diseases of muscle. In Adams JH, Duchen LW (Eds) *Greenfield's Neuropathology*, 5th edn. Edward Arnold, London, Chapter 21.

Morris CS, Esiri MM, Sprinkle TJ, Gregson N. 1993. Oligodendrocyte reactions and cell proliferation markers in human demyelinating diseases. *Neuropath Appl Neurobiol* **20**, 272–81.

Perry VH, Andersson PB, Gordon S. 1993. Macrophages and inflammation in the central nervous system. *Trends in Neurosci* **16**, 268–73.

Thomas PK, Landon DN, King RHM. 1992. Diseases of the peripheral nerves. In Adams JH, Duchen LW (Eds) *Greenfield's Neuropathology*, 5th edn. Edward Arnold, London, Chapter 18.

4   Biopsies

General considerations

Neuropathologists are expected to tackle the interpretation of biopsy specimens from the CNS and its surroundings, peripheral nerves and muscles. They may also be faced with smears, i.e. wet-film preparations from the operating theatre, from tumours, or from brain tissue, for instant diagnosis, and with CSF for cytology.

Clinicians show a proper reluctance to resort to biopsy for the diagnosis of disease of the CNS. Muscle and nerve biopsies are taken more frequently now than in the past, but brain biopsies other than tumour biopsies, are becoming less frequent as new, non-invasive methods of diagnosis are developed. When a brain biopsy has been decided on, it is very important to obtain as much useful information from it as one possibly can. For this, good communication between clinician and pathologist is essential. In practical terms, pathologists should attend ward rounds, and be readily available for discussion of cases. They should take the trouble to inform themselves about findings at operation, and be prepared to demonstrate their own material to clinicians. The clinician, in turn, should be urged to: provide adequate clinical information along with specimens; give due notice to the laboratory about planned operations which may result in biopsy; and learn what kinds of question pathologists can be expected to answer, and which are beyond their scope. The risk of a missed diagnosis and of an unprofitable or unnecessary operation is greatly lessened if both parties adhere to these guidelines.

When specimens arrive in the laboratory, what is done with them will depend on the nature of the specimen and the likely diagnosis (Fig. 4.1). In order to cover all eventualities it is often best to take a sample to freeze in liquid nitrogen, another for EM following fixation in glutaraldehyde, and to fix the rest in formalin. This allocation does not allow for microbiological culture, however, and if this is thought necessary, fresh samples in dry, sterile bottles should be sent rapidly to the microbiological laboratory. Remarks made in Appendix C should be heeded when handling unfixed biopsy specimens.

Biopsies of tumours

Tumour diagnosis is one of the main tasks of neuropathologists. In biopsy work, a fairly confident early diagnosis can be made in about nine cases out of ten. Among the rest, there is the occasional totally baffling case. Between these extremes, partial or imprecise reports may be helpful to the surgeon. The first question often to be answered is 'is this tumour?'. If the answer is 'no', it is usually possible to describe the tissue as (i) normal brain, (ii) reactive brain, (iii) necrotic debris, or (iv) inflammatory tissue. If the surgeon is convinced, on other grounds, that he is dealing with a tumour (or an abscess), a report of any of these four may help him to decide on his next step. For instance, if the radiology shows a brain tumour, the finding of necrotic debris in a smear makes it almost certain that the tumour is malignant. If the immediate answer is 'yes, this is tumour, but I am not sure what type of tumour', such an answer will usually suffice until further investigations have been carried out, or outside opinions sought. It can be particularly helpful if an indication of a tumour's likely benign or malignant nature can be provided.

An important ingredient in good understanding between surgeon and pathologist is that both parties should

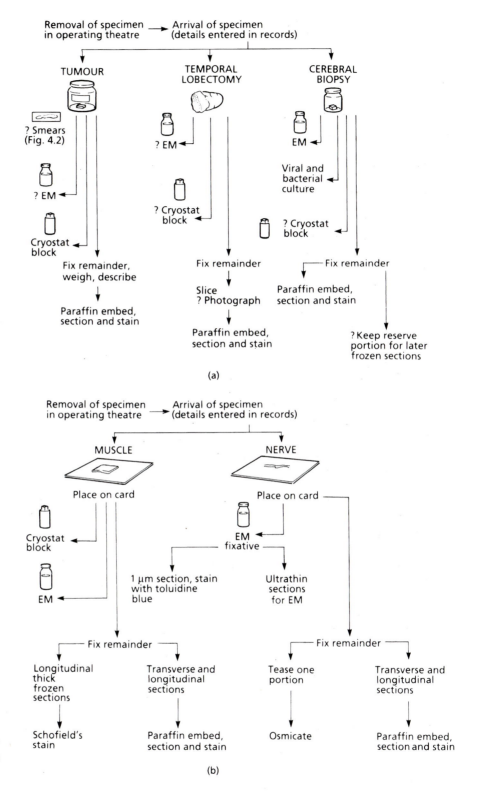

Fig. 4.1 Recommended procedures to adopt when dealing with tumour, temporal lobectomy and cerebral biopsy specimens (a), or with muscle and nerve biopsies (b).

be fully aware of the common diagnostic pitfalls. For instance, if the pathologist reports on a small biopsy specimen as 'low-grade astrocytoma', the surgeon should be aware that the sample may come from the periphery of a highly malignant glioma; and the pathologist has to remember that not all expanding lesions of the brain are neoplasms, and that it is often difficult to distinguish between reactive and neoplastic astrocytes. In any case of doubt they should confine themselves to writing an honest report on what they have actually observed, rather than extrapolate from this to what they think they *might* have seen if the surgeon had provide more material.

In dealing with the difficult cases the use of antibodies to relatively cell-specific antigens may be of value (see below). An important practical point arises from the fact that some of these antibodies need to be applied to cryostat sections, necessitating the use of fresh frozen tissue. As one does not know in advance which tumours are going to give rise to diagnostic difficulty, it is advisable to arrange for the rapid transport from the operating theatre to the laboratory of all tissue in an unfixed state, in a screw-topped container to prevent drying out. The pathologist can then decide how best to divide the tissue available for routine histology, cryostate sectioning and smears for rapid diagnosis. EM may also provide diagnostically useful information, and a sample can be appropriately fixed for this purpose if sufficient tissue is available. After the main specimen has been fixed, it is described, weighed and embedded, entire or in representative blocks, in paraffin wax.

Choice of stains to perform on paraffin sections will vary according to the supposed nature of the tumour, but H&E is used together with a PTAH stain for presumed gliomas and a Van Gieson stain for meningeal tumours and schwannomas. The PAS stain is helpful for showing mucinous material in carcinomas, choroid plexus tumours, myxopapillary ependymomas and chordomas, and stains for reticulin are helpful in the examination of meningeal tumours, pituitary specimens when there is doubt about whether they contain gland or tumour, and lymphomas. Pituitary tumours are traditionally examined with a combined PAS and Orange G or similar stain. Less commonly used but helpful at times are pigment stains for melanin and iron, and nerve fibre stains. Melanin may be present in a number of tumours including meningioma, nerve sheath tumour, ependymoma, medulloblastoma and choroid plexus tumour, as well as melanoma. The use of immunohistological techniques in tumour diagnosis is discussed on p.88, and the histological diagnosis of tumours in Chapters 12 and 13.

Smears in tumour diagnosis (Table 4.1)

For urgent tumour diagnosis there is a choice between smears and frozen sections, or a combination of these. This to some extent depends on personal preference and experience, but with some tumours the choice is largely dictated by their texture. Very soft tumours are best smeared, but with tough tumours frozen sections are to be preferred, though touch preparations, made by dabbing a portion of tough tumour firmly against a glass slide, may contain useful diagnostic features, such as whorl formations from a meningioma. Frozen sections and smears are often comple-

Table 4.1 Questions to answer in smear analysis.

If obvious tumour is present:
Is tumour readily identifiable?
If tumour is readily identifiable:
    is it benign-looking?
    is it malignant (necrosis, mitoses)?

If there is doubt about whether tumour is present, consider distinctions between:
fibrillary astrocytoma and gliosis?
glioma and acute MS?
necrotic tumour and brain?
necrotic tumour and pus?
lymphoma and chronic inflammation?
cerebellar tumour and normal/squashed cerebellum?
papilloma and choroid plexus?

If there is no tumour present:
is there normal brain (caution on cerebellar cortex)?
is there reactive brain (swollen astrocytes, etc.)?
is there inflamed brain (cuffed vessels, etc.)?
is there purulent inflammation, or acute infarction?

MS, multiple sclerosis.

mentary. Frozen sections provide valuable information about the architecture of a tumour but less cytological detail than smears; blood vessels and their relation to tumour cells are seen clearly in transverse section in frozen sections, while smears provide a good display of considerable lengths of vessels.

Smears are made by placing a small piece of tumour, 2–3mm across, at one end of a clean glass slide and pressing a second slide firmly across it (Fig. 4.2). Three or four smears can be prepared from different parts of the specimen. They are dried in air, fixed in absolute alcohol for a minute or so and stained with methylene blue (30 seconds) or H&E. Excess stain is washed away in tap water (distilled water is not necessary), taking care not to dislodge the smeared tissue. The slide is then dehydrated, cleared and mounted in the usual way. The whole procedure should take less than 5 minutes. Frozen sections are usually stained with H&E.

Many surgeons, faced with the clinical and radiological evidence of a malignant brain tumour, do not engage in open brain surgery. Instead, they approach the site of the tumour with a blunt hollow needle, via a burr-hole, and make smears of the tissue thus obtained. If the tissue proves malignant, no further surgery is undertaken. If the appearances are inconclusive, or if the tumour looks benign, they may proceed to formal surgery. It is particularly on these occasions that the pathologist needs to be circumspect in making a diagnosis, since the smear is all he has to go on. Recently, in some neurosurgical centres, the technique of using multiple CT-directed or magnetic resonance

Tumour fragment placed on lower slide

2nd slide placed over tumour fragment and moved smartly to left

Repeat to produce 3 – 4 separate smears, air-dry

Fix smears in abs. alcohol 1 min

Transfer to slide rack and place in tap water bath – few secs

Smear processing

Careful tap water wash (few secs)
1% methylene blue (30 secs)
Tap water wash (few secs)
Dehydrate
Clear
Mount

Fig. 4.2 Procedure for making smears of fresh biopsy (or post mortem) tissue.

image-directed biopsies has been evolved. This may result in great difficulties for the pathologist in reaching a firm diagnosis on multiple, very tiny specimens of tissue sent for immediate smears. On other occasions, smears are sent from the theatre with a request for an immediate opinion, and are followed by one or more solid specimens, usually in formalin. In these circumstances it may have to be pointed out that the smear diagnosis is only provisional. Occasionally, however, it is a smear which provides the answer, whereas the stained sections do not.

The following points are offered as guidelines to the diagnosis of tumours based on their appearance in smears. Further information of the appearance of CNS tumours in smears can be found in the monographs by Adams *et al.* (1981), Bigner and Johnston (1994) and the article by Barnard (1981), listed at the end of this chapter.

Reading a smear (see also Table 4.1)

First of all *check the source of the tissue* (cerebrum, cerebellum, meninges, pituitary fossa, etc.), *assess its overall cellularity* and *decide whether or not it contains tumour*. Bear in mind that 'cellularity' depends on the thickness of the smear, which can be gauged by focusing up and down with the high-power objective. This avoids being deceived into thinking a smear is 'cellular' merely because it is thick.

If no tumour is evident at first, search the slides carefully, as the tumour cells may be confined to one corner of one of several slides. If tumour is not present the tissue will consist of normal or 'reactive' brain, or contain some other pathology such as inflammation or infarction, or necrotic, uninterpretable debris. The appearance of normal or reactive brain depends on the site. Two normal ingredients of brain are particularly liable to be mistaken for tumour tissue. The first is cerebellar cortex, where the densely packed granule cells may mimic tumour, especially if the cells have been distorted by rough smearing (Fig. 4.3a). Smears of cerebellar cortex, but not tumour, should contain a few large Purkinje cells, and the granule cells should have regular nuclei without mitotic figures. The second is choroid plexus (Fig. 4.3b), which may be mistaken for adenocarcinoma. 'Reactive' brain contains plump, reactive astrocytes and possibly some lipid-filled macrophages, other inflammatory cells and prominent capillaries (Fig. 4.4).

If tumour is present, examine it at *low power* to gain an idea of the *general arrangement of the cells*. Carcinoma cells tend to form adherent clumps (Fig. 4.5), meningioma cells frequently form whorls (Fig. 4.6), ependymoma and neuroblastoma cells rosettes (Fig. 4.7), and choroid plexus papilloma forms papillary fronds reminscent of normal choroid plexus (Fig. 4.8). The tumour cells of gliomas,

Fig. 4.8 Appearance of a smear preparation from a benign choroid plexus papilloma. Methylene blue, ×170.

Fig. 4.9 Low-power view of lymphoma tumour cells in a smear preparation. Many tumour cells remain adherent to vessel fragments, while elsewhere they smear diffusely. H&E, ×150.

Fig. 4.10 A smear of astrocytoma tumour cells frequently shows a disorderly arrangement of cells. Methylene blue, ×180.

Figs 4.11–4.18 Nuclear morphology in methylene blue-stained smear preparations (×400) apart from Figs 4.14 and 4.15 H&E; Fig. 4.18 Orange G/PAS.

Fig. 4.11 Malignant astrocytoma.

Fig. 4.12 Medulloblastoma.

Fig. 4.13 Carcinoma.

of reactive astrocytosis. Nucleoli are prominent in ependymomas, some carcinomas, melanomas, pituitary adenomas, and some meningiomas and lymphomas (Figs 4.13–4.15), but are usually inconspicuous in other cerebral tumours. Glycogen-containing vacuoles in nuclei are a prominent feature of some meningiomas.

Various *miscellaneous features* may be present, providing useful clues to the nature of the tumour.

1 Normal, or nearly normal, brain occurring in close juxtaposition with clumps of frankly malignant cells—carcinoma.

2 Extracellular, finely fibrillar, metachromatic material (staining pink with aniline blue dyes)—gliomas, especially ependymomas (Fig. 4.19); other metachromatic material—chondrosarcoma or chordoma (Fig. 4.20).

3 Psammoma bodies—meningioma (benign).

Fig. 4.14 Lymphoma.

Fig. 4.15 Metastatic melanoma.

Fig. 4.16 Myeloma.

Fig. 4.17 Low-grade astrocytoma (note variation in nuclear size; nucleoli are unusually prominent).

Fig. 4.18 Pituitary adenoma.

Fig. 4.19 Smear preparation of a malignant glioma illustrating the appearance of characteristic metachromatic, extracellular fibrillary material (purple). Methylene blue, ×400.

4 Melanin pigment—melanoma or (occasionally) melanocytic meningioma, nerve sheath tumour, ependymoma, medulloblastoma or choroid plexus tumour. (If in doubt whether pigment is melanin or haemosiderin it may be necessary to perform a Perls' stain on another smear.)

5 Many large, multinucleate cells—glioblastoma, osteoclastoma (or osteoclastic reaction), malignant fibrous histiocytoma, carcinoma, reaction to craniopharyngioma or epidermoid/dermoid cyst, inflammatory condition (e.g. tuberculosis).

6 Distinct large and small cell populations—germinoma, lymphocytic reaction in a carcinoma, some lymphomas.

7 Keratin—craniopharyngioma, squamous cell carcinoma, epidermoid/dermoid cysts.

8 Frank tumour necrosis—malignant tumour.

9 Endothelial hyperplasia—malignant glioma (Fig. 4.21), cerebellar astrocytoma; rarely, bronchial oat cell carcinoma.

10 Calcium deposits—oligodendroglioma, astrocytoma, pituitary adenoma, meningioma.

11 Numerous mast cells—cerebellar haemangioblastoma.

Fig. 4.20 Abundant, wispy, extracellular, metachromatic strands and scanty, ill-defined cells in a smear preparation of a chordoma. Methylene blue, ×200.

12 Plasma cells—myeloma (especially if abnormal forms present; Fig. 4.16), plasma cell reaction to tumour, infection, etc.

13 Haemosiderin—meningioma, malignant glioma, cerebellar astrocytoma, angioma, schwannoma, cerebellar haemangioblastoma; also, tissue around aneurysms and arteriovenous malformations, and in infarcts.

14 Intense inflammatory cuffing of vessels accompanied by features of 'reactive' brain—encephalitis (Fig. 4.22); rarely, MS.

Finally, smears frequently contain contaminating material, such as bone dust, and especially glove powder (Fig. 4.23). It is almost impossible to try to identify every item in a smear, and it is time wasting and distracting to try to do so.

Immunohistological approach to the diagnosis of CNS tumours

Antibodies are now available to a number of antigens which display some degree of specificity for particular lines of cellular differentiation. A number of monoclonal antibodies to common or restricted antigens expressed by neuro-ectodermally derived mature cells and tumours are described by various groups, for example, Carrel *et al.* (1982). Other antibodies recognize antigens which are common to tumours and fetal neural tissues (Wikstrand *et al.* 1983). A third group of monoclonal antibodies is directed against antigens shared by CNS and haemopoietic cells (de Tribolet *et al.* 1984; Budka & Majdic 1985). At present there is what seems, to the outsider, a bewildering array of antibodies described by different groups of workers; most of these are not as yet widely available. Individual laboratories have raised antibodies to antigens present in tumour cells, which are suitable for diagnosis, but there is still no

Fig. 4.21 Smear preparation of a malignant glioma, demonstrating hyperplasia of endothelial cells (arrowed). Methylene blue, ×400.

Fig. 4.22 Intense inflammatory cell cuffing of a small blood vessel in a smear preparation from a case of encephalitis. Methylene blue, ×195.

Fig. 4.23 Appearance of glove powder (talc) in a smear preparation. Birefringent particles are visible at the centre of some of them (arrowed). Methylene blue, ×250.

generally available 'library' of such antibodies. Such a 'library' would be of great value to neuropathologists, particularly if they could be used on paraffin-embedded tissues, and it is to be expected that something of the sort will soon exist. Meanwhile, a summary of the range of available antibodies is given below. Both polyclonal and monoclonal antibodies to some antigens are now available. Where choice exists, there are practical and theoretical arguments for preferring the use of monoclonal antibodies (Gatter & Mason 1986). Some antibodies require the use of fresh frozen sections (e.g. the anti-macrophage and microglial antibody, EBM11, mentioned below), but most of those described here can be applied to formalin-fixed, paraffin sections. Reactions for some antigens may be improved by pretreatment of paraffin sections with enzymes or microwaving; thus the suppliers' instructions need to be carefully followed. It must be emphasized that antibodies cannot at present be used as tumour-specific reagents, and adjacent sections of a puzzling tumour need to be treated with a panel of antibodies. It is important for each laboratory to become familiar with the appearances obtained in normal tissues and well-differentiated tumours with each antibody before they are tried out on a puzzling tumour.

Immunohistology is most useful in tumour diagnosis in three circumstances: firstly, if the information obtained from an examination of the tumour's architecture and cytology is conflicting, e.g. there may be some features of one type of tumour, and some of another; secondly, if the tissue available is very limited in amount, or too fragmented or distorted to be capable of providing much morphological information; and thirdly, if the tumour is poorly differentiated. To these three circumstances might be added another: where more precise information on the proliferative potential of the tumour is needed than can be provided by conventional histology. This requirement may now be met with the use of antibodies to proliferative cell nuclear antigens. These antibodies label the nuclei of cells that have entered the proliferative cell cycle. Some of them

Table 4.2 Immunoreactivity of some human CNS tumours with a panel of antibodies (prepared in collaboration with Dr CS Morris).

	GFAP	EMA	CK	LCA	NF/SYN	NK	VIM	S-100	NSE
Astrocytoma	+	−	−	−	−	+	+/−‡	+/−‡	−/+‡
Carcinoma	−	+	+	−	−	+/−	−/+	−/+	−/+
Choroid plexus tumour	+/−	+	+	−	−	+/−	+	+	+
Ependymoma	+	+/−*	+/−	−	−	+	+	−/+	−/+ (focal)
Ganglioneuroma	−	−	−	−	+	−	ND	+	+
Ganglioglioma	+/−	−	−	−	+	−	+/−	+/−	+
Glioblastoma	+	−/+	+/−	−	−	+	+ (focal)	+	+ (focal)
Haemangioblastoma	+/−	−	−	−	−	−	+	−/+ (focal)	+/−
Lymphoma	−	−	−	+	−	−	±	±	−
Medulloblastoma	+/−	−	−	−	+/−	+/−	+ (focal)	+ (focal)	+
Melanoma	−	−	−/+†	−	−	−	+†	+	+ (focal)
Meningioma	−	+/−	+/−	−	−	−	+	+ (focal)	+ (focal)
Myeloma	−	+/−	+/−	+/−	−	−	±	−	−
Neuroblastoma	−	−	−	−	+	+	−	+/−	+
Neurocytoma	−	−	−	−	+	−	−	+/−	+
Neurofibroma	−	−	−	−	+/−**	+	+	+	−
Oligodendroglioma	+/−	−	−	−	−	+	−/+	+	+
Schwannoma	−	−	−	−	−	+	+	+	−/±§
Subependymoma	+	−	−	−	−	+/−	+	+	+

GFAP, glial fibrillary acidic protein; EMA, epithelial membrane antigen; CK, cytokeratin; LCA, leucocyte common antigen; NF/SYN, neurofilament synaptophysin; NK, natural killer cell/Leu 7; VIM, vimentin; NSE, neuron-specific enolase; ND, not done; +/−, usually positive, occasionally negative; −/+, usually negative, occasionally positive.
* positive, in our experience, in benign tumours, and negative in malignant ones.
† may show dual expression of CK and VIM.
‡ dependent on degree of malignancy/anaplasia.
§ NSE may be present in Antoni B areas.
** axons, not tumour cells, are positive.

are commercially available and can be applied to paraffin sections, particularly after microwave pretreatment (Cuevas *et al.* 1994).

Some of the specificities of widely available antibodies likely to be of use to neuropathologists when examining tumours are summarized below (see also Table 4.2, Bonnin & Rubinstein 1984; Weller 1985 and Perentes & Rubinstein 1987).

Antibodies to epithelial cell antigens

Most of these antibodies are directed against cytokeratin or epithelial membrane antigen (EMA). A positive reaction is obtained with carcinomas (Fig. 4.24), normal choroid plexus and choroid plexus tumours. Meningiomas may also give a focally positive reaction with some of these antibodies (Kepes 1986; Theaker *et al.* 1986) (Fig. 4.25). Myeloma and some lymphomas may give a focally positive reaction for EMA, and rarely for cytokeratin. Most gliomas usually give negative reactions with these antibodies, but the focal expression of cytokeratin antigens has been described in some glioblastomas, and benign, but not malignant, ependymomas show some reactivity for EMA (Fig. 4.26). Markers of specific carcinomas such as prostatic alkaline phosphatase and prostatic−specific antigen for prostatic carcinoma and thyroglobulin for thyroid carcinomas are occasionally of use when examining metastatic carcinoma deposits.

Antibodies to vimentin

Vimentin filaments are present in mesenchymal cells and also in glial cells. Gliomas, meningiomas, melanomas, schwannomas, lymphomas and sarcomas give a positive reaction for vimentin. Some carcinomas may also do so. In some studies, though not in all, there has been an inverse relation between the perceived degree of differentiation of astrocytomas and the intensity of reaction for vimentin.

Antibodies to glial fibrillary acidic protein (GFAP)

GFAP is a major cytoplasmic protein which is present in normal and reactive astrocytes. It is also present in gliomas with astrocytic differentiation, and in some cells in glioblastomas, subependymomas and ependymomas (Figs 4.27–4.29). Mixed gliomas containing both oligodendrocytes and astrocytes may show a positive reaction in both cell types (Fig. 4.30). Carcinomas, lymphomas, meningiomas, nerve sheath tumours and neuroblastomas do not react for GFAP. Haemangioblastomas, medullo-

Fig. 4.24 Positive reacton for epithelial membrane antigen (EMA) on cells of a metastatic carcinoma. Immunoperoxidase with haematoxylin counterstain, ×250.

blastomas and choroid plexus papillomas may contain a few positively reacting cells. Most cells in subependymal giant-cell tumours associated with tuberous sclerosis do not react for GFAP, but do react for neuron-specific enolase.

Antibodies to S-100 protein

S-100 protein is present in glial cells and cells derived from neural crest. It also occurs in small amounts in other cell types, which restricts its value for tumour diagnosis. The following tumours react, at least in some parts of the tumour, with S-100 antibodies; gliomas, benign nerve sheath tumours, melanomas, granular cell myoblastomas, choroid plexus papillomas, some carcinomas and lymphomas. Malignant nerve sheath tumours are not invariably reactive.

Antibodies to neuron-specific enolase

Neuron-specific ($\gamma\gamma$) enolase is found in neurons in the CNS and neuro-endocrine cells in other parts of the body. A strong positive reaction with this antibody is obtained with neuroblastomas, melanomas, APUDomas (carcinoids) and oat-cell carcinomas. Subependymal giant-cell tumours in subjects with tuberous sclerosis also react for this antigen. These antibodies are not helpful in distinguishing between different types of 'primitive' tumour, such as neuroblastoma and medulloblastoma, as some reaction tends to be present in all such tumours.

Fig. 4.25 Focal positive reaction for cytokeratin in cells surrounding hyaline bodies (unstained) in a meningioma. Immunoperoxidase with haematoxylin counterstain, ×350. (Courtesy of Dr J Theaker.)

drogliomas, and some medulloblastomas, also react with this antibody. Its antigen is thought to be myelin-associated glycoprotein. The pattern of staining produced frequently outlines the cell membranes.

Antibodies to pituitary hormones

These can be used to identify the hormones present in pituitary adenomas (p.242).

Antibodies to macrophages

α-1-anti-chymotrypsin is an antigen which can be used as a relatively specific cell marker for macrophages in the CNS in paraffin sections. Some recently introduced monoclonal antibodies, e.g. EBM11 (Esiri & McGee 1986), HAM56 (Adams & Poston 1990) and certain other macrophage antibodies (Franklin *et al.* 1986) react both with macrophages and with normal microglia in cryostat sections. Macrophages, among other leucocytes, also react for leucocyte common antigen, and for class 2 major histocompatibility complex (MHC) antigens.

Antibodies to embryonal cell markers

Germ cell tumours occasionally arise in the midline of the CNS and may give rise to diagnostic difficulty. They react positively for human chorionic gonadotrophin, placental lactogen and/or placental alkaline phosphatase (Fig. 4.32).

Other CNS biopsies

The use of biopsy in the diagnosis of non-neoplastic disorders of the CNS is limited to a few metabolic disorders, suspected viral encephalitis and other inflammatory conditions, and the investigation of dementia. Other conditions that may be found, though previously unsuspected, include acute MS, leucodystrophies and neuronal storage disorders. The extent to which use is made of biopsies for diagnosis of these conditions varies from one centre to another according to whether, in the clinicians' opinion, their diagnostic value outweighs any risk. In addition to diagnostic biopsies, there are opportunities to study surgical specimens when temporal lobes are partially resected or a hemispherectomy is performed for the relief of intractable epilepsy. These specimens and their management are discussed in Chapter 18.

Biopsies from cases of *suspected viral encephalitis* should be divided to provide samples for viral and bacterial culture, and, if indicated, animal inoculation studies, a sample for EM and a sample for routine light microscopy (Fig. 4.1a). By light microscopy the sections are scrutinized for changes described in Chapter 10. Snap-frozen tissue for cryostat sections may also be taken, but, as many microbial

Fig. 4.32 Germinoma from the parapineal region showing the typical dual population of large, anaplastic tumour cells and small, mature lymphocytes. The tumour cells show a reaction for placental alkaline phosphatase. Counterstained with haematoxylin, ×400.

antigens are now known to survive formalin fixation, they can be searched for more safely in paraffin sections. Smears can be made and treated with an anti-herpes simplex virus antibody, using the immunoperoxidase technique, if herpes simplex encephalitis is suspected (Fig. 4.33). If the results are negative the results of culture will have to be awaited. Toxoplasmosis can be diagnosed readily if typical cysts are present, but it may be useful to resort to antibodies if free organisms are all that are to be found (Fig. 4.34). CMV encephalitis is also readily confirmed using immunocytochemistry (Fig. 4.35). Success in detecting microbial antigens depends crucially on having a high-titre, specific antiserum or monoclonal antibody available. Positive and negative control sections or smears should be processed alongside the case under investigation whenever possible. A few infectious agents are more readily detected using *in situ* hybridization than immunocytochemistry, e.g. JC Papova virus in PML (Fig. 4.36) or measles virus in SSPE.

Cerebral biopsies from cases of *dementia* should be divided perpendicularly to the cortical surface, and one sample frozen for biochemical enzyme assay, another sample fixed in glutaraldehyde for EM, and the remainder fixed in formalin for light microscopy (Fig. 4.1a). After fixation, part of the latter sample is embedded in paraffin wax and sections cut and stained with H&E, Nissl, Congo Red or another amyloid stain, a myelin stain and a modified Palmgren (see Appendix A) or similar stain for neurofibrillary tangles. Most cases may be expected to

Fig. 4.33 Smear from a cerebral biopsy from a case of suspected herpes simplex encephalitis. A positive reaction in the nuclei of two neurons (arrowed) was obtained with a rabbit antiserum to herpes simplex type 1 virus. Normal rabbit serum gave a negative reaction on a second smear. Immunoperoxidase with haematoxylin counterstain, ×220.

Fig. 4.34 Immunocytochemical demonstration of toxoplasmosis in the brain. Cysts and free organisms are present. Counterstained with haematoxylin, ×220. (Slide prepared by Dr CS Morris.)

Fig. 4.35 Congenital cerebral cytomegalovirus (CMV) encephalitits. A multinucleated periventricular cell contains CMV antigen (red) as does the cell above. Counterstained with haematoxylin, ×1000. (Slide prepared by Dr CS Morris.)

show features of Alzheimer's disease (p.306). From such cases a cortical biopsy can be expected to contain several neurofibrillary tangles (Figs 3.14 and 17.8) and some amyloid deposition in leptomeningeal and cortical blood vessel walls (Fig. 3.35) and in the cores of plaques. Plaques are well displayed in paraffin sections with the methenamine silver stains (Fig. 3.16) or with an antibody to βA4 protein after formic acid treatment. (For precautions to take if Creutzfeldt-Jakob disease is suspected see p.445.) Some authorities regard the presence of argyrophilic plaques alone as an acceptable criterion for the diagnosis of Alzheimer's disease within certain age limits (at least 10 plaques per ×200 field at 66–75 years and at least 15 plaques per ×200 field over 75 years (Khatchachurian 1985). Other criteria rely on semi-quantitative estimates of the numbers of neuritic plaques, i.e. those containing tau-positive components (Mirra *et al.* 1991).

Site of injury

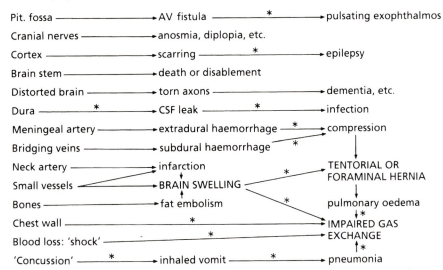

Pit. fossa ——————→ AV fistula ————*———→ pulsating exophthalmos

Cranial nerves ——————→ anosmia, diplopia, etc.

Cortex ——————→ scarring ————*————→ epilepsy

Brain stem ——————→ death or disablement

Distorted brain ——————→ torn axons ——————→ dementia, etc.

Dura ————*————→ CSF leak ————*——→ infection

Meningeal artery ——————→ extradural haemorrhage ——*——→ compression

Bridging veins ——————→ subdural haemorrhage ——*—↗

Neck artery ——————→ infarction ————*——↘ TENTORIAL OR FORAMINAL HERNIA

Small vessels ——————→ BRAIN SWELLING

Bones ——————→ fat embolism ————*——→ pulmonary oedema

Chest wall ————*——→ IMPAIRED GAS EXCHANGE

Blood loss: 'shock' ————*——→

'Concussion' ————*——→ inhaled vomit ————*——→ pneumonia

Fig. 5.1 Oversimplified diagram, showing some of the immediate and delayed effects of injury on the brain. Arrows indicate causal sequences. Asterisks show points at which medical or surgical intervention may be helpful. Capital letters indicate major immediate threats to life.

(a)

(b)

Fig. 5.2 Contusional haemorrhages. Woman aged 57, concussed for 20 minutes following a fall on the back of the head, causing a linear fracture of the left occipital bone. Fully conscious for 3 hours, then lapsed into coma. Acute subdural haematoma evacuated through a burr-hole, without improvement. Died 54 hours after injury. Post mortem findings of foraminal herniation: contusions of left cerebellar hemisphere and right frontal lobes, both giving rise to haemorrhages into the brain substance and subdural space. (a) Cerebellum, surface and slice. (b) Horizontal slice, showing massive haemorrhage into right frontal lobe, extending to the lateral ventricle. The right hemisphere is swollen, with subfalcine herniation and flattening of convolutions.

ploughing into tissue already suffering from ischaemic damage, giving rise to large subdural haematomas, and resulting in fatal herniation. The entire lesion, as displayed at post mortem, is commonly referred to as a 'contusion', whereas we think that a distinction should be drawn between the original contusion and the subsequent *contusional haemorrhage*. Our evidence for this view comes from the histological examination of a series of nine fatal head injuries, with survivals of up to 13 days. In those with more than 3 days' survival, there were cellular reactions, inflammatory and glial, datable to the time of injury. No such reactions were seen in relation to the major haemorrhages, which appeared to be terminal. The impression that the original lesions had been more or less trivial was

reinforced by the fact that most of the patients had talked coherently at some time after the injury.

Coup–contrecoup lesions

A further feature of these nine cases was that all of them had had a fall on the back of the head, and sustained a linear fracture of the occipital bone on the side of impact. Underlying this fracture was a contusion of the under-surface of the cerebellum; and a further contusion was present in the surface of the *opposite* frontal lobe (Fig. 5.2). In every case a massive haemorrhage had occurred from one or other of these contusions; in one case, from both. All nine cases were examples of the classical *coup–contrecoup* pattern of damage, described in detail by Courville in 1942. An example of the CT scan appearance of a coup-contrecoup pattern of injury is shown in Fig. 5.3.

Post mortem examination

In a case of head injury one is concerned with two main questions: (i) the mechanism of the injury, and (ii) the cause of death. These two are often related, as when the head injury is combined with a neck injury causing crushing of the cervical cord. Points of importance for the forensic aspects of the case are, first, the form and distribution of superficial bruises, scratches and lacerations, and second, the site and form of bony injuries to the skull, face, spinal column and elsewhere. Instructions on the examination of injured bodies (including the estimation of alcohol levels in the blood) and on the interpretation of one's findings are given in textbooks of forensic pathology. As to the immediate cause of death, this is to be found, in most cases, in the brain stem. In the most severe cases of acceleration injury of the brain, with instant death, one may find a tear running half-way through the midbrain, which is tethered within the posterior cranial fossa, and cannot withstand an extreme swirling movement of the cerebral hemispheres. In cases where death was not instantaneous, the cause is likely to be a tentorial or foraminal hernia, due to haemorrhage, or brain swelling, or a combination of these. If no hernia is present, it is well to look elsewhere for the cause of death: in the cervical cord, for instance, or in the chest.

(a)

(b)

Fig. 5.3 A 35-year-old male patient was unconscious having been involved in an RTA. (a) Axial cranial CT scan employing a bone window demonstrates a fracture (arrow) involving the left temporal bone and overlying scalp haematoma. (b) The underlying intracranial injury is well demonstrated at the same level using the conventional brain window setting. An extradural haematoma is seen beneath the fracture (arrow) as a lentiform extraaxial collection of high density. Two-thirds of extradural haematomas occur in the temporoparietal region as a result of damage to a branch of the middle meningeal artery. Extensive haemorrhagic contusion, caused by forcible contact between skull and parenchyma, is present in the right temporal lobe. This is a coup-contrecoup injury. There is also evidence of generalized cerebral swelling with loss of grey/white matter differentiation and effacement of the basal cisterns and sulci. Cranial CT remains the imaging modality of choice in the assessment of acute trauma. MRI provides more useful information regarding long term sequelae.

Fig. 6.1 Chronic subdural haematoma, in a man of 70. One year earlier he had suffered a minor blow to the head. The source of bleeding appeared to be a torn bridging vein running into the superior sagittal sinus.

brain. When the arachnoid is torn, as commonly happens in cases of head injury, or when an aneurysm ruptures outwards, subdural and subarachnoid blood are found together. The commonest sources of subarachnoid blood are traumatic contusions, ruptured aneurysms, and haemorrhages into the brain substance, either above or below the tentorium. The latter may reach the subarachnoid space either by direct eruption at the surface of the brain or by irruption at some point into the ventricular system, reaching the subarachnoid space by way of the fourth ventricle and the foramina of Luschka and Magendie, where blood may be seen emerging (Fig. 6.2) even before the brain is dissected.

Aneurysms

When the suspected source of subarachnoid blood is a ruptured aneurysm, it is advisable to look for the aneurysm before the brain is fixed. Formalin transforms a clot, with the consistency of red-currant jelly, which can be easily cleared away by superficial dissection in the post mortem room, to a hard, crumbly mass, which disrupts the brain tissue when it is sliced, and may make it very difficult to distinguish a thin-walled aneurysm from its surroundings. To start with, the likeliest situation of the aneurysm may be guessed at, after observing where the blood is most

dura and arachnoid. The membrane is thicker on its inner aspect, and is adherent to the arachnoid in one or more places. Histological examination of the membrane usually reveals a laminated structure, with alternate layers of connective tissue and blood residues, indicating that the bleeding has been episodic (Fig. 3.36). In places the tissue is highly vascular, and contains many thin-walled sinusoid vessels which are probably the source of the repeated haemorrhages. Chronic subdural haematomas are typically found either in young children suffering from some form of brain damage, or in old people with more or less atrophic brains, as in Fig. 11.1. The latter do not necessarily have a history of recent head trauma. It would therefore seem that when the brain has shrunk away from its membranes it is liable to small subdural bleeds during the course of everyday head movements.

Subarachnoid blood

This is readily distinguished from subdural blood by the fact that it cannot be simply wiped off the surface of the

Fig. 6.2 Blood in the basal cisterns, A large aneurysm, seen in the upper part of the picture, had ruptured into the anterior horn of a lateral ventricle, and the whole ventricular system had filled with blood. The blood at the base had escaped from the fourth ventricle via the foramina of Luschka.

abundant. After cutting through the arachnoid at this point, the clot may be cleared away piecemeal by blunt dissection until the aneurysm, and its point of rupture, have been identified. Even when angiography has already demonstrated an aneurysm, it is best to identify the source of bleeding in this way. Aneurysms are often multiple, and the offending lesion is not necessarily the one most obvious in the angiogram. In any case, it is worth locating the actual point of rupture, if only for the interest of the clinicians concerned with the case. Figure 6.3 gives an indication of the most usual sites for the formation of aneurysms. In general, they form at points of bifurcation of cerebral arteries. There is as yet no general agreement as to their causes. Some examples are shown in Figs 6.4–6.8 and the CT, MRI and angiographic appearances in Figs 6.9–6.12.

Apart from subarachnoid haemorrhage, ruptured aneurysms are a major cause of *intracerebral bleeding*. When the point of rupture faces the surface of the brain, blood at arterial pressure is pumped directly into brain tissue. This is particularly likely to happen when the aneurysm is embraced on two sides by cerebral cortex, as is the case with aneurysms of the anterior communicating and middle cerebral arteries. In the former, blood may even irrupt into the

Fig. 6.4 Dissected anterior circle of Willis with anterior communicating artery aneurysm (arrow).

anterior horn of a lateral ventricle; in the latter, into the inferior horn. Intracerebral haemorrhage due to rupture of an aneurysm is also more likely after an initial subarachnoid bleed has resulted in perianeurysmal subarachnoid adhesions and tethering of the aneurysm to the adjacent brain. Reports on long series of cases of fatal intracerebral haemorrhage have indicated that in about a fifth of the cases the cause of the haemorrhage was a ruptured aneurysm (Weller 1992).

Complications

Subarachnoid bleeding, whatever its source, may give rise to two complications, both of clinical significance: *ventricular dilatation* and *arterial spasm*. The former has been ascribed to impaired absorption of CSF in the arachnoid granulations, leading to back-pressure and raised intracranial tension (see Fig. 8.1). It is usually transient in non-fatal cases. The latter is a well-recognized feature in angiograms following subarachnoid haemorrhage. It can be severe and prolonged enough to cause areas — often multiple, often small — of cerebral infarction. These are commonly, but not exclusively, areas supplied by branches of the main artery bearing the ruptured aneurysm. Various histological changes may be seen in vessels which have undergone spasm. The most conspicuous of these changes, in cases with survival of a month or more, is a reduction of the lumen, due to proliferation of the tunica intima (Fig. 6.13). In the histological examination of fatal cases it is worth looking for areas of infarction, and for evidence of earlier bleeds, in the form of haemosiderin deposits in the meninges. In cases of ruptured aneurysm, histological sections of the aneurysm itself will show the transition from

Fig. 6.3 Diagram of the basal arteries, including the circle of Willis. The commonest sites for aneurysm formation are ringed. Of these the commonest are the neighbourhood of the anterior communicating artery (top of diagram) and the middle cerebral arteries.

(a)

(b)

Fig. 6.5 Giant aneurysm of left middle cerebral artery. Male, aged 58. (a) Base of of brain. (b) Aneurysm cut open. The mass consists almost entirely of organized thrombus, with very little liquid blood. The basal arteries, including the one carrying the aneurysm, are irregularly dilated and calcified.

Fig. 6.6 Aneurysm of the posterior cerebral artery in a 15-year-old (an unusual finding at this age).

Fig. 6.7 Bilateral middle cerebral artery aneurysms (arrowed) in a 49-year-old man. A clip had been applied to the one on the the right of the picture. The temporal poles have been cut away.

Fig. 6.8 Transverse section of vertebral artery aneurysm indenting the lower medulla. Male, aged 57.

Fig. 6.9 Axial cranial CT scan demonstrates extensive subarachnoid haemorrhage. The distribution of blood, which is concentrated in the left Sylvian fissure, suggests a bleed from a left middle cerebral artery aneurysm. The temporal horns of the lateral ventricles are dilated due to the onset of a communicating hydrocephalus. (CT remains the initial imaging modality of choice for subarachnoid haemorrhage.)

Fig. 6.10 Towne's projection of a left internal carotid artery digital subtraction angiogram of the patient in Figure 6.9. This confirms the presence of a bifurcation left middle cerebral artery aneurysm (arrow). This patient also has a left termination internal carotid artery aneurysm. The CT scan was useful to indicate the aneurysm responsible for the haemorrhage.

Fig. 6.11 Lateral projection of a right internal carotid artery digital subtraction angiogram of a 60-year-old female patient who presented with a complete, painful third nerve palsy involving the pupil, demonstrates the presence of a large lobulated aneurysm arising from the distal internal carotid artery in the region of the origin of the posterior communicating artery. The aneurysm projects posteriorly, inferiorly and laterally where it impinges upon the oculomotor nerve. Note also the narrowing due to spasm in the distal internal carotid artery as a result of recent haemorrhage.

Fig. 6.12 T1W coronal MR image in a 34-year-old male patient demonstrates a largely thrombosed giant termination right internal carotid artery aneurysm. The chronic thrombus within the aneurysm is seen as a complex, heterogeneous mass of multilaminated clot with low signal due to the presence of organized clot and haemosiderin together with areas of high signal methaemoglobin. The aneurysm is associated with mass effect and is compressing the foramina of Munro with resultant obstruction and dilatation of the lateral ventricles. There is also distortion of the optic chiasm.

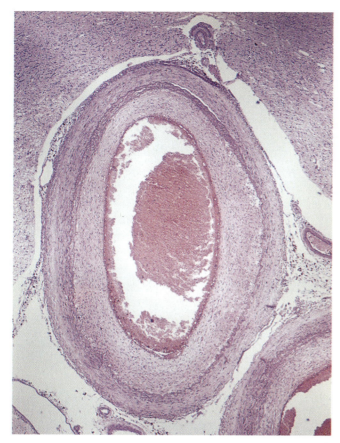

Fig. 6.13 Intimal thickening in a pericallosal artery, three months after a subarachnoid haemorrhage. Angiograms at that time showed severe and widespread arterial spasm. Note that the other coats of the artery are perfectly healthy. There is no surrounding haemorrhage or exudate. H&E, ×35.

the wall of the artery, which possesses an elastic lamina, and that of the aneurysm, which does not.

Intracerebral bleeding

When the source of bleeding lies inside the brain, it is often wise, before fixation, to extract as much of the clot as can conveniently be dislodged without disrupting the brain. This makes it easier to slice the brain after fixation. If the size of the clot is of interest, it can be weighed on its own. (Of course, if the only purpose of the post mortem is to satisfy a coroner as to the cause of death, it is an economy to slice the brain on the spot). After slicing, the following should be looked for: vascular malformations, tumours, aneurysms lurking in secluded places, and traces of earlier haemorrhages. Abnormally dilated veins should be looked for, as these may be the only evidence of an *arteriovenous malformation* which has destroyed itself in an explosive rupture. Most vascular malformations, however, are immediately recognizable from their strange tangles of ves-

sels surrounded by haemosiderin deposits (Figs 16.15 and 16.16), and often from their gritty resistance to the knife. The different types of malformation – telangiectases, cavernous angiomas, arteriovenous fistulae and the rest – are well described by Russell & Rubinstein (1989) and are briefly discussed in Chapter 16. Venous angiomas are not uncommonly the origin of 'spontaneous' haemorrhage in the region of the cerebellar vermis.

In what follows we discuss intracerebral haemorrhage in adult brains. Those occurring around the time of birth are discussed in Chapter 21.

'Spontaneous' cerebral haemorrhage

The commonest site of 'spontaneous' intracerebral haemorrhage is the *lentiform nucleus* (Fig. 6.14). A relevant factor here may be the normal disposition of the branches of the lateral striate (lenticulostriate) group of arteries (Fig. 6.15). These, after reaching and supplying the putamen, make a right-angled turn inward and upward to supply the caudate nucleus. It has been suggested that the intravascular stresses at the bend may result in (i) the formation of microaneurysms (the so-called Charcot–Bouchard aneurysms) and (ii) actual rupture of the vessel, particularly in those who are hypertensive. There is as yet no generally accepted view on the frequency and distribution of micro-aneurysms, and on the causal connections between micro-aneurysms, spontaneous bleeding and arterial hypertension. The subject is discussed, with admirable restraint, by McCormick & Schochet (1976).

In the brains of patients who have in the past made a good recovery from a hemiplegic stroke, it is not unusual to see a well-defined cavity, containing tarry fluid, in one putamen (Fig. 7.1). In such cases it is reasonable to suppose that the patient's hemiplegia was caused by oedema surrounding the haematoma and involving the posterior limb of the internal capsule, and that recovery was related to the subsidence of the oedema. An important, because treatable, cause of spontaneous, sometimes recurrent, cerebral haemorrhage is bleeding from a cavernous angiona (Fig. 6.16). The blood in the dilated sinusoidal spaces is not under raised pressure and therefore the extent of the bleeding is not large. Small leakages have an instant effect on neighbouring cortex and may cause epilepsy. These lesion are readily spotted on MRI (Fig. 6.16b).

Thalamus, brain stem, cerebellum

Apart from the lentiform nucleus, the commoner sites of spontaneous haemorrhage include the *thalamus* (Fig. 6.17), the vermis of the *cerebellum* (Fig. 6.18), and the *pons* (Fig. 2.14). Haemorrhages within the spinal canal are rare; the arteriovenous fistulae, or 'angiomas' of the cord, usually present with infarction and paraplegia rather than with

(a)

(b)

(c)

Fig. 6.14 (a) Acute haemorrhage into the lentiform nucleus, erupting into the ventricular system, in a 60-year-old woman. (b) A smaller, non-fatal haemorrhage in the left putamen. (c) Axial cranial CT scan demonstrates an acute haematoma (acute haemorrhage is high density: white) involving the right lentiform nucleus. There is some surrounding oedema (low density: dark) and mass effect manifest by compression of the frontal horn of the right lateral ventricle. Note the presence of fluid level within the haematoma (arrow). Fluid levels within a haematoma suggest a coagulopathy. This patient was taking warfarin.

subarachnoid or intramedullary haemorrhage (see p.34). Haemorrhages in the pons may originate in at least three ways, which may be rather difficult to distinguish. Firstly, there are 'spontaneous' haemorrhages, generally fatal, sometimes producing a dramatic onset of hyperthermia. Some of these may arise from vascular anomalies, which are destroyed in the course of the haemorrhage. Secondly, they may be the direct result of trauma. A characteristic

Fig. 6.15 X-ray photograph of a centimetre-thick coronal slice at level A1, following post mortem injection of a radio-opaque fluid into the aorta. Note in particular the nearly right-angled upward bend of the lateral striate group of arteries as they pass through the putamen on their way to the caudate nucleus. (Preparation by Dr Michael Dunnill.)

(a)   (b)

Fig. 6.16 Cavernous angiona. This example was removed at operation after the patient had presented with epilepsy. (a) Dilated, thin walled blood spaces separated by gliotic brain in which there is haemosiderin (blue) deposited following previous leakage of blood. Perls' stain for iron. (b) Proton density coronal MR image demonstrates the typical appearance of a cavernous angioma in the right posterior frontal lobe in a patient with focal epilepsy. This is the typical MRI appearance and is manifest by rounded foci of methaemoglobin (high signal-white) surrounded by a hypointense rim (black) of haemosiderin.

traumatic lesion is a tear, with consequent haemorrhage, in one or other superior cerebellar peduncle (Fig. 2.13). The third, and almost certainly the commonest, cause of bleeding in the pons is distortion of the upper brain stem, with rupture of its intrinsic vessels, in the course of transtentorial herniation (Fig. 2.12). In a case of head injury the second and third causes may be combined.

Fig. 6.17 Right thalamic haemorrhage in an elderly, hypertensive woman.

Phlebothrombosis

Among the more dramatic types of cerebral haemorrhage are those due to *thrombosis of major collecting veins* or dural venous sinuses (Fig. 6.19). The patterns of bleeding are characteristic of the vessels involved; for instance, thrombosis of an internal cerebral vein causes bleeding in the thalamus and basal ganglia on the same side, while if the great vein of Galen is affected, these lesions are bilateral. At the vertex, thrombosis of a major bridging vein causes haemorrhage in the parasagittal cortex and white matter, and with thrombosis of the superior sagittal sinus the lesions are bilateral. When such thromboses occur, there is almost always an underlying systemic disorder, severe dehydration, or a nutritional defect. They are particularly associated with marasmus in children, and taking an oral contraceptive in women.

Blood disorders

Massive or *multiple intracerebral haemorrhages* may be found in a variety of blood disorders, including *haemophilia*. They occur in various types of *leukaemia*, especially the more acute forms. *Thrombocytopenia*, however caused, predisposes to haemorrhage. In addition, cerebral haemorrhage is a well-recognized hazard of the therapeutic use of *anticoagulants*.

Fig. 6.18 Cerebellar haemorrhage in a woman aged 64, under treatment with an anti-coagulant for deep leg vein thrombosis.

Fig. 6.19 Haemorrhages in left temporal and inferior frontal areas, due to cortical venous thrombosis, in a woman aged 40.

Fig. 6.20 Haematoma, partly encapsulated, in the right parietal lobe of a demented woman aged 81 with cerebral congophilic angiopathy.

Vascular diseases

Diseases of blood vessels giving rise to brain haemorrhages include various types of cerebral *amyloid (congophilic) angiopathy* (for details, see Tomlinson 1992; Esiri and Plant 1996). In one of these, a rare familial form first reported from Iceland, fatal apoplectic strokes occur in previously healthy middle-aged subjects. In another familial form, severe changes in cerebral arteries, giving rise to infarcts and/or haemorrhages throughout the central nervous system, are coupled with peculiar 'plaque' formations resembling, but not identical with, the 'plaques' associated with either Alzheimer's disease or the Gerstmann–Sträussler syndrome (pp.306–11 and p.312). A sporadic form of cerebral amyloid angiopathy unassociated with systemic amyloidosis is said to account for up to 20% for 'strokes' due to cerebral haemorrhage in elderly subjects (Fig. 6.20). As in Alzheimer's disease, the affected vessels are situated

Fig. 7.4 Acute infarction in the territory of the anterior cerebral arteries. Man aged 47, with severe vasospasm following rupture of an aneurysm of the anterior communicating artery.

Fig. 7.5 Widespread laminar necrosis of cerebral cortex in a man aged 63, who suffered a postoperative cardiac arrest. Resuscitated, but remained in deep coma, on artificial ventilation, for 6 weeks.

Fig. 7.6 Laminar cortical necrosis following perinatal asphyxia.

either ischaemic or haemorrhagic, is nearly always due to tentorial herniation, with compression and distortion of the upper brain stem (see p.9). The infarcted tissue is either pale, as in Fig. 7.1, or more or less haemorrhagic, as in Fig. 7.3. The reason for this difference is not always clear; but in some cases haemorrhage may ensue when arterial pressure is re-applied to softened tissue—for example, when an embolus impacted in an artery is lysed or broken up and reflow of blood established.

The 'respirator brain'

Advances in techniques of intensive care led to a new pathological entity—the so-called 'respirator brain'. After 20 minutes or so of cardiac arrest, the whole brain is dead; but the heart can be restarted, and artificial respiration will keep the rest of the body alive. When the brain comes to be examined, it is discoloured, dark and rather soft. Histologically, it shows universal coagulative necrosis, with recognizable anatomical features, but no living cells. Today, as the clinical diagnosis of brain death is made with more confidence, the respirator is turned off before these changes develop and, the respirator brain is less frequently seen.

Causes of hypoxia

A great many factors, several of which may act in conjunction or additively, may be operative in producing local or generalized hypoxia in the brain.

Affecting oxygenation of blood

1 Lack of oxygen in inhaled air (e.g. self-asphyxiation by a child playing with a plastic bag).
2 Paralysis of, or mechanical interference with, breathing movements (e.g. motor neuron disease, pulmonary collapse).
3 Impaired gas exchange (e.g. in pneumonia, pulmonary oedema, emphysema).
4 Blocked airway (e.g. tumour, inhaled foreign body, oedema of glottis).

(a)

(b)

Fig. 7.7 Photographs of left hippocampus, in coronal section, at level P2; Nissl, ×5. (a) Normal. (b) Severe cell loss and shrinkage in the Sommer sector (H1; see Fig. 2.32), following repeated cardiac arrests, in a man aged 50.

Affecting oxygen-carrying power of blood

1 Anaemia, chronic or acute, from blood loss.
2 Carbon monoxide poisoning.

Affecting circulation of blood to head

1 Arterial hypotension (e.g. in shock or heart failure).
2 Partial or total occlusion of arterial lumina (e.g. coarctation of common carotid, atherosclerosis and other arteriopathies, thrombosis, embolism).
3 Vasospasm (especially after subarachnoid haemorrhage).
4 Venous occlusion, with back-pressure.

Affecting oxygen uptake by CNS tissues

1 Increased demand for oxygen ('consumptive hypoxia'). It is believed by some that this is a major cause of cell loss in the hippocampus and cerebellar cortex following protracted epileptic fits.
2 Hypoglycaemia (e.g. insulin overdose, islet-cell tumour).
3 Toxic or metabolic disorders (e.g. hyperammonaemia, avitaminosis (vit B_1)).

Although any of these factors may affect the severity and distribution of a cerebral infarct, the major causes of infarction are those causing blockage of arterial lumina — namely atheroma, thrombosis and embolism, and combinations of these. All three are included, along with spontaneous or hypertensive haemorrhage, under the commonly used heading of 'cerebrovascular disease'.

Infarction due to atheroma

The commonest and most easily identified site at which the arterial supply of the brain is compromised is the bulbous lower end of the internal carotid artery. Atheroma is rarely seen in the common carotid, which runs straight from its origin upwards. At its bifurcation, the blood flow becomes turbulent; and atheromatous narrowing of the origins of the internal and external carotids is exceedingly common in later life (Fig. 7.8). From time to time one is astonished to find that both internal carotids are more or less occluded, although the cerebral hemispheres show no significant softenings. In such cases it is supposed that the cutting-off of the cerebral arterial supply has been gradual, allowing time for expansion of alternative routes, including the vertebral/basilar system, and certain anastomotic pathways from the external carotids. Part of the explanation may lie in the observation that there is a rough inverse relationship between the degree of atheromatous narrowing of the internal carotids and the severity of atheroma of the anterior part of the circle of Willis. This suggests that high arterial pressure is conducive to atheroma, and that narrowing of the internal carotids in the neck protects the cerebral arteries.

The process of compensating for narrowing of this or that artery may take place from a very early age. Gross, presumably congenital, inequalities of size between the two internal carotids, and even more commonly between the two vertebral arteries, are not unusual in young subjects, and are matched by compensatory asymmetries in the circle of Willis, which in any case has a very variable pattern.

Fig. 7.8 Transverse section through the left internal carotid artery close to its origin, from a man aged 60 with a recent right-sided hemiplegic stroke. The internal carotid is almost totally occluded by atheroma and thrombus.

Sites of atheroma

Selection of sites for the development of atheroma in arteries supplying the brain may depend on factors other than turbulence and blood pressure. Atheroma is rarely seen in those parts of the internal carotid and vertebral arteries which are encased in bony canals. This suggests that atheroma may be encouraged by the artery's freedom to wriggle with each pulse wave.

Atheroma of the arteries at the base of the brain is very common in elderly subjects—at least, in over-fed populations. Any vessel may be affected; but severe narrowings, which can be held responsible for infarcts, are most commonly seen around the bifurcation of an internal carotid, in the more proximal parts of the middle and posterior cerebral arteries, and in the basilar and vertebral arteries (Fig. 7.9). Histological changes in these vessels are much the same as those seen in small- and medium-sized arteries elsewhere in the body. Less commonly, arteries of the vertebral/basilar system are not narrowed but elongated, tortuous, expanded, and irregularly calcified (Fig. 7.10). These changes are reminiscent of the disease of the abdominal aorta that commonly gives rise to aortic aneuryms. It is by no means clear whether these two forms of atherosclerosis belong to the same spectrum of disease.

'Cerebral thrombosis'

In clinical parlance, the term 'cerebral thrombosis' is used freely in cases of non-haemorrhagic infarction of parts of the brain, whether the cause of the infarct is thrombosis, atheroma or embolism, or a combination of these. In prac-

Fig. 7.10 Calcification of basal arteries. The pattern of arteries is highly asymmetrical (for instance, the basilar is supplied almost entirely by one vertebral), and there are several fusiform aneurysms. Being brittle, the basilar artery has snapped at its upper end during dissection.

tice, it is often not possible to be sure of the cause, even after a careful post mortem examination and histological examination of suspect vessels. For instance, one may find an atheromatous narrowing near the origin of a middle cerebral artery, with the residual lumen blocked by thrombus, and be unable to decide whether the thrombus had formed locally, or been lodged as an embolus from the heart or from the carotid sinus. Clotting may, of course, occur over a large extent of the artery *distal* to an occlusion.

Embolism

Embolization of the brain commonly occurs from one of two sites: the heart and a carotid sinus. On the left side of the heart thrombus may form and become loosely attached to the endocardium overlying a myocardial infarct. It may also form, in a fibrillating heart, in the left atrium. Small

Fig. 7.9 Multiple brain stem infarcts, due to atheroma of the basilar artery, in a hypertensive 83-year-old woman.

Fig. 7.11 Embolic infarct in the right thalamus (arrow) from a patient with a left atrial myxoma.

Fig. 7.12 Fool's plaques'. These are well-defined grey areas of infarction, superficially resembling plaques of MS, in the central white matter (arrow). 92-year-old man, with 3 weeks' history of confusion and right hemiparesis. At post mortem the heart was enlarged and scarred, with fragments of thrombus in the left ventricle. The lesions in the brain are attributable to a shower of small emboli from this source.

Fig. 7.13 T2W coronal MR image in a 87-year-old male diabetic patient without neurological deficit demonstrates patchy high signal in the periventricular white matter and basal ganglia bilaterally due to white matter ischaemia. The periventricular lesions appear identical to those seen in multiple sclerosis and are the MRI equivalent of 'Fool's plaques'.

emboli may also arise from vegetations, infected or otherwise, on the mitral or aortic valves or from a left atrial myxoma (Fig. 7.11). In bacterial endocarditis, these may give rise to mycotic aneurysms, most commonly at some point in the course of a middle cerebral artery (p.159). Emboli from the carotid sinus may be either dislodged chunks of atheromatous debris, or fragments of thrombus overlying a raw area of the intima. In either case, the embolus is likely to be impacted, according to its size and friability, at the bifurcation of the internal carotid artery, or at some point in the course of the middle cerebral artery, the artery in most direct continuity with the internal carotid. Sometimes (presumably when the embolus is very friable) a shower of small emboli may lodge in the lumina of penetrating arterioles, giving rise to multiple softenings in the cerebral white matter and basal ganglia. In the acute phase, these softenings, with their sharply defined edges, may suggest a diagnosis of MS, and have been called 'fool's plaques' (Figs 7.12 and 7.13).

Cerebral emboli originating in the lungs appear to be uncommon, apart from fat emboli in cases with broken bones, and metastases from malignant tumours and septic foci. Very rarely, phlebothrombosis in a systemic vein gives rise to a 'paradoxical' embolism via a patent foramen ovale. An initial pulmonary embolism may increase the pressure on the right side of the heart, and so divert a second embolus into the left atrium (Gleysteen & Silver 1970). We have encountered one such case.

Embolization in the territory of the vertebral arteries appears to be rare. Infarcts in the brain stem and cerebellum are usually readily accounted for by atheroma of a vertebral artery. An occluded vertebral artery is the usual finding in the condition known to clinicians as the lateral medullary syndrome (see p.424), which is due to infarction in the territory of a posterior inferior cerebellar artery (PICA), an artery that acts as an end artery for the vertebral artery on its own side (Figs 7.14 and 24.3). We have encountered only one case of embolization (other than malignant) in the hindbrain. This was in a case of (presumably traumatic) thrombosis at the origin of a vertebral artery. The case is briefly described on pp.111–2.

(a)

(b)

Fig. 7.14 (a) Lateral medullary infarction, due to thrombosis of the left vertebral artery (lower left), in a 62-year-old woman. (b) A series of four consecutive T2W axial MR images (A–D) through the posterior fossa demonstrate thrombotic occlusion of the left vertebral artery including its PICA origin (arrow). Normal 'flow void' (black) is present within the right vertebral artery. Abnormal signal is seen in the left lateral medulla and inferomedial cerebellar hemisphere representing infarction.

Arterial spasm

Arterial spasm, lasting long enough to cause infarction, is a well-documented complication of massive subarachnoid bleeding, whether from trauma or from rupture of an aneurysm. It is discussed above. In this connection, it is worth remembering that a direct neurosurgical approach to an aneurysm entails the risk of trauma, and subsequent thrombosis, in the artery bearing the aneurysm, giving rise to a large and, on occasion, disastrous infarct. More controversially, spasm may very rarely precipitate stroke in subjects with severe migraine.

Patterns of infarction

There are certain commonly occurring patterns of cerebral infarction, which can be fairly satisfactorily accounted for on the basis of the normal distribution of cerebral arteries and points of anastomosis between them. Figures 7.15–7.17 show the normal distribution of the brain arteries. There are various points to note.

1 There are anastomoses between the terminal branches of the anterior, middle and posterior cerebral arteries on the surface of the brain, but not in the interior. The penetrating arteries, including those supplying the thalamus and basal ganglia, are end-arteries, with clearly defined territories.

2 The anterior communicating artery usually has a fair-sized calibre. If the first part of, say, the right anterior cerebral artery is clipped in the course of surgery, the left anterior cerebral artery will usually take over the supply of its territory via the anterior communicating artery.

3 There is a reciprocal relationship in the size of the posterior communicating artery and the first part of the posterior cerebral artery on the same side. When the former is large and the latter small, the posterior cerebral territory is supplied mainly by the internal carotid artery, and the basilar artery is smaller than usual. There is a similar reciprocal relation in the sizes of the left and right vertebral arteries.

4 The blood supply of the cerebellum is variable. Usually the superior cerebellar artery supplies the rostral third, the anterior inferior cerebellar artery (AICA) is small, and the PICA supplies about two-thirds of the cerebellar hemisphere. Quite often, however, the AICA is large, and the PICA correspondingly small, on one or both sides.

Figure 7.18 shows the effect of occlusion of a middle cerebral artery (MCA) when the anterior (ACA) and posterior (PCA) cerebral arteries are fully patent. The central part of the MCA territory—part of the lentiform nucleus, insula, and opercula of the lateral fissure—are softened, while the border zones are kept alive by the ACA and PCA via surface anastomoses.

In Fig. 7.1 the entire MCA territory is infarcted. This is usually the result of an occlusion, by embolism, of the

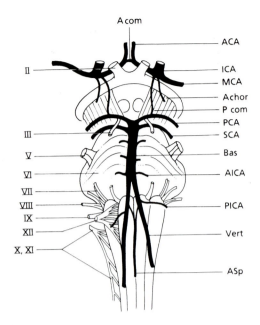

Key

ACA	Anterior cerebral artery
Acho	Anterior choroidal artery
A com	Anterior communicating artery
AICA	Anterior inferior cerebellar artery
ASp	Anterior spinal artery
Bas	Basilar artery
ICA	Internal carotid artery
MCA	Middle cerebral artery
PCA	Posterior cerebral artery
P com	Posterior communicating artery
PICA	Posterior inferior cerebellar artery
SCA	Superior cerebellar artery
Vert	Vertebral artery

Fig. 7.15 The basal arteries of the brain. The circle of Willis comprises the proximal parts of the anterior and posterior cerebral arteries, and the anterior and posterior communicating arteries.

upper end of the internal carotid artery. The ACA territory is supplied, via the anterior communicating artery, from the opposite ACA. The territory of the lateral striate arteries, which arise from the MCA in the lateral fissure, is softened; that of the medial striate, coming from the recurrent branch of the ACA, is firm, with a clear line of demarcation. Figure 7.19 shows the effect of acute internal carotid occlusion when take-over by the ACA is not achieved. Figure 7.20 shows a long-standing infarct in the territory of the PCA.

Arterial blood pressure falls continuously between the aorta and the capillary bed. In the cerebral arteries, the pressure is at its lowest at the termination of their branches, i.e. at the points where they form anastomoses with the

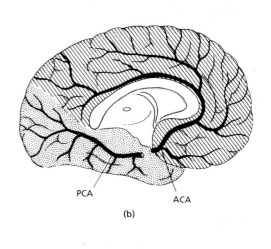

ACA

MCA

PCA

Fig. 7.16 (a) The superficial distribution of the left middle cerebral artery. (b) The anterior and posterior cerebral arteries.

ACA

MCA

PCA

penetrating arteries from circle of Willis

Fig. 7.17 The territories of the anterior, middle and posterior cerebral arteries (a) in a coronal slice at level A1, and (b) in a horizontal slice at mid-thalamic level.

Fig. 7.18 Infarct of 6 months' standing, due to an embolus originating in the left carotid sinus, affecting the left insula and inferior frontal gyrus, in a 59-year-old diabetic man.

Fig. 7.19 Acute infarction of the territories of the left anterior and middle cerebral arteries, due to thrombotic occlusion of the left common and internal carotid arteries, in a 57-year-old woman. The horizontal slice shows swelling, with subfalcine herniation, of the anterior two-thirds of the left hemisphere.

Fig. 7.20 Long-standing infarction of the territory supplied by a branch of the left posterior cerebral artery. The artery itself can be seen winding around the lateral surface of the midbrain. (In passing, note the close relationship between the posterior cerebral arteries and the oculomotor nerves (arrowed). In the presence of a diencephalic downthrust, the nerve is kinked by the artery, giving rise to the important clinical sign of the fixed dilated pupil.)

Fig. 7.21 Border-zone ('watershed') infarcts, in a 47-year-old woman with aortic valve disease leading to heart failure. Confusion and coma for one month before death. There is haemorrhagic softening in the border zones of the middle and anterior cerebral arteries on both sides, and of the middle and posterior cerebral arteries on the left side. There were similar softenings in the border-zones of the superior and inferior cerebellar arteries on both sides.

Fig. 7.22 Acute haemorrhagic infarction of part of the territory of the left posterior cerebral artery. Man, aged 53, with rupture of an aneurysm of the anterior communicating artery.

terminations of neighbouring arteries. This supplies a very plausible explanation of the common association of border-zone infarcts (Fig. 7.21) with severe or protracted heart failure. Similar border-zone infarcts may be seen in the same cases at the junction of the territories of the superior and inferior cerebellar arteries.

Cerebral infarcts may result from *pinching* of arteries, rather than from occlusion of their lumina. This can be caused by distortion, as from a tumour; but the most familiar instance is in cases of unilateral cerebral swelling or compression, with tentorial herniation. On the same side or on the side opposite the swelling, the backward-directed branches of the PCA are squeezed against the free edge of the tentorium. This interrupts the supply to the under-surface of the temporal and occipital lobes, and of the calcarine cortex. If the patient survives (a rare occurrence) he is left with a homonymous hemianopia. The infarct itself is almost always haemorrhagic (Fig. 7.22). Even more dramatic haemorrhage occurs in infarcts due to venous occlusion (Fig. 6.19). These are discussed on p.122. Infarcts due to traumatic tearing of vessels are discussed on pp. 111–12.

Lacunes

On slicing the brain of an elderly person, one commonly sees multiple small rarefactions (so-called *lacunar state*) in the thalamus and basal ganglia—most conspicuously in the lentiform nucleus (Fig. 7.23). On close inspection, small vessels can usually be seen at the centres of these lacunes (Fig. 7.24). They are regarded by some as mini-infarcts, but their causes are still uncertain. They are associated with

(a)　　　　　　　　　　　　　　　　　(b)

Fig. 7.23 (a) Rarefactions ('lacunes') in the corpus striatum (arrows). Man, aged 65, with long-standing hypertension (heart weight, 500 g) and 18 months' progressive dementia. (b) Axial cranial CT scan demonstrating multiple bilateral lacunar infarcts seen as small well defined foci of low density in the basal ganglia (arrows).

Fig. 7.24 Rarefactions related to small vessels in the corpus striatum of a hypertensive woman aged 85, suffering from general debility and mental confusion. H&E, ×35.

atheroma of the small arteries at the base. Clinically, they are suspected of playing a part in senile tremor and other Parkinson-like disturbances. Much more rarely, one finds multiple softenings and rarefactions in the cerebral white matter, associated with hyaline, thickened arterioles. The patients are usually elderly, hypertensive, and more or less demented. The condition is sometimes referred to as *Binswanger's disease* (p.315), although it is not very clear what Dr Binswanger originally described.

'Strokes' and hypertension

Whereas the association of cerebral haemorrhage with chronically raised blood pressure seems to be well estab-lished, the part played by hypertension in cerebral infarction is not yet clear. A causal link between raised blood pressure and atheroma may well exist, but there are objections to most of the simple theories of the nature of such a link. The arteriolar changes seen in Binswanger's disease are common in other parts of the body in chronic hypertensives; but whereas hypertension is common, Binswanger's disease is rare.

An enlarged heart is regarded as good evidence of chronic hypertension. It is therefore prudent to record the weight of the heart at post mortem in all cases suspected of cerebral circulatory disorder.

Hypertensive encephalopathy

This, in contrast, is a rare, fulminating, usually fatal condition associated with *sudden* elevation of the blood pressure, such as may occur in malignant hypertension and toxaemia of pregnancy. In the brain, the characteristic finding is of fibrinoid necrosis of small vessels, with petechial haemorrhages, and a variable amount of oedema of white matter.

Infarcts in the spinal cord

These are not very common, and when they occur the causes are generally different from those of infarcts in the brain. The main artery is the anterior spinal, which is continuous from its origin from the two vertebral arteries to the conus medullaris, and is fed by two or three major radicular arteries. If any of these feeding arteries is occluded, some part of the cord is likely to be infarcted.

Common causes of occlusion

1 *Compression of the nerve root* carrying a major radicular artery as it passes through an intervertebral foramen. The compressing agent is usually a tumour, benign or malignant. Benign offenders include schwannomas and meningiomas; malignant ones include carcinomas (especially Pancoast's tumour of the lung), myelomas, lymphomas and neuroblastomas. As causes of paraplegia, these are probably at least as common as tumours inside the spinal canal.

2 *Occlusion of a radicular artery* at its origin from an atheromatous aorta, causing a reduction in perfusion pressure.

3 *Trauma.* This includes unfortunate cases where surgery at the back of the abdomen (for instance, in the course of a lumbar sympathectomy) results in damage to a relevant nerve root and artery.

4 *Nitrogen embolism.* In divers, too rapid decompression may result in release of bubbles of nitrogen into the bloodstream, giving rise to decompression sickness (caisson disease, the 'bends'). In fatal cases, fresh softenings may be found, especially in the white columns of the thoracic cord. With longer survival, upward and downward tract degeneration occurs.

5 *Spinal 'angioma'.* An uncommon condition, known at various times as 'subacute necrotizing myelitis', 'angiodysgenetic necrotizing myelopathy', 'Foix–Alajouanine disease' and 'angiomatosis of the spinal cord', is now generally regarded as the result of a fistulous communication between the arterial supply and the venous drainage of the lower part of the spinal cord. How the fistula arises is not known. The disease presents, in adult life, as a progressive motor and sensory paraplegia. Exposure from behind shows the lower half of the cord covered with what looks like a tangled mass of dilated veins (Fig. 2.23), but careful dissection shows that this mass is composed of a single, extremely tortuous, thick-walled vein. Similar, but much smaller, tortuous veins may be seen running along the roots of the cauda equina. Under the microscope, the affected veins are seen to be 'arterialized', with thick, fibrous walls, devoid of the smooth muscle fibres and elastic laminae characteristic of arteries—a change liable to occur wherever veins are subjected to near-arterial pressures. Their lumina are more capacious than those of normal superficial veins. The small intrinsic vessels of the cord, on the contrary, have thick, hyaline walls, and the lumina are either diminished or abolished. The cord tissue itself shows a mixture of infarction, gliosis and wallerian degeneration, often with a few surviving nerve cells in the central parts. Thrombosis may be seen in both extrinsic and intrinsic vessels.

Arterial disease

Diseases of arteries, other than atheroma, causing ischaemic lesions in the CNS, include polyarteritis nodosa, temporal (giant-celled) arteritis, systematic lupus erythematosus, and endarteritis obliterans (Heubner's arteritis). The first of these, when it occurs in the brain, spinal cord or meninges, does not differ histologically from the same disease in other parts of the body. The second is more often encountered by neuropathologists in the shape of temporal artery biopsies than in post mortem material. Briefly, it is a granulomatous panarteritis characterized by giant cells of Langhans type. It is very rarely seen in intracranial vessels.

In systematic lupus erythematosus small arteries and arterioles in the leptomeninges and brain show evidence of platelet antigens incorporated in their walls, suggesting that platelet thrombi are largely to blame (Fig. 7.25) (Ellison *et al.* 1993).

Endarteritis obliterans

Endarteritis obliterans is a condition associated with meningitis, especially with *chronic* meningitis—syphilitic, tuberculous or fungal (see Chapter 9, p.155). It affects small- and medium-sized superficial arteries which lie bathed in purulent or granulomatous exudate (Fig. 7.26). The characteristic histological feature is that although the medial coat and elastica are well preserved, the intimal coat is thickened—sometimes to the point of complete occlusion of the lumen—by new-formed connective tissue. Why this should happen is a mystery, but there may well be a common causal link between this intimal thickening and that seen following subarachnoid haemorrhage (see p.114). Infarcts due to endarteritis may be extensive, and

Fig. 7.25 Small leptomeningeal arteries from a case of systematic lupus erythematosus. The red staining material is immunoreactive for platelet-derived antigens shown up with monoclonal antibody JC70 (anti CD-31). Counterstained with haematoxylin, ×120. (Courtesy of Dr D Ellison.)

Fig. 7.26 Endarteritis obliterans (Heubner's arteritis). Woman aged 36, with a 4-week history of tuberculous meningitis, × 35.

(a)

(b)

Fig. 7.27 Familial congophilic angiopathy. Case 1 of Griffiths *et al.* (1982). (a) Vessels in cerebral cortex, showing varying degrees of obliteration. (b) Vessels in cerebellum, one occluded by organized thrombus, with leakage into surroundings. Accumulations of siderin phagocytes are indicated by arrows. (a) PAS, ×75. (b) Congo Red, ×100.

may involve important areas of central grey matter. They, along with the effects of obstructive hydrocephalus (see p.142), take the blame for poor results following successful treatment of the infection in cases of tuberculous meningitis.

Congophilic angiopathy, mentioned above (p.123) as a cause of intracerebral bleeding, may also be complicated by thrombosis of diseased vessels, with consequent infarction (Fig. 7.27) (see Griffiths *et al.* 1982).

Effects of blood disorders

In general, any blood disease in which spontaneous intravascular clotting occurs is liable to produce infarction— anaemic if it affects arteries or arterioles, more or less haemorrhagic if it occurs in veins or venules. In *thrombotic thrombocytopenic purpura* both blood and small blood vessels are affected. (For the pathology of this condition, see Graham and Adams 1992).

Recommendations

In conclusion, we would make the following recommendations for the post mortem examination in a case of clinically diagnosed cerebrovascular disease.

1 In the post mortem room, examine the heart carefully; in particular, weigh it, as this may provide the best evidence for chronic arterial hypertension. Take, and preferably fix for later dissection, as much as is accessible of the common and internal carotid arteries. If the cord is involved in the disease, and if circumstances permit, take and fix the vertebral column, with the abdominal aorta attached.

2 At post mortem and in the subsequent cut-up, check the patency of the carotid and vertebral arteries in the neck. Examine the circle of Willis, observe its anatomical pattern, and note points of narrowing by atheroma or thrombus. If infarcts are found, compare their outlines with those of arterial territories.

3 Take blocks for histology, not only from areas of obvious disease but from areas (e.g. hippocampus and cerebellum) known to be vulnerable to hypoxia. Take sections of selected arteries and look for changes not only of atheroma, but also of other arteriopathies.

4 When infarcts are found, aim at giving a plausible account of their causation, and how they produced the recorded clinical features.

Further reading and references

Brierley JB, Graham DI. 1992. Hypoxia and vascular disorders of the central nervous system. In Adams JH, Duchen LW (Eds) *Greenfield's Neuropathology*, 5th edn. Edward Arnold, London.

Chester EM, Agamanolis DP, Banker BQ, Victor M. 1978. Hypertensive encephalopathy: a clinicopathologic study of 20 cases. *Neurology*, **28**, 928–39.

Choi DW. 1988. Glutamate neurotoxicity and diseases of the nervous system. *Neuron*, **1**, 623–34.

Ellison D, Gatter K, Hevyet A, Esiri MM. 1993. Intramural platelet deposition in cerebral vasculopathy of systemic lupus erythematosus. *J Clin Pathol*, **46**, 37–40.

Gleysteen JJ, Silver D. 1970. Paradoxical arterial embolism: collective review. *Am Surg*, **36**, 47–54.

Griffiths RA, Mortimer TF, Oppenheimer DR, Spalding MK. 1982. Congophilic angiopathy of the brain. *J Neurol Neurosurg Psychiat*, **45**, 396–408.

8　Hydrocephalus, Cysts and Syrinxes

Hydrocephalus

Hydrocephalus (in the vernacular, water on the brain) in practice means enlarged cerebral ventricles. The term 'external hydrocephalus', which denoted enlargement of the cerebral subarachnoid spaces, has dropped out of use, as it is no more than an aspect of cerebral atrophy. The terms 'communicating' and 'non-communicating' hydrocephalus are still used. They denote the presence or absence of communication, via the apertures of the fourth ventricle, between the ventricular system and the subarachnoid space. Mention has already been made (pp.26–8) of naked-eye changes in cases of hydrocephalus, and of some of the causes of ventricular enlargement.

The most important of these causes (important because it may threaten life) is interference with the circulation of CSF, leading to back-pressure. A short account of the CSF pathways is given below, with particular mention of the points where such interference may occur, and which therefore need attention when examining a hydrocephalic brain. Obstruction at several points may occur, as in cases of congenital hydrocephalus due to the Chiari type 2 malformation, which is discussed on p.288.

CSF pathways: points of obstruction

The main source of CSF is the choroid plexus of the lateral ventricles, with contributions from the plexuses of the third and fourth ventricles. Resorption of fluid occurs, on a small scale, at many points on the cerebral and spinal arachnoid; but the main site of resorption is in the arachnoid granulations (Pacchionian bodies) associated with the superior longitudinal sinus and bridging veins on the vertex of the brain. When production of CSF outruns absorption, pressure builds up in the lateral ventricles, which expand in consequence.

The only recognized cause of CSF over-production is a functioning *papilloma of the choroid plexus* (p.218), which may arise within any of the four ventricles, producing a symmetrical hydrocephalus, most marked in the lateral ventricles. Defective absorption of CSF, thought to be due to blood corpuscles choking the arachnoid granulations, is a common effect of subarachnoid haemorrhage—usually, but not always, transient (Fig. 8.1).

Between the choroid plexus and the arachnoid granulations there are various points where the flow of CSF may be obstructed, of which the first are the *interventricular foramina* (of Monro). A rare benign (but potentially fatal) lesion, which may obstruct one or both foramina, often transitorily, is the so-called *colloid cyst of the third ventricle*. This invariably arises in the roof of the ventricle, close to the foramina, where it dangles from a short stalk (Fig. 8.2). When the brain is sliced, it may become detached. It should be looked for in cases with a history of recurrent severe headache, especially if the onset and cessation are sudden. The third ventricle itself may be blocked by tumour—in particular, by *ependymomas*, *craniopharyngiomas*, and *teratoid tumours* (including germinomas in the pineal region (see pp.215, 240, 252–5).

A more frequent site of obstruction is the *aqueduct*. Kinking of the aqueduct is probably the main reason for the association of hydrocephalus with posterior fossa tumours (see Fig. 8.3). Surgical removal of the tumour often suffices to relieve the hydrocephalus. Compression of the aqueduct occurs with expanding pontine gliomas and with pineal tumours. Actual blockage of the lumen may occur acutely, from intraventricular haemorrhage, or gradually, as a result of progressive granular ependymitis (see p.60), in the condition generally known as *aqueduct stenosis* (Fig. 8.4). There are also cases of congenital atresia, or 'forking' of the aqueduct (Russell 1949; see Fig. 8.5). In all these conditions, the lateral and third ventricles are dilated, but not the fourth; and there is an associated flattening of the cerebral convolutions.

Narrowing or obliteration of the lateral and median apertures of the fourth ventricle (foramina of Luschka and Magendie) is almost always due to fibrosis following a subacute or chronic (or inadequately treated) meningitis

Fig. 8.1 Hydrocephalus following repeated subarachnoid bleeding from an aneurysm of the right posterior communicating artery, in a woman aged 77. Note flattening of the convolutions, indicating that the hydrocephalus is due to obstruction rather than to cerebral atrophy.

(a)

(b)

Fig. 8.2 (a) Colloid cyst of third ventricle. Incidental finding in a 55-year-old man. Note proximity to interventricular foramina. (Courtesy of Dr TH Moss.) (b) T1W coronal MR image demonstrates the presence of a hyperintense (white) colloid cyst in its characteristic location, at the anterosuperior aspect of the third ventricle, between the columns of the fornices. Their appearance is variable on MRI due to different concentrations of water, mucin and paramagnetic substances.

(a)

(b)

Fig. 8.3 (a) Undersurface of the brain in a woman of 82 with a recurrent tumour (schwannoma) of the left acoustic nerve. Much of the left cerebellar hemisphere was removed at the time of operation, about 10 years earlier. (b) Obstructive hydrocephalus resulting from distortion of the brain stem.

(Fig. 8.6). In such cases the fourth ventricle shares in the general dilatation. A chronic meningitis—in particular, tuberculous meningitis—may also result in dense fibrous adhesions between the edge of the tentorial opening and the surface of the midbrain, blocking the subarachnoid pathway of the so-called *cisterna ambiens*. Finally, there is a danger that the flattening of the cerebral convolutions, caused by raised intraventricular pressure, may interfere with the passage of fluid through the cerebral sulci on its way to the arachnoid granulations, creating a vicious circle. Blockage of the intercellular channels in the granulations by blood cells is mentioned above (p.142).

The patency or otherwise of the interventricular foramina and aqueduct is easily observed in brain slices. The lateral apertures are likewise easily displayed, if they have not already been exposed. They are recognizable by their glossy ependymal lining. The median aperture may be hard to distinguish because of post mortem tearing of the delicate velum overlying the lower end of the fourth ventricle. For similar reasons the patency of the cisterna ambiens may be hard to determine if the brain has been removed from the skull in the customary fashion.

Fig. 8.4 Proliferation of neuroglia, with new vessel formation, in the aqueduct of a patient with tuberculous meningitis. The aqueduct is totally blocked. The remains of the ependyma can be seen in the form of tiny canaliculi (arrowed) around the edge of the blockage. The stimulus to glial proliferation was probably haemorrhage from repeated needling of the lateral ventricles. PTAH, ×40.

(a)

(b)

Fig. 8.5 (a) Aqueduct stenosis presenting as hydrocephalus in childhood. No lumen can be identified naked eye. (b) In a similar case presenting in the newborn period, the aquaduct is represented only by a series of small ependymal-lined, unconnected, ducts. H&E, ×100.

Fig. 8.6 Severe obstructive hydrocephalus in a 20-year-old man, treated in childhood for tuberculous meningitis. The site of obstruction was the cisterna ambiens (i.e. the subarachnoid space surrounding the midbrain). Note the preferential loss of white matter, as against grey.

Non-obstructive causes of ventricular enlargement

The pathology of so-called '*normal-pressure hydrocephalus*' is still in dispute. It seems that in some such cases the intracranial pressure is not consistently normal, but is raised during certain periods of the day or night. Also, there has sometimes been an alleviation of symptoms of gait disturbance, dementia and incontinence, and a decrease in ventricular size, following a shunting procedure. In any case coming to post mortem, a meticulous search for possible obstructive lesions should be carried out. Deep white and grey matter vascular lesions commonly occur with normal pressure hydrocephalus. For a recent review see Pickard (1992).

Enlargement of the lateral ventricles, without signs of raised intraventricular pressure, may be due to *loss of brain*

Fig. 8.7 Loss of central white matter in the right hemisphere of a 76-year-old mental defective, with spastic left hemiplegia from infancy. The lesion, which may occur on one side or both, is a characteristic result of perinatal circulatory disturbance.

Fig. 8.8 Loss of cerebral white matter on both sides, in a 13-year-old girl whose mother suffered from toxaemia in pregnancy. The child was retarded, quadriplegic and epileptic. Note the virtual disappearance of the corpus callosum; also the relative sparing of the crowns of the gyri, as compared with the sulci (*ulegyria*; see p.295 and Fig. 16.14).

Fig. 8.9 Coronal slice at level A1 from a man aged 52 with Huntington's chorea. The ventricles are large because of atrophy of the corpus striatum. There is no obvious wasting of cortex or white matter, and the corpus callosum is of normal bulk.

Fig. 8.10 Coronal slices, at levels A1 and P1, from the left hemisphere of a man aged 67 with Pick's disease. In this individual there was atrophy of the caudate nucleus, compensating with enlargement of the frontal horn of the ventrical. The other main visible abnormality is an extreme atrophy of the temporal cortex and white matter, with compensatory dilatation of the inferior horn of the ventricle.

Fig. 8.11 Enlarged fourth ventricle in a woman aged 76 with pontocerebellar atrophy.

tissue, from a variety of causes. One of these is perinatal cerebral hypoxia or ischaemia, which produces characteristic lesions in the central cerebral white matter on one or both sides (see pp.366–70). Not uncommonly, the brains of lifelong mental defectives, or of sufferers from so-called cerebral palsy, show a deficiency of cerebral white matter on one side or both, compensated by a lateral and upward extension of the body of the lateral ventricle (Fig. 8.7).

These extensions tend to have a roughly square outline, unlike the rounded shape of ventricles subjected to raised internal pressure. In general, loss of cerebral tissue is reflected in a visible thinning of the corpus callosum (Fig. 8.8).

Infarcted brain tissue, having been swollen in the acute phase, thereafter shrinks as the necrotic material is removed by macrophages. *Old infarcts* are probably the commonest cause of local compensatory dilatation of the ventricles. Other common causes include *demyelination*. Myelin constitutes more of the brain's bulk than do nerve cells, glial cells and their processes. In some cases of severe MS, much of the cerebral myelin is destroyed, and the ventricles may be conspicuously enlarged (Fig. 14.10). In *Huntington's chorea* the caudate nuclei lose their neurons and shrivel, causing symmetrical compensatory dilatation of the anterior horns of the ventricles (Fig. 8.9). The same may occur in *Pick's disease*, with the additional feature of dilatation of the inferior horns, due to atrophy of the temporal cortex and white matter (Fig. 8.10). Similar dilatation of the fourth ventricle is seen in cases of 'system' degenerations of the brain stem and/or cerebellum (Fig. 8.11). Unilateral enlargement of a temporal horn may be seen in cases of temporal lobe epilepsy (see Chapter 18).

Intracranial cysts

Intracranial cysts are of various kinds. Cystic cavities in the centra ovalia, alongside the lateral ventricles, are generally the end-result of perinatal circulatory disturbances (see pp.366–70). They are commonly referred to as *porencephalic cysts* (Fig. 21.8). Among the commoner causes of cysts in the brain are *tumours*, in particular those of the astrocytic series, ranging from the benign cerebellar astrocytoma of childhood to the more malignant types of glioma in the cerebral hemispheres of adults (Fig. 11.6; see pp.193 and 205). Cysts of large and life-threatening size are associated with haemangioblastomas of the cerebellum (p.239). In these, progressive enlargement of the cyst is often responsible for the patient's symptoms, which can be relieved temporarily by drawing off the contained fluid.

A rare cause of intracerebral cysts is *sequestration* of some part of a lateral ventricle—in particular, of a temporal horn, with inclusion of a frond of the choroid plexus. This may give rise to the clinical features of an expanding lesion, whereas loculation of the tip of an occipital horn, containing no choroid plexus, does not cause symptoms.

Not uncommonly one finds, on slicing a brain, that the septum lucidum is split, with a fluid-filled cavity between the two leaves (Fig. 16.10a). The cavity, referred to as a *cavum septi*, is said to be relatively common in professional boxers. It is lined with neuroglial fibres, whereas loculated ventricles are at least partially lined by ependyma.

Arachnoid cysts

These consist of clear fluid enclosed between reduplicated layers of arachnoid membrane. They may cause symptoms by pressure on underlying structures, or appear as incidental post mortem findings. They are commonly called 'congenital', but are very rarely found in the brains of newborn babies; their origin is obscure. They are found in various sites above and below the tentorium, but are commonest within a lateral fissure, lying between the frontal and temporal lobes (Fig. 8.12). Fortunately, they are seldom encountered within the spinal dura, where their expansion might result in an irreversible paraplegia. The subject is reviewed by Shaw & Alvord (1977).

Subdural fluid collections (other than haematomas) overlying the brain have been attributed either to valvular traumatic tears in the arachnoid, with leakage of CSF, or to

Fig. 8.12 Large collapsed arachnoid cyst in the region of the right Sylvian fissure, an incidental finding at the post mortem examination of a 20-year-old male.

(a)

(b)

Fig. 8.13 Syringomyelia. (a) Seen in the transverse section of the cord. A 60-year-old woman who had an obstructive hydrocephalus due to a vascular hamartoma in the fourth ventricle, and a syrinx extending from the second to the fifth cervical segment. There was also an exaggerated lordosis of the cervical spine. (b) T2W axial (A) and sagittal (B) images through the cervical cord demonstrate that the cord is expanded at C2 and C3 by a large cystic cavity compatible with a localized syringohydromyelia. There is no evidence of a Chiari malformation nor a prior history of trauma and no evidence of a cord tumour.

imbibition of fluid by chronic haematomas. Both types are referred to as *subdural hygromas*.

Hydromyelia and syringomyelia

From childhood onward the 'central canal' of the spinal cord is for the most part not a canal at all, but a rather irregular column of ependymal cells, Among these there may be short stretches of an ependyma-lined tubule, less than 1 mm in diameter, and of no known clinical or pathological significance. Where the contained fluid comes from is not known. A longer stretch, of greater calibre, wholly or partially lined with ependyma, is dignified by the term *hydromyelia*. A longitudinal cavity in the cord, unconnected with the central canal, having no ependymal lining, is referred to as a '*syrinx*', and the condition is called *syringomyelia* (Fig. 8.13). Occasionally one may find a syrinx as well as a patent canal in a single transverse section. In such cases, upward and downward exploration may reveal a communication between the two cavities. One is then tempted to suppose that fluid secreted into a hydromyelic canal has erupted into the cord substance, and proceeded to track upward and downward along fibre tracts. More often, no such communication is found.

Pathology

Before interference, a spinal syrinx is an extended longitudinal cyst, blowing out the cord to about double its normal cross-sectional area. The lower cervical and upper thoracic segments are the most commonly affected. After interference by surgeon or pathologist, the cord collapses; being tethered at the sides by the denticulate ligaments, it undergoes anteroposterior flattening. The wall of the cavity consists of glial fibres, sometimes reinforced with collagen fibres. The thickness of the wall is thought to correspond to the age of the lesion. Examination of transverse sections shows that the cavity grows mainly at the expense of grey matter; the white columns are also reduced in area, but here, as in other instances of the effects of pressure, the reduction appears to be largely due to demyelination, with relative preservation of axis cylinders. The amount of destruction of grey matter can be roughly assessed from the degree of fibre loss in anterior roots at the affected levels; loss of pyramidal tract fibres at levels below the syrinx is some indication of the severity of damage to the spinal white matter. Damage to the white commissure, which is believed to be responsible for dissociated sensory loss, with defective painful and thermal sensation over a few segments, is hard to assess histologically.

The *routine examination* of a syringomyelic cord should include an attempt to account for the patient's recorded disabilities in terms of damage to the grey matter of the

cord and interruption of fibre tracts It must also include a careful search for *associated lesions*, particularly in the form of *tumours* or evidences of past *trauma*. Intrinsic tumours with associated cysts, which may track up and down the cord, including ependymomas and haemangioblastomas, may sometimes be the actual source of the cyst fluid; but there is also an unexplained association of syringomyelia with extrinsic spinal tumours such as meningioma and schwannoma, and even with tumours in the posterior fossa. In some cases of spinal trauma, a syrinx appears, usually above the level of the lesion, and slowly enlarges. A wide variety of *congenital deformities* of the skull, vertebral column and neuraxis have been associated with syringomyelia; the mechanisms involved are generally

(a)

(b)

Fig. 8.14 Syringobulbia. Man aged 22, with bony deformity of upper cervical spine, associated with Chiari type 1 malformation, syringobulbia and cervical syringomyelia. Presented with 3-month history of paraesthesiae. (a) Upper medulla. (b) Lower medulla. The patient's left side is on the left side of the pictures. Myelin stain. The main cavity extends from the fourth ventricle to the pial surface on the left.

as obscure as in cases of 'primary' or 'idiopathic' syringomyelia. One of the more plausible theories envisages a valvular opening at the point of entry of a posterior nerve root into a syrinx which has extended into the posterior grey horn, with inward leakage of subarachnoid fluid caused, perhaps, by lengthening, shortening and twisting movements of the cord. For reviews of the subject see Netsky (1953), Gardner (1973) and Barnett, Foster & Hudgson (1973).

Syringobulbia

The term syringobulbia seems to imply that a similar pathological process occurs in the lower brain stem, but this is not necessarily the case. Commonly the lesions in question are not enclosed cysts, but slits, extending from the floor of the fourth ventricle into the substance of the medulla oblongata (Fig. 8.14). The lesions may be on one side or both. Whether or not they communicate with the ventricle, it seems that they do not present as expanding lesions, but produce disturbances by destruction of nerve cells and interruption of fibre tracts. Their cause is unknown. There are several reported cases in which syringobulbia and syringomyelia coexisted, but we know of none in which there was a demonstrable continuity between the two lesions. Even so, it is advisable in such cases to make a very careful search, at microscopic level, for evidence of such continuity; in any and every case of syringomyelia a hunt should be made for possible communications between the syrinx and the subarachnoid space. The classsical work on syringobulbia by Jonesco-Sisesti (1932), is available in English translation.

Further reading and references

Barnett HJM, Foster JB, Hudgson P (Eds). 1973. *Syringomyelia*. WB Saunders, Philadelphia.

Gardner WJ. 1973. *The Dysraphic States*. Excerpta Medica Foundation, Amsterdam.

Jonesco-Sisesti N. 1932. *Syringobulbia: a contribution to the pathophysiology of the brainstem*. Translated by RT Ross, 1986. Praeger, New York.

Harding BN. 1992. Malformations of the nervous system. In Adams JH, Duchen LW (Eds) *Greenfield's Neuropathology*, 5th edn. Edward Arnold, London, Chapter 10.

Netsky MG. 1953. Syringomyelia: a clinicopathological study. *Arch Neurol Psychiat* **70**, 741–75.

Pickard JD. 1992. Normal pressure hydrocephalus. In Swash M, Oxbury JO (Eds) *Clinical Neurology*. Churchill Livingstone, London, pp.151–54.

Russell DS. 1949. *Observations on the pathology of hydrocephalus*. Medical Research Council Report Series no 265. HMSO, London.

Shaw CM, Alvord EC. 1977. 'Congenital' and arachnoid cysts and their differential diagnosis. In Vinken PJ, Bruyn GW (Eds) *Handbook of Clinical Neurology*. North-Holland, Amsterdam, **31**, 75–135.

9   Pyogenic Infections and Granulomas

When faced with the neuropathological examination of a case of possible CNS infection the main aims are to establish (i) the *cause* of the infection (Table 9.1; Figs 9.1, 9.8, 9.18); (ii) the *route* by which the nervous system was reached by the organism, and (iii) the *effects* the infection has had on the nervous system itself. This may be a relatively straightforward task, for example in a case of classical acute leptomeningitis due to pneumococcal infection with associated pneumonia and bacteraemia. On the other hand, in another case infection may not have been considered in the differential diagnosis, the naked-eye appearances at post mortem examination may be unremarkable, and the organism may be a relatively uncommon one. The pathologist needs to be particularly alert for infection when examining material from patients who, for one reason or another, may be suspected of being immunodeficient.

Routes of infection

Bacteria reach the nervous system and its membranous coverings either via the bloodstream or by spread from a nearby focus of infection. Blood-borne spread of bacteria to the nervous system may occur from a focus of established infection elsewhere (e.g. osteomyelitis, septic arthritis, endocarditis, bronchiectasis, skin sepsis). Common local sources of infection are the paranasal air sinuses, middle ears and bones of the skull and spine. Infection arising in a middle ear may spread backward and laterally into mastoid air cells, upward into the ipsilateral temporal lobe or backward into the ipsilateral cerebellar hemisphere, and in a frontal sinus may easily reach the adjacent frontal lobe. It is remarkable how readily bones of the skull may be eroded by pus under raised pressure. Infection may also gain direct access to the CNS in patients with malformations, such as a meningomyelocele, a skull fracture, particularly at the base of the skull, or with a shunt inserted in a ventricle. Acute meningitis, cerebral abscess, epidural

abscess or subdural empyema may all develop from local spread of infection. The virulence of the invading organism, the effectiveness of the host defences, and the speed of commencing appropriate antibiotic therapy all influence the outcome. Highly virulent pneumococci, on reaching the brain, are liable to cause a focal purulent encephalitis rather than an abscess because there is no time available for capsule formation to take place to contain the infection. Many organisms can multiply rapidly in the CSF, which provides an excellent culture medium, relatively removed from immune defences. Organisms in the subdural space are difficult to eradicate because of the low vascularity of the dura, and the poor penetration of antibiotics unless these are instilled directly. Organisms of relatively low virulence, such as cryptococci and other fungi, and toxoplasmosis, are generally encountered in immunosuppressed, very young, or elderly and debilitated patients, and may evoke little in the way of an inflammatory response.

Consequences of infection

There are important secondary effects of infections in and around the nervous system that may complicate the picture. They include oedema, acute, possibly fatal, vascular events such as sagittal sinus thrombosis with venous infarction, cerebral arterial infarction due to arteritis, and hydrocephalus.

Several important practical considerations listed below, follow from the foregoing comments.

1 As far as possible, an *aseptic technique* should be adopted when performing a post mortem examination on cases suspected of having an infective aetiology, at least until specimens have been taken for microbiological investigation. These should be sent to the laboratory with sufficient information to ensure that appropriate media are used for culture. Additional samples of CSF and serum may be stored

(a)

(b)

(c)

(d)

Fig. 9.1 Examples of organisms seen in the brain or meninges in cases of meningitis (a) Listeria, gram stain, (b) Nocardia, gram stain, (c) cryptococcus, PAS stain, (d) coccidiomyces, PAS stain.

Table 9.1 Organisms causing meningitis and/or granulomas in and around the brain (commoner organisms are indicated in bold).

BACTERIA
Actinomyces (Gram + branching filaments)
Bacillus anthracis (Gram + rods)
Borrelia burgdorfii (spirochaetes)
Brucella species (Gram − cocco-bacilli)
Coliforms (Gram − rods)
Haemophilus influenzae (Gram − rods)
Klebsiella species (Gram − rods)
Listeria monocytogenes (Gram + rods)
Meningococcus (Gram − cocci in pairs)
Mycobacteria tuberculosis (Gram +, acid-fast rods)*
Other mycobacteria (Gram +, acid-fast rods)*†
Nocardia species (Gram + branching filaments)
Pneumococcus (Gram + cocci in pairs)
Proteus species (Gram − rods)
Pseudomonas (Gram − rods)
Serratia species (Gram − rods)†
Staphylococci (Gram + cocci)
Streptococci (Gram + cocci in chains)
Treponema pallidum (spirochaetes)*

FUNGI
Aspergillus (septate hyphae)*†
Blastomyces (yeast)*
Candida albicans (yeast)*†
Cladosporidium (septate hyphae)*
Coccidiomyces (yeast)*

Cryptococcus (yeast)*†
Histoplasma (yeast)*
Zygomycetes (mucor) (non-septate hyphae)*
  (especially in diabetics)

PROTOZOA AND METAZOA
Amoebae* (some)†
Cysticercus (with cysts)*
Echinococcus and other tapeworms (with cysts)*
Micronemiasis
Onchocerca
Paragonimus
Schistosoma*
  S. japonicum mainly in the brain
  S. haematobium and *mansoni* mainly in the spinal cord
*Strongyloides**
*Toxocara**
Toxoplasma*† (and infants)
*Trichinella**

VIRUSES
Enteroviruses
Herpes simplex type 2 virus
HTLV1 (see p.178)
HIV† (see p.176)
Lymphocytic choriomeningitis virus
Paramyxoviruses (especially mumps)

*May be associated with granulomas.   †Opportunistic infections.

Fig. 9.2 Base of the brain from a case of acute meningitis. There is a thin film of pus obscuring the under-surface of the brain.

deep-frozen in case they are needed for estimation of microbial antibody titres at a later stage.

2 Observations need to be made regarding the source of infection. In cases of bacterial infection the frontal air sinuses and middle ears must be carefully entered and inspected, and swabs taken from them for culture. A track leading from the sinus to the meninges may be identifiable. Sources of infection need also to be sought elsewhere in the body (e.g. lungs, pleural and peritoneal cavities, heart valves, joint spaces, bones). Skull bones need to be inspected for fractures, particularly at the base following head injury.

3 A careful search needs to be made for evidence of systemic diseases that are associated with immunodeficiency, such as Hodgkin's disease or other lymphoma, sarcoidosis or acquired immune deficiency syndrome (AIDS). It should be remembered that previous splenectomy predisposes to pneumococcal infection.

Leptomeningitis

Acute meningitis

In classical cases this diagnosis is easily made. There is a purulent exudate readily visible in the subarachnoid space (Fig. 9.2). This may be more marked over the vertex or at the base. The brain itself often appears congested and swollen, and occasionally these features, together with the presence of a few petechial haemorrhages, may be all there is to note on naked-eye examination (Fig. 9.3). Death in such fulminating cases can result directly from the cerebral swelling and associated brain stem compression.

Small penetrating vessels at the surface of the cortex and brain stem are surrounded by acute inflammatory cells which occupy the superficial perivascular spaces. Acute hypoxic (homogenizing) changes (p.51) may be seen in cortical and hippocampal neurons. The subarachnoid space and leptomeninges contain a neutrophil polymorph infiltrate. Fibrin strands are also frequently seen. Organisms may be demonstrated with appropriate stains, unless

Fig. 9.3 Base of the brain from a case of fulminating pneumococcal meningitis. Petechial subarachnoid haemorrhages and severe brain swelling with foraminal herniation are evident. Frank pus formation has not occurred, though microscopy showed a neutrophil polymorph infiltrate throughout the subarachnoid space.

treatment with antibiotics during life has largely eradicated them. Outside the CNS there may be adrenal or skin haemorrhages, and evidence of more widespread intravascular coagulation.

Chronic meningitis

When the inflammatory process in the subarachnoid space continues for more than a week or two, secondary effects on the brain are liable to develop. One of these is hydrocephalus, caused by interruption of the normal CSF circulation by fibrin and, later, granular ependymitis at the aqueduct, gliosis or fibrosis around the outlet foramina of the fourth ventricle, and fibrosis in the subarachnoid space. The degree of hydrocephalus may be quite gross (Fig. 8.6). A second important complication is the development of multiple cerebral infarcts (Fig. 9.4), due to narrowing of, and thrombosis in, arteries affected by endarteritis obliterans (p.139; Fig. 7.26). This consists of intimal proliferation, and inflammation of all layers of the arterial wall, but particularly of the adventitia. The hydrocephalus and infarcts are readily visible to the naked eye, as is the collagenous thickening of the leptomeninges, chiefly at the base (Figs 9.5 and 9.6). The endarteritis requires microscopy to be appreciated (Fig. 7.26). With infection due to organisms producing chronic meningitis, there are also likely to be microscopic granulomas. These contain lymphocytes, macrophages, plasma cells, epithelioid cells and multinucleate giant cells (Fig. 9.7). Some organisms produce more diffuse, mononuclear inflammation. Cerebral infarction is particularly common in fungal infections, when it may be due to invasion of artery walls by hyphal growth, followed by local thrombosis (Fig. 9.8). The organisms themselves can be identified with appropriate stains (Gram for bacteria, Ziehl–Neelsen for *Mycobacteria*, PAS and methenamine silver stains for fungi, Giemsa for protozoa, Levaditi for spirochaetes).

Cranial and spinal nerve roots are often inflamed and damaged in chronic meningitis (Fig. 9.9). Dorsal spinal root involvement is particularly characteristic of tertiary syphilis, and gives rise to *tabes dorsalis*. Cases of tabes are still seen, and the characteristic finding in the spinal cord is of patchy secondary degeneration of posterior column nerve fibres (Fig. 2.25b). Residual inflammation in treated cases is either sparse or absent.

A granular *ependymitis* is almost invariably present in cases of chronic meningitis, since the inflammatory process reaches all the regions lying close to the CSF. The foci of granulomatous inflammation and gliosis form small nodules on ependymal surfaces (Fig. 9.10). Initially these contain inflammatory cells and reactive astrocytes (Fig. 9.11). Later on, the inflammatory cells disappear, leaving a small gliotic nodule. These nodules are caused not only by previous inflammation, but also by a variety of irritants, including blood or high-protein exudates reaching the CSF.

Chronic spinal arachnoiditis

Occasionally symptoms and signs of spinal root compression are found to be due to an *adhesive arachnoiditis* in which collagenous thickening and chronic inflammatory cell infiltration of the arachnoid occur (Fig. 9.12). In some subjects

Fig. 9.4 Coronal slice across the cerebrum from a patient with a 6-week history of tuberculous meningitis. There is infarction of the left thalamus, left hippocampus and right caudate nucleus (haemorrhagic) due to arteritis. Hydrocephalus is also present. Note also inflammatory exudate in hippocampal fissures.

this develops after injection of radiological contrast medium, particularly Myodil, into the subarachnoid space. Sequestered remains of such material may be evident lying free or in macrophages if the opportunity arises to examine the arachnoid membrane microscopically. In other cases there is no obvious predisposing cause. Organisms are not usually identifiable.

Subdural empyema

Pus in the subdural space usually spreads from a focus of local osteomyelitis or paranasal sinus infection. There may also be associated acute meningitis. In contrast to the

Fig. 9.5 Base of brain from a case of tuberculous meningitis. Anatomical features and the basilar artery are largely obscured by an opaque, gelatinous exudate in the subarachnoid space.

Fig. 9.7 Subarachnoid granulomas in chronic meningitis due to tuberculosis. Inflammation takes the form of coalescing, caseating granulomas. H&E, ×200.

Fig. 9.6 Close-up view of the ventral surface of the pons from a case of tuberculous. meningitis (same case as in Fig. 9.5). An arrow marks the stump of the right trigeminal nerve at the lateral border of the pons.

Fig. 9.8 Transverse section of a segment of artery wall from a case with arteritis due to aspergillus infection. Hyphal structures, many of them radially orientated, are shown with the methenamine silver stain. ×70. (Slide courtesy of Dr P Gallagher.)

Fig. 9.9 Chronic meningitis due to sarcoidosis with inflammation and fibrosis around cranial nerve roots (left) at the base of the brain. H&E, ×60.

Fig. 9.10 View of the lateral ventricular surface from a case of tabes dorsalis in which there was, in addition to spinal root damage, a marked ventriculitis. Granulomatous nodules project above the normal ependyma-lined surface.

Fig. 9.11 Low-power view of a section through an ependymal granulation (see Fig. 9.10). The ependyma is disrupted and inflammatory and glial cells contribute to the cellular nodule projecting into the ventricular cavity above. PAS, ×120.

Fig. 10.3 Coronal slice through the frontal and temporal lobes of the brain from a case of subacute sclerosing panencephalitis (SSPE) in which the disease lasted 7½ years. Note marked, generalized atrophy with ventricular enlargement, grey discoloration of cerebral white matter, severe narrowing of the corpus callosum and leptomeningeal thickening (arrowed).

Fig. 10.5 Focus of neuronophagia in the dentate nucleus of the cerebellum from a patient with a renal transplant, on immunosuppressive therapy. The clinical history did not suggest any neurological disease, but post mortem examination of the brain showed scattered foci such as this in the cerebrum and cerebellum, one of which was associated with a typical CMV inclusion body in a neuron (Fig. 10.9). H&E, ×180.

Fig. 10.4 Measles virus antigen demonstrated in neuron nucleus, cytoplasm and processes by application of a rabbit antiserum to measles virus to a paraffin section of cerebral cortex from a case of SSPE. Peroxidase reaction with weak haematoxylin counterstain, ×570.

neuronophagia (Fig. 10.5). Neuronophagic cell clusters should be carefully searched for in grey matter. They are most conspicuous when considerable numbers of large neurons are killed more or less simultaneously, as occurs, for example, in acute poliomyelitis. When cell death is less

selective, involving not only neurons but also glial cells, frank tissue necrosis is seen, as in acute herpes simplex encephalitis. Cell death may also occur on a relatively small scale and over an extended period of time, as in subacute sclerosing panencephalitis (SSPE), or in the glial nodule encephalitis which occurs in some immunosuppressed patients (Fig. 10.5). In these cases neuronophagia may be found only after prolonged searching.

Cell structure may be altered without cell lysis in some forms of encephalitis. Examples of such change are the development of neurofibrillary tangles in some neurons in SSPE, and of bizarre changes in astrocyte nuclei in progressive multiforcal leucoencephalopathy (PML) (Fig. 10.6).

Inclusion bodies

These are also alterations of cell structure which occur in a number of viral infections. They usually contain virus-coded material. Most characteristic are Negri bodies, cytoplasmic inclusions found in neurons in rabies. They consist of one or several hyaline eosinophilic bodies lying close to the nucleus (Fig. 10.7). Round or oval, intranuclear, eosinophilic inclusion bodies, larger than nucleoli, and usually surrounded by a halo of clear nucleoplasm, are found in neurons and oligodendrocyte nuclei in SSPE and 'immunosuppressive' measles encephalitis (Cowdry type A inclusions) (Fig. 10.8). They are also sometimes present in neurons in herpes simplex encephalitis. Large intranuclear inclusion bodies are seen in the brain in adult and congenital CMV infection (Figs 10.9 and 21.15; see p.371). Basophilic, enlarged oligodendrocyte nuclei are present in PML (Fig. 10.10).

Inflammation

Inflammatory cell infiltration, oedema and congestion occur in the brain in all forms of acute viral encephalitis. Initially the infiltrating cells are neutrophil polymorphs, but these are replaced within two or three days by

mononuclear inflammatory cells. Some petechial or larger haemorrhages are also common, particularly in herpes simplex encephalitis. After 10–15 days plasma cells become prominent in addition to lymphocytes and macrophages. These inflammatory cells form dense cuffs of cells in perivascular spaces and also extend into neighbouring brain parenchyma (Figs 3.21 and 10.11). The leptomeninges also contain some inflammatory cells (Fig. 10.12). Inflammation persists for months or even years after an episode of acute encephalitis, though in diminishing amount. In persistent infection, such as in SSPE, the cuffing continues to be prominent. In immunosuppressed patients it is reduced or absent even in the presence of abundant viral antigen.

Fig. 10.6 Bizarre multinucleate astrocytes in cerebellar white matter from a case of PML. H&E, ×450.

Fig. 10.8 Intranuclear eosinophilic inclusion bodies surrounded by a pale halo in a cortical neuron from a case of immunosuppressive measles encephalitis. H&E, ×650.

Fig. 10.7 Negri body (arrowed) in the cytoplasm of a hippocampal pyramidal cell from a case of rabies. H&E, ×760.

Fig. 10.43 Perivenous inflammatory infiltrate in perivenous encephalitis. Particularly characteristic is the manner in which the inflammatory cells fan out into the neighbouring parenchyma, rather than remaining as dense cuffs, largely confined to the Virchow–Robin spaces. H&E, ×130.

mononuclear inflammation with demyelination (Chapter 14), and therefore closely resemble those of PVEM. The clinical histories of these two diseases are, however, usually different, and histologically the lesions of acute MS extend further from the vein walls and show more evidence of a glial reaction. This reflects the usually longer duration of disease in MS. However, occasional cases show features of both diseases (Fig. 10.49). Experimental forms of allergic encephalitis resembling MS have now been produced in some laboratory animals.

Other forms of encephalitis and myelitis

Purulent encephalitis is discussed in Chapter 9, and parenchymal syphilitic lesions in Chapters 9 and 17.

Rickettsial encephalitis

Rickettsial diseases are acute, systemic infections, caused by bacterium-like organisms, usually transmitted to man by insect vectors. The organisms have a predilection for invading and multiplying in the endothelial cells of small blood vessels. A skin rash usually develops. Neurological involvement results if vessels of the nervous system or leptomeninges are colonized. Lesions consist of a focal vasculitis affecting small blood vessels, sometimes accompanied by small infarcts. The diagnosis is usually made on the basis of serological tests demonstrating a rise

in antibody titre to one of the Rickettsiae, coinciding in time with the systemic illness.

Parasitic infections

Most parasitic infections of the brain and leptomeninges provoke formation of granulomas (Chapter 9). *Toxoplasmosis* in neonates or immunosuppressed adults may, however, cause an encephalitis reminiscent of viral encephalitis, with inflammation, glial nodules, focal necrosis and late calcification (Fig. 10.50). Toxoplasma cysts can usually be identified in the lesions (Fig. 10.51 and Fig. 4.34). In *cerebral trypanosomiasis* (sleeping sickness) there is a diffuse meningoencephalitis with cuffing of vessels by lymphocytes and plasma cells and with some reactive astrocytosis in cerebral white matter. Cerebral and cerebellar white matter, basal ganglia and brain stem tend to be the areas most affected, and the cerebral cortex is relatively spared. Morula cells (plasma cells distended with immunoglobulin) occur in perivascular spaces and in the brain.

Cerebral malaria results chiefly from infection with *Plasmodium falciparum*. The diagnosis is made on the basis of acute neurological disease in a subject whose blood contains malaria parasites. The lesions in the brain in fatal cases are widely distributed and centred on small blood vessels, many of which can be seen to contain large numbers of parasitized red blood cells (Fig. 10.52). In addition

(a)

(b)

Fig. 10.44 (a) Intense perivenous inflammatory cell cuffing from the cerebrum of a case of perivenous encephalitis. Nissl, ×120. (b) Myelin-stained section demonstrating the perivenous loss of myelin. ×120.

to the congestion and presumed stasis of blood in capillaries and other small vessels, the vascular endothelium appears swollen, and extravasated red cells and proteinaceous fluid may be seen around them (Fig. 10.53). There is also necrosis of the perivascular brain parenchyma, with focal loss of myelin staining in white matter, and accumulation of reactive microglia and astrocytes in the vicinity.

Encephalitis of undefined aetiology

Rasmussen's encephalitis

Rare cases of chronic encephalitis, with epilepsy as one of the chief presenting features, were first described by Rasmussen (1978). Almost all those affected have been children. Histopathological studies have been made on surgi-

Fig. 10.45 Axon stain in perivenous tissue from a case of perivenous encephalitis. Many axons remain intact in the inflamed zone. ×150.

Fig. 10.46 Late effects of perivenous encephalitis. Inflammation has largely subsided, but there is fibrosis in the perivascular space, and intense gliosis in the surrounding neuropil. PTAH, ×120.

Fig. 10.47 Perivenous inflammatory cell infiltrate in acute haemorrhagic leucoencephalitis. The majority of cells are neutrophil polymorphs. H&E, ×220.

cally removed tissues, including temporal lobectomy and hemispherectomy specimens. They show a subacute or chronic meningoencephalitis affecting chiefly cerebral cortex, but also white matter, with perivascular mononuclear inflammatory cells, microglial nodules and foci of neuronophagia. Inclusion bodies have not been seen, and viral culture and EM studies have failed to reveal viruses or other organisms in the brain. It has been suggested that the disease may be due to an auto-immune reaction against

a receptor for the neurotransmitter, glutamate (Rogers *et al.* 1994).

Behçet's disease

Behçet's disease is characterized clinically by recurrent ulceration of the mouth and genitalia, and iridocyclitis. In some cases there are also neurological abnormalities, the pathology of which consists of multiple, focal, ill-defined

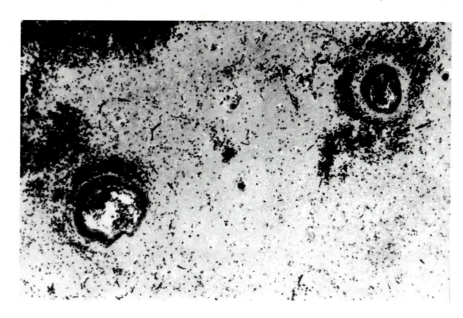

Fig. 10.48 Intense congestion, perivenous and more diffuse haemorrhages in cerebral white matter from a case of acute haemorrhagic leucoencephalitis. PTAH, ×100.

(a)

(b)

Fig. 10.49 Myelin-stained sections of the cerebrum (a) and medulla (b) from a case of perivenous encephalitis in which, in addition to the characteristic perivenous inflammation and demyelination, seen in (a), there were also more extensive plaques of demyelination resembling those seen in MS (a and b). (a) ×2, (b) ×4.

areas of congestion and softening. The commonest sites affected are the brain stem, especially the midbrain, basal ganglia, hypothalamus and internal capsule. These areas should be included among those examined microscopically in this disease. Both grey and white matter are affected, and contain inflammatory, necrotic foci with perivascular lymphocytes, microglial nodules in grey mat-ter, and a more diffuse microglial and astrocytic reaction (Figs 10.54 and 10.55). There is loss of myelin and to a lesser extent of axons and neurons. Vessels show relatively little pathological change. The leptomeninges adjacent to affected parenchyma are mildly inflamed. The cause of the disease is not known.

Occasional cases of encephalitis occur in which *no definite diagnosis* can be made. The inflammation may predominate in grey or white matter, with or without neuronophagia, and in the absence of perivenous demyelination or inclusion bodies. Provided these distinguishing features have been carefully searched for, and microbiological studies have been taken far enough to exclude identifiable causes of encephalitis, the pathologist will have taken the matter as far as can be expected.

Fig. 10.50 Intense diffuse and perivascular inflammation in cerebral toxoplasmosis. H&E, ×80.

Fig. 10.52 A focus of white matter oedema and rarefaction with veins packed with parasitized erythrocytes in a case of cerebral malaria. H&E, ×200.

Fig. 10.51 Toxoplasmosis cyst, one of several widely distributed in the lesion illustrated in Fig. 10.50. H&E, ×400.

Encephalitis associated with carcinoma (Paraneoplastic encephalitis)

Subacute or chronic encephalitis occurs in some patients with carcinoma, particularly oat-cell carcinoma of the bronchus. The primary tumour in such cases is almost invariably small, and metastatic spread is limited to regional lymph nodes. The brain shows little abnormality externally. In slices there may be a suggestion of ill-defined softening and discoloration in grey matter at almost any level of the neuraxis. The regions that merit particular attention in any individual case are those to which the clinical signs and symptoms were referable, and samples for microscopy should be taken from these areas and also from other major subdivisions of the nervous system (cerebral cortex, white matter, basal ganglia, thalamus, several levels of the brain stem and spinal cord and dorsal root ganglia). The areas predominantly affected are grey matter and they show perivascular cuffing with mononuclear inflammatory cells, chiefly lymphocytes, loss of neurons and neuronophagia (Fig. 10.56). Microglia proliferate, and astrocytes are variably reactive. Inflammation and neuron loss do not always go hand in hand. There tends to be a predominant area of damage, for example in the cerebral cortex, where the hippocampus and medial temporal lobe are particularly likely to be involved, or in the basal ganglia, thalamus, brain stem, or spinal cord. Mild inflammation is more widely spread. The sensory ganglia may show loss of neurons with satellite cell proliferation accompanying involvement of the CNS or in isolation. This ganglioradiculitis is accompanied by secondary degeneration of nerve fibres in posterior columns of the spinal cord. Such cases usually show evidence of a sensory neuropathy clinically. Cases with ataxia show one of two

Fig. 10.53 Pericapillary haemorrhages in the cerebellar subcortical white matter in cerebral malaria. H&E, ×100.

Fig. 10.54 Microscopic focus of rarefaction (arrowed) in the cerebral cortex from a case of Behçet's disease. H&E, ×80.

Fig. 10.55 Behçet's disease. Lymphocytic perivascular cuffing in the brain. H&E, ×230.

rather different lesions in the cerebellum: inflammation and loss of neurons in the dentate nuclei, or severe depletion of Purkinje cells and to a lesser extent of granule cells, without inflammation. Serum or CSF of some cases of the latter type have been shown to contain an antibody which reacts with cerebellar Purkinje cells.

Encephalitis lethargica

A world-wide epidemic of encephalitis lethargica (von Economo's encephalitis) occurred during, and in the decade after, the First World War. No aetiological agent was identified, but the epidemiology and pathology were consistent with a viral cause. The epidemic overlapped in time with a world-wide outbreak of influenza, and this has led to speculation that a neurovirulent strain of influenza virus may have been involved. Occasional sporadic cases that fit the clinical pattern of the disease have continued to be described, but again no agent has been identified. Fever, somnolence and impaired oculomotor function characterize the acute phase of the disease. In a significant proportion of the survivors parkinsonian symptoms and oculogyric crises occurred. Patients who died in the acute phase of the disease had a polioencephalitis more or less limited to the brain stem, particularly the midbrain and diencephalon, with conges-

11   Space-occupying Lesions

Types of expanding lesion

In the earlier chapters stress is laid on the importance of tentorial and foraminal herniations as causes of death. In this chapter we discuss the various causes of such herniations. Inevitably, there will be some repetition of points made in other chapters. We also discuss some lesions within the spinal canal, which by their expansion cause paraplegia or tetraplegia rather than sudden death.

The effects of expanding lesions depend on several factors, including their position, their size and their rate of expansion. In general, the effects of intracranial expanding lesions differ according to whether they lie above or below the tentorium. Treating the supratentorial lesions first, the following has to be considered.
1 Haematomas, intrinsic or extrinsic.
2 Neoplasms, intrinsic or extrinsic.
3 Abscess.
4 Obstructive hydrocephalus.
5 Cerebral oedema.

Intracranial haemorrhage

Intracranial haemorrhage is discussed in Chapter 6. In general, the effects of a massive supratentorial haemorrhage, whether in the brain substance or outside it, will be: to shift midline structures to the opposite side, producing a subfalcine hernia (Figs 2.8c and 11.1), with compression and distortion of the lateral ventricles; to force diencephalic structures downward through the tentorial opening (Figs 2.8 and 2.9); to apply lateral compression to the midbrain via the ipsilateral uncus and parahippocampal gyrus (Fig. 2.12); to press the opposite cerebral peduncle against the free edge of the tentorium (Fig. 2.10), and to kink one or both oculomotor nerves where they cross the posterior cerebral arteries. Branches of the opposite posterior cerebral artery may be pinched, causing infarction of occipital cortex, including the striate area (Fig. 7.22).

Brain tumours

These act similarly, but as a rule more slowly. A slowly-growing tumour such as a meningioma may be accommodated by demyelination of central white matter, which thus loses bulk while keeping most of its axons intact (Fig. 11.2). A fast-growing tumour, on the other hand—a glioblastoma, say, or secondary carcinoma—may enhance its deadly potential by causing an oedematous reaction in the surrounding brain tissue (Figs 11.3 and 11.4) or, occasionally, bleeding (Fig. 11.5). With some tumours—notably with gliomas of the astrocytic series—space occupation is as much due to the formation of an associated cyst (Fig. 11.6) as it is to expansion of the solid tumour tissue. The tumours most commonly met with are *gliomas*, which are described in the next chapter. The commonest of these, alas, is the fast-growing malignant *glioblastoma*. This occurs mainly in men and women over 50 years of age. Among younger adults, the slower-advancing diffuse *astrocytoma* is commoner. *Lymphomas* are less common, but often highly malignant. Of the extrinsic tumours, the relatively benign meningioma is the most frequent in elderly people: in young people, pituitary adenomas and craniopharyngiomas are relatively common. In some parts of the world non-neoplastic tumours such as tuberculomas are all too frequent.

Abscesses (see Chapter 9) may be blood-borne, most commonly from an infected lung, or arise by inward extension from an infected frontal sinus or middle ear (Fig. 9.14).

Obstructive hydrocephalus

Obstructive hydrocephalus may be due to tumours (see p.142). The aqueduct may be partially or totally blocked even by small tumours in the tectum or in the pineal region, or merely by kinking due to other posterior fossa lesions. Here it should be noted that an expanding lesion in the posterior fossa tends to resist a transtentorial downthrust, and herniation, when it occurs, is likely to

Fig. 11.1 Effects of a large chronic subdural haematoma. The brain has been sliced coronally, with much of the dura, and the underlying haematoma, in place. There has been a remarkable degree of displacement of midline structures to the right, and the left cingulate gyrus has virtually wrapped itself around the free edge of the falx. In contrast, the convolutions are not flattened, and the ventricles appear to be of normal size. Explanation: the brain was already atrophic at the time of injury, and there was ample room for the haematoma to expand without causing a fatal transtentorial hernia.

Fig. 11.2 Large meningioma indenting the right parietal lobe in a woman aged 52, with a 9-month history of headaches. Died in operating theatre. Loss of white matter is mainly attributable to demyelination of axons in white matter, owing to compression. The tumour is histologically benign, and non-invasive.

Fig. 11.3 Oedema of the right frontal lobe, associated with a malignant astrocytoma, situated anteriorly to this, in a man aged 30, with a 2-month history of headaches; final state, mute and incontinent. Note the midline shift, subfalcine hernia, flattening of convolutions, and grooving and bruising of the right parahippocampal gyrus. The corpus callosum, here and in Fig. 11.4a, is tilted downward on the right, indicating that swelling is more intense in the upper than in the lower part of the hemisphere.

(a)

(b)

Fig. 11.4 Metastatic tumours. (a) Bronchial carcinoma. Deposits are seen in the right thalamus and middle frontal convolution. There is severe associated oedema, with midline shift and subfalcine hernia. (b) Carcinoma of the lung. Deposits are widely dispersed in cortex, white matter and thalamus; but there is no apparent oedema or displacement.

take place at the foramen magnum. Tentorial herniation is the natural result of acute distension of the lateral ventricles due to aqueduct stenosis or an impacted cyst of the third ventricle.

Cerebral swelling: oedema

Acute cerebral swelling has a variety of causes. The old distinction between *dry swelling*, in which there is extra fluid in blood vessels or within brain cells, and *cerebral*

Fig. 11.5 Acute haemorrhage into a diffuse bilateral frontal astrocytoma causing tentorial herniation and sudden death.

oedema, in which fluid seeps into intercellular spaces, may be theoretically sound, but it is very difficult to apply in individual cases. In practice, it seems that the former, but not the latter, may be reduced by intravenous osmotic agents such as mannitol and urea. It is oedema which constitutes the biggest threat to life in the neurosurgical and acute neurological wards. The patient, for instance, who dies in the acute phase of non-haemorrhagic stroke is killed not by the loss of vital brain tissue, but because of distortion of his upper brain stem by a herniated parahippocampal gyrus propelled downward by swelling of the infarcted tissue (see p.126).

Among the causes of acute dry swelling of the brain the most familiar are *hypoxaemia* and *hypercapnia*. When the brain is exposed at operation, trouble with the airway is quickly betrayed by congestion and darkening of pial vessels and a tendency of brain tissue to rise out of the wound. The process can usually be quickly reversed. Oedema, on the other hand, implies an increase in the water content of the brain, which is less easily controlled. The physiology of the process has been studied intensively in recent years; and at present the prevailing view is that there are two main types of cerebral oedema: the *vasogenic*, which affects white matter more than grey, and the *cytotoxic*, which affects mainly glial cells and neurons. The two may both occur, it seems, in the same brain. For further discussion, see Miller & Adams (1992).

Cerebral oedema occurs in many different conditions. It is one of the main bugbears of surgeons concerned in the management of head injury. In acute infarction, it affects

Fig. 11.6 Cyst associated with a relatively small right frontal malignant astrocytoma, in a woman aged 50. Main complaints, headaches and epileptic fits. (The congealed cyst fluid, which would normally be yellow or colourless, is darkened by haemorrhage.)

Fig. 11.7 Acute MS, of Balò type, in a 21-year-old woman, with a total history of 5 weeks. The dark lesion in the left hemisphere is a haemorrhagic needle-track. The whole brain is swollen, with flattened convolutions and compressed ventricles.

the tissue adjacent to the infarct, and it may be difficult to determine the boundary between the softening due to irreparable loss of blood supply and that due to oedema of the surrounding tissue. Oedema due to toxic and metabolic disturbances is particularly apt to occur in young children,

and is the main neuropathological finding in, for instance, Reye's syndrome (p.346). It occurs in the neighbourhood of many tumours, including benign growths such as meningiomas, and malignant ones such as secondary carcinomas (Fig. 11.4). It occurs in association with inflammatory lesions, both focal and diffuse, and in this context it is worth noting that the lesions of acute MS have an inflammatory character, and may give rise to intense swelling (Fig. 11.7).

Both before and after fixation, oedematous brain is unnaturally soft. In slices of fixed brain, the affected white matter is slimy to the touch, and often yellowish in colour. If it is adequately fixed, the tissue, though softer than normal, is still resilient: unfortunately, formalin is slow to penetrate oedematous tissue, and without special precautions (see p.7) the result may be a sour-smelling, almost fluid, substance resembling toothpaste.

In histological preparations the affected areas stain poorly for myelin (Fig. 11.8); it is not always clear to what extent this is due to actual myelin breakdown. If oedema has persisted for more than a day or so, one sees numerous swollen-bodied astrocytes, presumably engaged in the business of laying down the fibres which form the meshwork of post-oedematous gliosis (Fig. 11.9). (These cells, incidentally, may be very conspicuous in a diagnostic smear preparation; the pathologist has to be cautious in making the diagnosis between reactive astrocytosis and gemistocytic astrocytoma.)

Fig. 11.9 Postoedematous spongy state. Myelin stain on a section of cortex from another case of acute MS, of Schilder type, in a 12-year-old girl dying after an illness lasting 5 months. In this case, and in the one illustrated in Figs 11. 7 and 11.8, the clinical diagnosis was of a rapidly-growing tumour. Here, the oedema had subsided by the time of death, leaving a spongy tissue in which, surprisingly, many demyelinated axons remained. In the picture, a few patches of surviving subcortical myelin are seen (arrowed). ×2.2.

Fig. 11.8 Same case as in Fig. 11.7. A myelin-stained section of the left frontal lobe shows two distinct demyelinated areas in the central white matter. Around the smaller of these is a wide area of oedema, in which myelin is not destroyed, but stains feebly.

Effects of expanding lesions in the head

In general, the effect of expanding *supratentorial lesions*, including cerebral oedema, is, first, to drive fluid out of the lateral ventricles and subarachnoid spaces, then to thrust the diencephalon downward, and finally to cause transtentorial herniation and distortion of the upper brain stem. There are three important exceptions to this rule. Firstly, in young children, whose cranial sutures have not yet closed, the cranial cavity may be expanded by pressure from within, so that transtentorial herniation is avoided. Secondly, if the expanding lesion involves the posterior parts of the hemispheres, the whole tentorium will be pressed downwards, in which case pressure is transferred to the posterior fossa, favouring a foraminal rather than a tentorial herniation. Thirdly, a very slowly expanding lesion—a meningioma, for instance, or hydrocephalus due to a partial or intermittent occlusion of the aqueduct—may result in diffuse demyelination of white matter, i.e. compensatory brain shrinkage.

Expanding lesions in the posterior fossa

These include tumours arising in the base of the skull (chordoma, chondroma, chemodectoma), meningiomas and nerve sheath tumours (especially schwannoma of the eighth cranial nerve) (pp.228–9) and cerebellar abscesses. Intrinsic tumours include *diffuse astrocytoma* of the brain stem (a condition at one time referred to as 'hypertrophy of the pons'), the relatively benign *circumscribed astrocytoma* of the cerebellum (p.202) and the highly malignant *medulloblastoma* of the cerebellum (p.223). The first two of these tend to occur in children or young adults, the third in infants and young children. The commonest cerebellar tumour in elderly people is probably *secondary carcinoma*; middle-aged people are more liable to develop a cerebellar *haemangioblastoma* (p.239). This, in spite of its sinister-sounding name, is usually a benign tumour, completely removable by surgery if caught in time. Although it is a tumour of vasoformative tissue, and so presumably unrelated to the glioma family, it has a close similarity to the benign astrocytoma of the cerebellum, in that it produces symptoms mainly through the formation of an expanding cyst, which is usually much larger than the tumour itself. *Ependymomas*, of various degrees of malignancy, arise in the aqueduct, fourth ventricle and lateral aperture (foramen of Luschka), whereas they are relatively rare in the lateral and third ventricles. They are apt to send tongues of tumour out through the foramina into the subarachnoid space (Fig. 12.33). At operation it may be possible to peel these away cleanly, so that the free passage of fluid is re-established; the tumour, however, is usually adherent at some point to a structure which it would be imprudent to disturb. A benign variant, sometimes encountered in routine examination of the medulla, is the *subependymoma*, or subependymal astrocytoma (p.217). This is usually a small nodule, harmlessly tucked into the lower end of the fourth ventricle, and only rarely growing to a size capable of obstructing the lateral apertures.

Lhermitte–Duclos disease is a rare but interesting condition, presenting clinically as a posterior fossa tumour. In this the granule cells in a circumscribed area of cerebellar cortex undergo gross hypertrophy. The resulting expansion is increased by myelination of the axons of the granule cells. Purkinje cells, and cerebellar white matter, are squeezed out of existence; what remains is a thick, much-folded blanket of soft pale tissue. The condition is described on p.220.

In general, the effects of expanding lesions in the posterior fossa are threefold, with differences of emphasis in different cases. First, there is the damage to cells and fibre tracts due to infiltration or to pressure. (In cases of diffuse astrocytoma, in which the whole brain stem is infiltrated by hyperplastic or neoplastic astrocytes, it is sometimes astonishing how little interference with function seems to have occurred. In the case of the cerebellum, a great deal of tissue may be lost before clinical ataxia becomes troublesome.) Second, there is in most cases some obstruction of CSF pathways, causing dilatation of the lateral and third ventricles (see p.142). The presence of a small tumour in one cerebellar hemisphere may be enough to produce a kink in the upper brain stem, impeding the flow of fluid through the aqueduct. Children appear to be particularly at risk in this respect: almost any tumour in the posterior fossa of a child is likely to cause raised pressure and papilloedema.

The third effect is to promote *herniation*, which may be either upward or downward (see pp.21–6). In either case, life is threatened. Of the two, downward displacement, with impaction of the lower medulla and cerebellar tonsils in the foramen magnum, is by far the commoner. This may well be because in many cases upward pressure is countered by a downward thrust due to high pressure in the lateral and third ventricles.

The risk of foraminal herniation is enchanced if there is already a congenital prolongation of one or both cerebellar tonsils (Chiari type 1 malformation) or if the capacity of the posterior fossa is reduced by a congenital or acquired deformity of the base of the skull, such as platybasia or Paget's disease.

Expanding lesions in the spinal canal

These may lie in the spinal cord, subarachnoid space, meninges, or extrathecal space, or in the vertebral column. The effects are exerted on the cord, or nerve roots, or both.

Intrinsic neoplasms of the cord

These are mostly *gliomas*, of which the commonest is an ependymoma or subependymoma arising from the central canal (Fig. 11.10). Some of these are well circumscribed, and can even be shelled out by the surgeon through an incision between the posterior white columns. Diffuse astrocytomas are less common, and secondary carcinomas, though they occur, are rare. Ependymomas are also found growing from the *filum terminale*, which normally consists of little more than pia and ependyma. These are usually benign, and can be dissected cleanly away from the surrounding roots of the cauda equina. They are hard to distinguish from schwannomas by the naked eye. *Haemangioblastomas* also occur in the substance of the cord, but not as commonly as in the cerebellum.

Whereas the brain can expand at the expense of ventricular and subarachnoid spaces, and is finally restricted by the folds of the dura mater, the cord is contained in a relatively inelastic tube of pia mater. It can increase its volume somewhat in the cervical region by becoming more circular and less elliptical in cross-section (Fig. 11.11); beyond this, as the intrapial pressure increases, the circulation of blood is embarrassed, and necrosis may ensue. The other recourse

Fig. 11.10 Myelin-stained section from the cervical cord of a woman aged 53 with a two-year history of progressive tetraparesis. The tumour is a cystic ependymoma. The tissue surrounding it shows a mixture of necrosis and oedema. The white columns are reduced in bulk, but still contain axons. The grey matter of the anterior horns (arrowed) is fairly well preserved.

prolapsed intervertebral discs and *cervical spondylosis*. In younger people traumatic *fracture-dislocations* are more frequent. Other lesions of the vertebral column which may cause narrowing of the spinal canal include tuberculous *spinal caries*, *rheumatoid arthritis*, *spondylolisthesis*, *Paget's disease*, and congenital deformities affecting the atlas and axis vertebrae. For a satisfactory post mortem examination of such cases, a careful study of the vertebral column, preferably combined with X-rays of the relevant part, as well as of the cord itself, should be carried out.

In the lumbosacral region, *disc protrusions* may compress nerve roots near their point of entry into intervertebral foramina, and even affect the calibre of the spinal canal. Thoracic disc protrusions tend to be small, limpet-shaped midline excrescences, and seldom cause disability. Protrusions in the cervical region are commoner (no doubt because of the greater mobility in the neck), and more of a threat to life. Not only is the cord itself at risk from anteroposterior compression, but its blood supply may be compromised by pressure on the anterior spinal artery. In *cervical spondylosis*, stripping of anterior and posterior longitudinal ligaments in the vicinity of degenerate discs gives rise to formation of new bone – *osteophytosis*. Anteriorly, this is a comparatively harmless process; posteriorly, the osteophytes encroach on the spinal canal (Fig. 2.21), and thus decrease the margin of safety in the face of sudden movements—especially that of over-extension of the neck. A further effect of posterior osteophytes is that they form fibrous adhesions with the theca, thus hampering up-and-down movements of the spinal cord, and adding to the risks from sudden movement of the neck. The effects of spinal trauma are discussed on pp.111–12.

The spinal cord may undergo compression by a variety of expanding *cystic lesions*, all of them rare, histologically benign, and for the most part developing from embryonic rests. They include *dermoids* and *epidermoids* (see p.242), *arachnoid cysts*, which occasionally protrude through the dura into the extrathecal space, and *enterogenous cysts*. The latter lie in the cervical or thoracic subarachnoid space in front of the cord, and are lined by a columnar epithelium, usually of gastrointestinal type or, very rarely, of bronchial type. In some cases, they communicate with a similar cystic lesion in the mediastinum.

In examining cases in which myelopathy is thought to have ensued from pressure on the cord, the general rule is to take sections from above and below the lesion, and to look for loss of fibres in the ascending (spinocerebellar and posterior column) and descending (pyramidal) tracts respectively (see Fig. 5.12).

Further reading and references

Miller J Douglas, Adams J. Hume. 1992. The pathophysiology of raised intracranial pressure. In Adams JM, Duchen LW (Eds) *Greenfield's Neuropathology*, 5th edn. Edward Arnold, London, Chapter 2.

12   Tumours Arising in the Brain and Spinal Cord

This chapter and the following one aim to provide an overview of tumours of the nervous system. It is not our intention to deal comprehensively with their natural history, incidence and aetiology. These can be found in reference works on tumours of the nervous system such as those listed at the end of the chapter. What we hope to provide in these two chapters is a guide to the diagnosis of tumours, indicating the signposts that we have found useful along the way. Management of surgical specimens, interpretation of smears, and brief consideration of the role of immunohistological techniques in tumour diagnosis can be found in Chapter 4.

CNS tumour classification

The main requirement regarding surgical specimens is to provide the surgeon with a name for the tumour and some indication of its likely growth potential. This is not as straightforward as it might seem, for the classification of CNS tumours has long been a matter of debate, and small biopsies of gliomas do not always provide a reliable guide to prognosis. In any case, the surgeon, looking for guidance in management and treatment of the case, and for indications of the prognosis, will have other (and often more significant) clues than the histological report: the patient's clinical history, the neurological examination, radiological findings, and so on. If the neuropathologist merely reports on the most malignant features of the material examined, the surgeon should be satisfied. For post mortem diagnosis, on the other hand, the points of interest are not only the histological details of the tumour, but also its effects on the functions of the brain or spinal cord, the correlation of focal brain damage with clinical signs, and the evidence on the tumour's mode of spread and on the way in which it has contributed to the patient's death.

With regard to tumour classification, we have followed that proposed by the WHO (1992) (Table 12.1). The different tumours are considered below and in Chapter 13, items 1 and 4 being contained in this chapter and the rest in Chapter 13. Mention should also be made of the widely used classification and grading of gliomas proposed by Kernohan *et al.* (1949) and modified in various ways subsequently, which has commended itself to surgeons and others wishing to relate clinical outcome to histological findings in gliomas. This procedure is not without its pitfalls, largely on account of the tendency for some gliomas not only to contain different areas that would fit the criteria for different grades in the Kernohan classification, but also to become progressively less well differentiated with time. Despite these reservations, there is, of course, a need to provide the surgeon with as accurate a definition as possible of the nature of the tumour specimen received. A disputable system of tumour classification is a proposal to categorize many childhood tumours of the CNS as 'primitive neuroectodermal tumours' (Rorke *et al.* 1985; Rubinstein 1985). Whether this term may have some use when only a very small biopsy is available is open to debate. If there is sufficient evidence to indicate a more precise diagnosis, such as medulloblastoma, ependymoma or neuroblastoma, it is desirable that this should be stated in any report on a childhood CNS tumour.

Post mortem examination of cases of CNS tumour

When examining the CNS in cases with tumours at post mortem, the presence of midline shift, herniations, other consequences of intracranial space occupation (Chapter 11) and other associated CNS disease should be noted. If the tumour caused epilepsy, the brain may show pathological changes associated with this condition (Chapter 18). It is of course important to carry out a careful examination of extracranial viscera looking particularly for sources of metastatic deposits. These include carcinoma, lymphoma, leukaemia and sarcoma. In cases of malignant disease treated with chemotherapy or radiotherapy, and in diseases associated with immunosuppression, one has to look for the effects these may have on the CNS. There may also,

Table 12.1 Classification of CNS tumours based on WHO (1992).

1 *Tumours of neuroepithelial tissue*
  1.1 Astrocytic tumours (see Table 12.2)
  1.2 Oligodendrogliomas (benign/malignant)
  1.3 Ependymal tumours
     Benign, malignant, myxopapillary, subependymoma
  1.4 Mixed gliomas
  1.5 Choroid plexus tumours (papilloma/carcinoma)
  1.6 Neuroepithelial tumours of uncertain origin
     Astroblastoma, polar spongioblastoma, gliomatosis
     cerebri
  1.7 Neuronal and mixed neuronal-glial tumours
     (see Table 12.4)
  1.8 Pineal tumours
     Pineocytoma, pineoblastoma or mixed
  1.9 Embryonal tumours (see Table 12.5)

2 *Tumours of cranial and spinal nerves*
  2.1 Schwannoma
  2.2 Neurofibroma
  2.3 Malignant peripheral nerve sheath tumour

3 *Tumours of the meninges*
  3.1 Tumours of meningothelial cells
     Meningioma, (variants)
     Atypical meningioma
     Papillary meningioma
     Anaplastic (malignant) meningioma
  3.2 Mesenchymal, non-meningothelial tumours

  3.3 Primary melanocyte lesions
  3.4 Tumours of uncertain histogenesis
     Haemangioblastoma

4 *Haemopoeitic neoplasmas*
  Primary malignant lymphomas
  Plasmacytoma
  Granulocytic sarcoma

5 *Germ cell tumours*
  Germinoma
  Embryonal carcinoma
  Yolk sac tumour
  Choriocarcinoma
  Teratoma and variants
  Mixed germ cell tumours

6 *Cysts and tumour-like lesions*

7 *Tumours of the sellar region*
  Pituitary adenomas/carcinoma
  Craniopharyngioma

8 *Local extensions of regional tumours*
  Paragangliomas, chordoma, chondroma, chondrosarcoma,
    adenoid cystic carcinoma, others

9 *Metastatic tumours*

Items 1 and 4 are discussed in this chapter and the others in Chapter 13.

rarely, be evidence of: extracranial spread of primary CNS or pituitary tumour to other sites; endocrine effects of pituitary adenomas; and extracranial pathology associated with intracranial or spinal tumours such as von Recklinghausen's disease (p.230), tuberous sclerosis (p.299) or Lindau's syndrome (p.298).

The spinal cord should be examined along with the brain if there was any clinical suspicion of spinal cord disease or if tumours known to disseminate via CSF pathways have been earlier diagnosed. These include medulloblastoma, choroid plexus tumours, melanoma, ependymoma, and carcinomas, particularly those arising in the breast or stomach.

Macroscopic and microscopic features of intrinsic neuroepithelial tumours

Glial tumours

By definition, gliomas are tumours of neuroglial cells, that is, astrocytes, oligodendrocytes and/or ependymal cells. As all these cells are derived from the cells labelled 'spongioblasts' by embryologists, it is not surprising to find that in many neuroglial tumours there is a mixture of cell types and patterns reminiscent of two or even three of the normal types and patterns. In consequence, it is often difficult to classify a particular tumour as *an* astrocytoma, *an* oligodendroglioma, or *an* ependymoma, whereas there is no such difficulty in speaking of *a* glioma. This point should be borne in mind when reporting on a small sample of tumour from a biopsy. The fact that the fragment of tissue has the appearance of gemistocytic astrocytoma does not exclude the possibility that another part of the tumour may have the features of an oligodendroglioma, or (as is very often the case) that elsewhere in the tumour there are areas of anaplastic malignancy.

A remarkable characteristic — one might almost call it a virtue — of gliomas in general is their reluctance to metastasize, or perhaps the reluctance of other parts of the body to accept glioma metastases. Since there are no lymphatics in the CNS, this channel of spread is unavailable to gliomas; although they are well supplied with veins, reports of glioma metastases in lungs are exceedingly rare. Experimentally explanted tumours, on the other hand, are said to flourish. Even the kind of seeding through the CSF pathways so characteristic of medulloblastomas, which are generally regarded as primitive neural tumours, rarely occurs. Glioblastomas and oligodendrogliomas do indeed reach, and transgress, the pial membrane, and continue to grow for a certain distance in the subarachnoid space, whence they may re-invade the brain. Fragments of malignant glioma may also become detached and adhere to ependymal surfaces, whence they may grow back into the brain. What it is that inhibits their wider spread is not known.

Gliomas composed predominantly of astrocytes (Table 12.2)

It is unfortunate that one word – astrocytoma – is used to cover at least two very different tumours. The first is diffusely spread through a region of the CNS. It has no clearly defined boundaries (Fig. 12.1) and in most cases is inoperable, simply because its removal would entail an unacceptable loss of functioning nervous tissue (the exception is a glioma of an optic nerve; if it does not involve the chiasma, it can be removed at the expense of the already compromised sight in one eye). This diffuse type of astrocytoma is nevertheless regarded as relatively benign, in that it grows slowly, and is compatible with several years' useful life. In contrast, there are tumours composed of astrocytes, unmixed with nervous tissue, and having well-demarcated margins. Except in a few vital areas in the brain stem, these can be completely removed surgically with good hope that they will not recur. They are most commonly met with in the cerebellum in young people. On the assumption that they are true neoplasms, rather than local glial reactions to some congenital malformation, they constitute the benign end of the spectrum of malignancy in gliomas. They are often separated from the diffuse astrocytomas under the clumsy title of 'benign cerebellar astrocytoma of childhood'. Benign, in fact, they are, provided they are

Table 12.2 Classification of astrocytic tumours (WHO 1992).

Astrocytoma and variants (fibrillary, protoplasmic, gemistocytic)

Anaplastic (malignant) astrocytoma

Glioblastoma and variants (giant cell, gliosarcoma)

Pilocytic astrocytoma

Pleomorphic xanthoastrocytoma

Subependymal giant cell astrocytoma (in tuberous sclerosis)

(a)

(b)

Fig. 12.1 (a) Coronal brain slice from a case of diffuse astrocytoma of the left cerebral hemisphere. The left side of the cerebrum and diencephalon are diffusely enlarged, particularly the thalamus, and midline structures are pushed over to the right. Lateral and third ventricles are compressed. The corpus callosum is infiltrated with tumour on both sides and contains a cyst on the right (arrow head). Notice how the infiltrated structures in the left hemisphere retain their original form as they expand (e.g. hippocampus). (b) T2W coronal images (A–D: back to front) of an infiltrating glioma involving the left frontal lobe. The left frontal lobe is swollen and high signal is seen predominantly involving the white matter. The tumour has not extended across the corpus callosum.

(a)

(b)

Fig. 12.2 (a) Coronal slice across the frontal and temporal lobes and optic chiasm from a case with diffuse expansion of the optic chiasm by an astrocytoma (arrowed). (b) T1W coronal MR scan in a 7-year-old child with neurofibromatosis (NF 1) and poor vision demonstrates marked expansion of the optic chiasm by a glioma (arrow). (Compare with Fig. 2.6b, level A2). There was no evidence of retrochiasm extension but the glioma extended along both optic nerves.

removed; otherwise the child will die from the effects of mounting pressure in the posterior cranial fossa. This pressure is usually due not to the size of the tumour, which remains small, but to the expansion of an associated

Fig. 12.3 Nodular expansion of the pons by a diffuse glioma. The basilar artery lies in a groove surrounded by the asymmetrically expanded base of the pons.

cyst. In most cases it is this that causes the patient's symptoms.

A real and practical difficulty arises in making the distinction between low-grade astrocytoma and reactive gliosis. In one variety of glioma a region of the brain or spinal cord is expanded – sometimes grotesquely so – by the presence of vast numbers of well-differentiated astrocytes lying between and among nerve cells and their processes. This may occur in many parts of the CNS, including the optic nerves and brain stem (Figs 12.2 and 12.3). The clinical findings in such cases show that the nervous elements are functioning more or less normally. The histological appearance, one feels, could as well be designated 'pathological hyperplasia of astrocytes' as 'diffuse astrocytoma' – apart, that is, from the prognostic implication of the latter term, which is that the process will continue relentlessly until the space-occupying aspect of the condition kills the patient, or blinds him, as the case may be.

Gliosis, in the sense of astrocytic proliferation in response to a partial injury to CNS tissue, is distinguished from this by having an underlying cause (e.g. death of nerve cells, blood–brain barrier deficiency or demyelination), and by not being a progressive change. The distinction may, however, not be fundamental. Very little is known about the immediate causes of gliosis, and even less about those of astrocytoma; it is reasonable to suppose that the former is induced by chemical or hormonal influences arising in the area of damage, which cease to operate when the damage is repaired, and that the abnormal persistence of a similar hormone might account for the astrocytoma. In this connection it is worth mentioning the not-infrequent reports of gliomas arising in proximity with an older plaque of MS.

Returning from the theoretical to the practical, the diagnosis of astrocytoma on a biopsy specimen – especially on a smeared preparation – should always be guarded. We know of instances where the surgeon, on the evidence of angiograms or air encephalograms, has diagnosed a temporal lobe glioma; and the presence of an excess of astrocytes in the biopsy seemed to confirm the diagnosis. Later it has emerged that the temporal lobe was oedematous and gliotic as a consequence of a middle fossa meningioma. This counsel of hesitancy still applies even when many of the astrocytes appear abnormally large, or possess bizarre, polyploid nuclei. Bizarre astrocytes may be found in a variety of conditions, including hepatic failure, PML and acute MS. Before leaving this topic we should stress that difficulty in distinguishing between reactive and neoplastic astrocytes is not merely a pitfall for beginners. An experienced neuropathologist, examining the outskirts of a frankly malignant glioma post mortem, will not always be able to say whether the astrocytes in the border zone represent reaction or infiltration.

Microscopically, the commonest cell type in astrocytomas is the *fibrillary astrocyte* and its reactive form, the *gemistocyte*. Astrocytomas in which fibrillary astrocytes predominate are moderately cellular and are composed of cells diffusely arranged or displayed as bundles of elongated cells with ill-defined cell borders. In 'piloid' astrocytomas the processes are aligned in the direction of underlying nerve fibre tracts (Fig. 12.4). The cell processes are well shown with the PTAH stain (Fig. 12.5), or with antibodies to GFAP (Fig. 4.27). They may contain condensations of material forming hyaline PTAH-positive, elongated or globular bodies called *Rosenthal fibres* (Fig. 12.6), or more rounded granular bodies. Small foci of calcification may be seen in blood vessel walls or scattered in the fibrillary matrix. The cell bodies are usually inconspicuous and spindle-shaped, and the nuclei round or oval and moderately dense. Mitotic figures are rare or absent in well-differentiated tumours of this type. Slight variation in nuclear size is common, and provides a useful feature distinguishing a sparsely cellular astrocytoma from reactive gliosis (Fig. 12.7). Some tumours have a microcystic background matrix which, if present, also helps to distinguish benign astrocytoma from gliosis.

In contrast to astrocytomas containing mainly fibrillary astrocytes are rarer tumours in which *protoplasmic astrocytes* predominate. These tumours have a low or mod-

Fig. 12.4 Diffuse astrocytoma in which the bipolar neoplastic astrocytes are aligned parallel to the direction of the infiltrated fibre tract. H&E, ×175.

erate degree of cellularity and are composed of cells with multiple, fine processes which form a delicate network frequently interspersed with microcystic spaces containing eosinophilic fluid (Fig. 12.8). The fine processes take the PTAH stain. Nuclei show some variation in size. Mitotic figures are usually absent.

Gemistocytic tumour astrocytes have a distinctive microscopic appearance. They are large cells with a prominent, rounded cell body containing pale eosinophilic cytoplasm and an eccentric nucleus (Fig. 12.9). Short processes are given off from the margins of the cells and these stain with PTAH or with GFAP antibody. Many astrocytomas contain foci of gemistocytic astrocytes, but it is rare for a tumour to be composed solely of cells of this type. However, they may predominate in a biopsy specimen. Their presence in an astrocytic tumour is generally associated with a poor prognosis.

The distinctive *astrocytic gliomas* arising in the *cerebellum* have already been referred to. Most contain intermingled areas of fibrillary astrocytes and microcystic foci in which the cell bodies of the neoplastic cells cluster around blood vessels and project fine processes to form a sketchy, web-like pattern interspersed among the cysts. Foci of calcification and haemosiderin deposition are common, and a moderate degree of vascular hyperplasia may be present without the implied malignant potential that this feature imparts to cerebral astrocytomas (see p.207). Leptomeningeal invasion is also common and does not influence the usually benign outcome following removal of this tumour. Features that are correlated with a poor outcome are only rarely seen and consist of a high overall degree of cellularity and frequent mitotic figures (Fig. 12.10). Nuclear pleomorphism may be found even in benign tumours.

Fig. 12.5 Fibrillary astrocytoma stained with PTAH to show up the processes as well as the cell bodies of the tumour cells. ×400.

Fig. 12.6 Rosenthal fibres in a fibrillary astrocytoma, examples arrowed. PTAH, ×340.

Fig. 12.7 Diffuse astrocytoma infiltrating cerebral white matter. The overall cellularity is hardly increased, but the presence of neoplasia is revealed by the pleomorphism of some of the nuclei (arrow heads). Note, however, that there are other conditions giving rise to pleomorphic astrocyte nuclei (see p.203). H&E, ×160.

Fig. 12.8 Low-power view of a section of a protoplasmic astrocytoma containing microcysts. H&E, ×90.

Fig. 12.9 Gemistocytic astrocytoma composed of cells with abundant, eosinophilic cytoplasm and eccentrically placed nuclei. The processes of these cells are inconspicuous, but can be shown up with the PTAH stain. There are hyperplastic endothelial cells also present in this field — a feature emphasizing the malignant character of these tumours despite a relatively bland appearance to the tumour cells. H&E, ×300.

Subependymal giant cell tumours may occur in subjects with tuberous sclerosis (p.299), *formes frustes* of that condition, and in a number of cases in isolation. These tumours occur around the lateral ventricles and are relatively slow-growing and circumscribed (Fig. 16.19b). Microscopically they contain conspicuous large cells with abundant cytoplasm and short processes. Nuclei are large, often bizarre, and are eccentrically situated (Fig. 12.11). Some of the cells resemble gemistocytic astrocytes, but others are larger and may have two or more nuclei. Foci of calcification are frequently present. These tumours are considered to be related to the bizarre astrocytes found in the cortex in tuberous sclerosis, and their immunoreactions (often GFAP-negative, usually NSE-positive, sometimes NF-positive) suggest an origin from dysplastic cells related both

to neurons and astrocytes. The unwary may take these tumours for glioblastomas, but they differ from these in the absence or rarity of mitotic figures, and absence of necrosis and of endothelial hyperplasia (p.208).

Foci of anaplastic change may occur in an otherwise better-differentiated astrocytoma. Microscopically, *anaplastic astrocytoma* is hard to differentiate from glioblastoma and, in terms of clinical outcome, the distinction is not great. Compared with well-differentiated astrocytoma (Table 12.3) anaplastic tumour shows greater overall cellularity, and fewer recognizable astrocytic features, though gemistocytic astrocytes may be present. The tumour cells are haphazardly arranged, and nuclei are pleomorphic (Fig. 12.12). Mitotic figures are present, and there is mild endothelial cell enlargement and

Fig. 12.10 Malignant cerebellar astrocytoma showing a high degree of cellularity, nuclear pleomorphism and mitoses. H&E, ×340.

Fig. 12.11 Subependymal tumour from a case of tuberous sclerosis. The cells are large, closely packed and contain several processes. Nuclei are large and pleomorphic, often with prominent nucleoli. Mitoses are not a regular feature of these tumours. H&E, ×370.

hyperplasia, and a high degree of vascularity in most tumours. Small areas of necrosis may be present. When infiltrating the cortex these tumours characteristically produce clusters of cells around neuron cell bodies, mimicking the satellitosis seen sometimes in the deep cortex late in life (Fig. 12.13).

An unusual variant of astrocytic glioma, warranting rec-ognition because of its relatively good prognosis compared with other variants of pleomorphic astrocytoma, is the *pleomorphic xanthoastrocytoma*. This is a tumour found superficially situated in the cerebrum in young adults. It is distinguished by the presence of lipid in the cytoplasm of many of the tumour cells (Fig. 12.14), and by the presence of reticulin around them (Fig. 12.15).

Fig. 12.12 Anaplastic astrocytoma showing closely packed cells of varying size and shape, some with mitoses. Nuclei are hyperchromatic and pleomorphic. H&E, ×300.

Table 12.3 Histological criteria for grading astrocytomas (after WHO 1992).

	Grade			
	I	II	III	IV(Glioblastoma)
Differentiated astrocytes	+	+	∓	−
Pleomorphic nuclei	−	∓	+	+
Mitoses	−	−	+	+
Necrosis	−	−	−	+
Endothelial hyperplasia	−	−	−	+

Well-differentiated astrocytoma reacts immuno-histologically with antibodies to GFAP (Fig. 4.27). A variable proportion of tumour cells in anaplastic astrocytoma do likewise (Fig. 4.28). However, this reaction is not specific for astrocytoma, since ependymoma, glioblastoma and oligodendroglioma may also show some GFAP-immunoreactivity. Even haemangioblastoma, medulloblastoma and choroid plexus papilloma may contain a few tumour cells reactive with GFAP antibodies. The majority of astrocytic tumours also react with anti-Leu 7 (NK cell) monoclonal antibody, but again this is not a specific reaction (see Table 4.2). Astrocytomas also contain vimentin, and some investigators have found an inverse relation between the intensity of staining for vimentin and the degree of differentiation of the astrocytoma.

Fig. 12.13 Cerebral cortex adjacent to an anaplastic astrocytoma of the white matter. Clusters of neoplastic astrocytes surround neuron cell bodies, producing an appearance resembling satellitosis. H&E, ×280.

Glioblastomas

The commonest kind of glioma lies, alas, at the most malignant end of the spectrum. Although the various cell types seen in this tumour bear little, if any, resemblance to

Fig. 12.14 Pleomorphic xanthoastrocytoma. The cells are haphazardly arranged and show considerable nuclear pleomorphism. Some cells possess pale, swollen cytoplasm containing lipid droplets. H&E, ×220.

Fig. 12.15 Section showing the abundant reticulin network throughout a xanthoastrocytoma. ×220.

embryonic glial cells, the tumour is generally known as glioblastoma (the adjective 'multiforme', which is traditionally attached to this term, is redundant, as it does not differentiate one type of glioblastoma from another). The most striking macroscopic feature is its variegated appearance on slicing, which is largely due to: scattered haemorrhages which show dark or red-brown; patches of necrosis showing yellow or white; and multiple, small cystic cavities, containing yellowish fluid, which coagulates on fixation and even on standing (Fig. 12.16). On palpation there is a similar variety, ranging from slimy through mushy, soft and rubbery, to tough and gristly. The tumours are commonest in elderly people, and arise most often in one or other cerebral hemisphere, but may occupy both hemispheres as so-called 'butterfly tumours', with a connection through the corpus callosum (Fig. 12.17). Their effect on the brain is exerted in four ways: they destroy, they expand, they give rise to cysts and, rarely, they may bleed extensively. Some glioblastomas seem, from the clinical and pathological evidence, to have been malignant and fast growing from the start. The illness lasts six months or less; on slicing the brain, the tumour is separated from more or less normal brain tissue by a margin only a centimetre or less wide, of infiltrated tissue. In other cases, with a longer history – a year or more – one finds a large area of diffuse astrocytoma containing a malignant patch

(a)

(b)

(Fig. 12.18). Such tumours might be referred to as 'astrocytoma-gone-bad'. Similarly, one may come across cases, again with somewhat longer clinical histories, of 'oligodendroglioma-gone-bad' and 'ependymoma-gone-bad'. The malignant areas in these are hardly distinguishable from 'bad-from-the-start' tumours. In a few cases glioblastomas appear to arise in more than one focus; they may then be misinterpreted clinically and in scans or radiographs as metastatic tumours.

Microscopic appearances in glioblastomas are varied. In some tumours there are foci of clearly recognizable astrocytes, fibrillary or gemistocytic, or of oligodendrocytes. In other areas there are densely packed, haphazardly arranged, nondescript, small cells with scanty wisps of cytoplasm and darkly staining nuclei (Fig. 12.19). Some fields contain markedly pleomorphic, larger cells

Fig. 12.16 Glioblastoma of the right parietal region. The main tumour mass occupies the white matter, but it extends into medial parietal cortex also. Note variegated, partially necrotic, cut surface appearance and relatively sharp margin to the tumour.

Fig. 12.17 Horizontal slice through a 'butterfly'-shaped glioblastoma massively expanding both cerebral hemispheres and the corpus callosum.

Fig. 12.18 Diffuse cerebral astrocytoma expanding the right cerebral hemisphere in the more rostral slice (a). A glioblastoma has arisen in this tumour more posteriorly (b).

with conspicuous, lobulated or multiple nuclei, and in a few tumours multinucleate cells are numerous (Fig. 12.20). Other fields consist of frankly necrotic debris. A very characteristic appearance, best appreciated at low power, is of 'pseudopalisading' of dense rows of nuclei around irregular or serpiginous patches of necrosis (Fig. 12.21). Some of these nuclei are those of tumour cells, but others belong to macrophages. Mitotic figures in the tumour cells are frequent, but are not always conspicuous, and may need to be carefully sought. The PTAH stain reveals positively stained neuroglial fibrils to a variable extent in the cells of a glioblastoma. Remnants of surviving neural structure, such as neurons and axons, are encountered in some tumours, testifying to the infiltrating character of the tumour growth (Fig. 12.22). The vasculature is striking. There are large, thin-walled, congested vessels, usually with evidence at some point of haemorrhage or thrombosis or both. The small vessels, particularly the capillaries, show a characteristic hyperplastic change which makes them appear tortuous, with thickened walls composed of enlarged endothelial cells, some containing mitotic figures, increased reticulin and reduplicated basal lamina. Zones of

Fig. 12.19 Glioblastoma composed of densely packed, small cells with dark-stained nuclei and scanty cytoplasm, with wispy processes. Several multinucleate cells are present. H&E, ×200.

Fig. 12.20 Glioblastoma in which many of the tumour cells are large and multinuleate. H&E, ×250.

Fig. 12.21 'Pseudopalisade' of nuclei surrounding a focus of necrosis in a glioblastoma. H&E, ×150.

Fig. 12.22 Surviving brain stem neuron surrounded by a dense infiltrate of tumour cells in a rare glioblastoma arising in the medulla. H&E, ×220.

hyperplastic change in small vessels are frequently prominent at the advancing edge of the tumour (Fig. 12.23), and explain the high degree of enhancement seen in CT scans at the margin of these tumours when the patient has been given contrast medium (Fig. 12.24). In some tumours this hyperplastic change becomes neoplastic (see section on gliosarcomas below). The factor responsible seems to be the production of an endothelial growth factor by the tumour cells.

Immunohistologically, glioblastomas usually contain some GFAP-positive cells and processes. Vimentin and Leu 7 antigen are also usually detectable in these tumours, and there may be a focal reaction for cytokeratins.

Gliosarcomas

A gliosarcoma is a malignant tumour containing both glial and mesenchymal neoplastic elements. The glial element has features of a glioblastoma, and the mesenchymal component appears to be derived from the hyperplastic

vascular structures seen in typical glioblastomas or from the leptomeninges. Up to 10% of tumours in published glioblastoma series have a sarcomatous element and the prognosis is unaffected. Macroscopically, these tumours are frequently seen reaching the meninges, and the sarcomatous areas are tough and (being relatively avascular) pale (Fig. 12.25). Microscopically, there are swathes of spindle cells with pleomorphic nuclei and mitotic figures, with reticulin and collagen deposition in the sarcomatous areas (Figs 12.26 and 12.27). Very occasionally, differentiation of the mesenchymal elements towards muscle or cartilage may be found.

A wealth of growth factors has recently been detected in malignant gliomas. These include transforming growth factor β, platelet derived growth factor, endothelial cell growth factor and basic fibroblast growth factor. Some of these factors are almost certainly produced by the tumour cells themselves and have the effect of accelerating their own proliferation; others may be produced by infiltrating macrophages. Several are capable of enhancing endothelial

Fig. 12.23 Zone of hyperplastic blood vessels in superficial cortex adjacent to subarachnoid and subpial glioblastoma. H&E, ×120.

Fig. 12.24 CT scan of a predominantly right-sided cerebral glioblastoma after the patient had been given intravenous contrast medium. There is contrast enhancement, reflecting the abundant blood flow in hyperplastic vessels, around the low-density area which consists of a zone of central tumour necrosis.

Fig. 12.25 Macroscopic appearance of a gliosarcoma in the right tempo-parietal region. The sarcomatous element appears pale and felt tough.

cell growth and proliferation, providing a ready explanation for the often florid endothelial cell hyperplasia that is seen so characteristically in malignant gliomas and sometimes spills over into sarcomatous change. However, the trigger to the increased production of these growth factors and the rapid acceleration of uncontrolled tumour growth that they allow is unclear. Scrutiny of the genes controlling certain tumour-associated antigens such as p53, (Louis 1994) has uncovered evidence of mutations that may be relevant in this context.

Fig. 12.26 Microscopic appearance of a gliosarcoma, with intermingled areas of glioma (purple) and sarcoma (pink). PTAH, ×220.

Fig. 12.27 Reticulin pattern in a gliosarcoma showing dense reticulin deposition in the sarcomatous regions of the tumour only. ×220.

Gliomas composed predominantly of oligodendrocytes

Tumours of oligodendrocytes are more often than not associated with astrocytoma. In their purer forms they are usually fairly well circumscribed, expanding rather than infiltrating, and tending to grow slowly (Fig. 18.4). They occur almost exclusively in the cerebral hemispheres. Peculiar features are, first, their tendency to evoke calcification (often visible on radiographs) in the surrounding brain tissue, and second, a way of fungating into the subarachnoid space, without widespread subarachnoid seeding. Some have associated cysts, whereas others do not.

Microscopically, these tumours are composed of diffusely arranged uniform cells with a centrally situated, more or less round nucleus, with coarse, stippled chromatin and small nucleolus. The surrounding cytoplasm is often swollen and empty looking (Fig. 12.28). The appearance of such cells has been aptly likened to that of fried eggs. Some areas of the tumours lack the cytoplasmic swelling, and then the cells appear more closely packed (Fig. 12.29). Processes are not visible on the cells with

Fig. 12.28 Microscopic appearances of an oligodendroglioma. Cells are uniform, polygonal or cuboidal, and have centrally placed, regular nuclei. The cells are divided into clusters by a delicate, vascular stroma. H&E, ×470.

Fig. 12.29 Microscopic appearance of an oligodendroglioma infiltrating cerebral cortex. The tumour cells are less swollen and their cytoplasm less 'empty' looking than those in Fig. 12.28. H&E, ×340.

routine stains, but can be shown up on some cells with silver stains. Calcospherites and calcification of blood vessel walls in and just beyond the tumour are common findings. Occasionally bone may form. There is an abundance of capillaries in most oligodendroglial tumours and these characteristically form a prominent net-work dividing the tumour cells into clusters (Fig. 12.30), or parallel rows. Endothelial hyperplasia may be seen in otherwise benign-appearing tumours. Nuclei usually show little pleomorphism and mitotic figures are rare in most tumours. Mucinous degeneration may occur in clusters of tumour cells and spill over into the background matrix of the tumour. As indicated above, mixed gliomas composed of oligodendrocytes and astrocytes are more common than tumours composed solely of oligodendrocytes. Malignant oligodendrogliomas are also well recognized. They have a higher cell density, greater nuclear pleomorphism and more numerous mitotic figures than the more benign tumours (Fig. 12.31).

Immunohistologically, oligodendrocytes are mainly characterized by the absence rather than the presence of recognizable antigens. They give negative reactions with antibodies to neurofilaments, epithelial membrane antigen and cytokeratins. However, they usually show some reaction with antibodies to GFAP (Fig. 4.30) and S-100 protein, and with the monoclonal antibody Leu 7.

Fig. 12.30 The capillary network in an oligodendroglioma. H&E, ×150.

Gliomas composed predominantly of ependymal cells

Ependymomas may arise wherever there are ependymal cells; in practice, they are commonest in the fourth ventricle (including Luschka's foramina). Other common sites are the so-called central canal of the spinal cord, the filum terminale, the third ventricle and the aqueduct. They are generally slow growing, although malignant varieties occur. In the third and fourth ventricles and aqueduct their main effect is to produce hydrocephalus by obstructing the flow of CSF. In the spinal cord the effect is to compress the surrounding tissues (Fig. 11.10) and in the filum terminale to compress the roots of the cauda equina (Fig. 12.32). The fourth-ventricle tumours are surgically accessible; if they arise from the roof of the ventricle a complete removal may be achieved, but if they arise from, or are closely adherent to, the floor of the ventricle, this is not practicable. Spinal ependymomas can sometimes be shelled out from behind, and those of the filum terminale can be dissected away entire.

Macroscopic appearances vary, but most tumours appear greyish in colour and are granular in texture. They are sometimes cystic and are usually circumscribed, but not encapsulated. They tend to spill irregularly, or in lobulated form, into the ependymal-lined cavity from which they arise (Fig. 12.33). Seeding of tumours into the CSF can give rise to metastatic CNS deposits.

Microscopic appearances show wide variation, but certain features usually allow *typical ependymomas* to be easily identified. The most characteristic of these is the occurrence of rosettes of cells arranged around a central space (Fig. 12.34), recalling the appearance of reactive ependymal cells buried beneath the ventricular surface. Sometimes the central spaces of the rosettes are enlarged to form microscopic or macroscopic cysts, and the arrangement of the tumour cells may then be papillary (Fig. 12.35). Even more common than rosettes are pseudorosettes, formed by elongated bipolar tumour cells orientated around blood vessels (Fig. 12.36). Nuclei of the tumour cells are placed well away from the vessel, the space between being occupied by the radially directed processes of the ependymal cells. These processes appear poorly defined and eosinophilic with

Fig. 12.31 Malignant oligodendroglioma. The tumour cells are packed closely together, are less uniform than those of a benign oligodendroglioma, and have pleomorphic nuclei. A few foci of capillary calcification are present. H&E, ×19420.

Fig. 12.32 Section across an ependymoma of the filum terminale.

Fig. 12.33 Macroscopic appearance of an ependymoma arising in the left foramen of Luschka. After incomplete surgical removal of the tumour there was a 6-year survival. The tumour is seen spilling out into the subarachnoid space, and invading the medulla.

Fig. 12.34 Ependymoma. Low-power view showing a pattern chiefly of pseudorosettes, with tumour cells orientated around blood vessels but with some rosettes also. H&E, ×100.

H&E, but are better appreciated with the PTAH stain. The PTAH stain will also sometimes reveal clusters of cytoplasmic bodies, blepharoplasts, the basal bodies to which the shafts of cilia are attached. Cilia themselves may be visible, but blepharoplasts are more widespread. At the ultrastructural level, microvilli occupy the central space in the rosettes and gap junctions can be found, reflecting the epithelial character of the cells. The nuclei of ependymoma cells are oval or round and darkly stained. They usually show little pleomorphism, and mitotic figures are rare or absent.

Myxopapillary ependymomas are virtually confined to the cauda equina region, where they appear to arise from the filum terminale. They form sausage-like, slightly irregular, discrete masses surrounded by compressed nerve roots. The microscopic appearance of these tumours is unusual

Fig. 12.35 Papillary pattern of growth in a cystic ependymoma. H&E, ×100.

(a)

(b)

Fig. 12.36 Pseudorosettes in an ependymoma. (a) Vessels are surrounded by a pale zone containing processes of tumour cells, which separate the vessel wall from the cell nuclei. H&E, ×100.

(b) With the PTAH stain radially orientated cell processes can be discerned. ×100.

and distinctive. They are composed of flattened cuboidal epithelial cells covering connective tissue cores containing blood vessels and abundant acellular, hyaline, matrix material (Fig. 12.37). The matrix reacts with stains for mucin. Nuclei are small and uniform, without mitoses. The prognosis for these tumours is usually very good, but occasionally they exhibit malignant behaviour.

A not uncommon tumour composed of an intimate mixture of ependymal cells with fibre-forming astrocytes, called *subependymoma*, occurs mainly in the fourth ventricle, where it may be an incidental post mortem finding (Fig. 12.38). For the most part these tumours belong to the benign end of the glioma spectrum.

Ependymomas with malignant features (patchy necrosis, invasive tendencies, pleomorphism and frequent mitoses; Fig. 12.39) occur most commonly in children, and are usually situated in the fourth ventricle. The differential diagnosis of such tumours includes malignant choroid plexus tumour, glioblastoma and medulloblastoma. At the malignant end of the spectrum is the ependymoblastoma, a rare childhood variant combining cellular anaplasia, a high mitotic incidence and a characteristic ependymal pattern.

In their immunohistological reactions, ependymomas usually show foci of positive reactivity for GFAP and to a lesser extent for Leu 7 antigen. Epithelial membrane antigen is focally expressed by the more benign forms, but not by malignant ones, a distinction of some diagnostic value (Fig. 4.26).

Fig. 12.37 Myxopapillary ependymoma of the cauda equina. The tumour is composed of cores of myxoid stroma surrounding blood vessels, and covered by a layer of flattened cuboidal epithelial cells. The epithelium appears as a dark layer enveloping the myxoid cores. H&E, ×100.

Fig. 12.38 A subependymoma arising in the floor of the fourth ventricle, which was discovered as an incidental finding at post mortem examination. The tumour is almost filling the cavity of the fourth ventricle, and might have been expected to cause hydrocephalus eventually.

Fig. 12.39 Malignant ependymoma showing a disorganized, but still recognizable, pseudorosette pattern. Nuclei are pleomorphic. H&E, ×210.

Choroid plexus tumours

Choroid plexus tumours are rare, occurring mainly in infants and children. Benign papillomas form discrete, papillary growths projecting into a ventricular cavity, most commonly the fourth ventricle. There may be associated hydrocephalus, attributable either to obstruction or to excess production of CSF. Microscopically, the pattern of growth of the papillae resembles that of normal choroid plexus, only the profusion of cells and a slight raggedness of the pattern distinguishing the tumour (Fig. 12.40). There are ribbons of cuboidal epithelial cells covering vascular stalk-like projections or papillae. Nuclei are regular and without mitoses. Some mucus production or cilia may be seen. Even such benign-appearing neoplasms may give rise to recurrent local or distant tumour on account of the readiness with which tumour cells seed into the CSF.

Anaplastic or malignant choroid plexus tumours still

Fig. 12.40 Choroid plexus papilloma. The papillary growth pattern is well developed, and the resemblance to choroid plexus easily appreciated. PAS, ×100.

Table 12.4 Neuronal and mixed neuronal–glial tumours (WHO 1992).

Gangliocytoma

Dysplastic gangliocytoma of the cerebellum (Lhermitté–Duclos disease)

Desmoplastic infantile ganglioglioma

Dysembryoplastic neuroepithelial tumour

Ganglioglioma

Anaplastic (malignant) ganglioglioma

Central neurocytoma

Paraganglioma of the filum terminale

Olfactory neuroblastoma/neuroepithelioma

bear a resemblance to normal choroid plexus. In contrast to benign papillomas, there tends to be a heaping up of epithelial cells into layers more than one cell thick. The fronds of cells are more disordered, nuclei more variable in size and staining properties, and mitotic figures are much more easily found than in benign papillomas (Fig. 12.41).

Immunohistological reactions of choroid plexus papillomas are mixed. They show some foci of positivity with antibody Leu 7, antibodies to epithelial membrane antigen, GFAP and carbonic anhydrase 2.

Tumours containing neurons (Table 12.4)

Tumours containing mature neurons are rare in the CNS, and uncommon elsewhere. In the CNS they must be distin-guished from the much more common finding of neurons surviving in an area of neural parenchyma extensively in-filtrated by a glioma (Fig. 12.22). Neurons forming part of the neoplastic process are found rarely in the CNS in neuroblastomas, gangliocytomas, dysembryoplastic neuroepithelial tumours and ganglioneuromas, and in the peripheral nervous system in neuroblastomas and ganglioneuromas.

Neuroblastomas have been described as rarely arising in the cerebral hemispheres in infants and children. These malignant tumours are generally quite well circumscribed and firm, and are sometimes cystic. Microscopically they are composed of dense collections of small cells with dark-staining nuclei, resembling those of a medulloblastoma. Rosette formations may be present and mitotic figures are plentiful. A well-developed fibrous connective tissue stroma is usually present, dividing the tumour cells into lobules. Some mature or immature ganglion cells may be identifiable in these tumours. These are large, polygonal cells with vesicular nuclei and prominent nucleoli. Cell processes may be detectable if silver stains are used.

Gangliocytomas and gangliogliomas are tumours composed predominantly of mature neurons in a stroma of non-neoplastic glia (gangliocytoma) or neoplastic glia (ganglioglioma). Such tumours outside the CNS have a stroma of Schwann cells and a few fibroblasts (ganglioneuroma). To identify such a tumour, it is neces-sary to be convinced of the neoplastic nature of the neurons. Indications of neoplasia include abnormal cellu-lar morphology and occurrence at sites not normally har-bouring ganglion cells (Fig. 12.42). Mitotic figures are not seen in the neurons. Astrocytes contribute to the stroma and may be frankly neoplastic, as in a fibrillary astrocytoma.

Fig. 12.41 Malignant choroid plexus papilloma. The papillary pattern is still discernible, but the cellular arrangement is much more dishevelled than in a benign papilloma. Cell nuclei are also more pleomorphic and there are frequent mitoses. H&E, ×100.

Neurocytomas are a recently recognized category of CNS tumour thought to be derived from neuronal stem cells (Nishio *et al.* 1988). They have been diagnosed most commonly in young adults and are located in the lateral or third ventricles. Long tumour-free intervals following removal have been recorded in most cases. Histologically the tumours bear a remarkable resemblance to oligodendrogliomas and in the past were probably diagnosed as such (Fig. 12.43). They are composed of small uniform cells with perinuclear haloes and central, round, regular nuclei. Mitoses are infrequent. The key diagnostic feature is the presence ultrastructurally of 100–200 nm diameter dense-core vesicles and occasional 20–25 nm diameter microtubules in cell cytoplasm (Fig. 12.44). Immunocytochemically they usually show some immunoreactivity for synaptophysin, S-100 and neuron-specific enolase (Table 4.2).

A good prognosis is also characteristic of the recently defined *dysembryoplastic neuroepithelial tumour* (Daumas-Duport *et al.* 1988), a tumour that is generally small and largely confined to the cerebral cortex of temporal or frontal lobe in children. It causes epilepsy. The tumour contains a mixture of disorganized neurons and neoplastic glial cells.

Certain other space-occupying lesions, not clearly neoplastic in nature, are occasionally seen. These include hamartomas in the region of the mamillary bodies or tuber cinereum (p.427), which are a cause of precocious puberty in children and the cortical tubers found in tuberous sclerosis (p.299).

Lhermitte–Duclos disease

A rare condition belonging to the twilight zone between malformation and neoplasia is the Lhermitte–Duclos disease, now classified as a dysplastic gangliocytoma of the cerebellum. This presents clinically as an expanding cerebellar tumour. The cerebellar lesion, exposed at operation or post mortem, consists of an area in which the folia are expanded and pale (Fig. 12.45). The lesion has a striking MRI appearance (Fig. 12.46). On section, the tissue is found to consist of two layers: an outer one, occupied by myelinated nerve fibres, and an inner one composed of rather large abnormal nerve cells (Fig. 12.47). At the margins of the abnormal tissue, the outer layer is seen to be continuous with the molecular layer, and the inner one with the granule cell layer. Silver impregnations show that the myelinated fibres in the outer layer have the orientation of normal granule cell axons, running vertically outward, bifurcating, and then running horizontally, parallel with the axis of the folium. In the affected area there is a total loss of Purkinje cells, and of central white matter. Outside the area, where normal-looking granule and Purkinje cells are present, there may be areas in which some of the

Fig. 12.42 A large, abnormal neuron (arrowed) in a tumour removed from the pituitary fossa of a patient with acromegaly. The tumour contained some areas of gangliocytoma, of which this was a small part, and other areas of eosinophil adenoma, which were reactive for growth hormone. Some nerve fibres are also present. Neuro filament antibody, counterstained with haematoxylin, ×200. (Slide prepared by Dr CS Morris.)

Fig. 12.43 Histological appearance of a neurocytoma. The resemblance to an oligodendroglioma is striking. H&E, ×100.

granule cell axons are myelinated, with attendant oligodendrocytes.

The fact that the lesion behaves as an expanding tumour has led some authors to classify it as a neoplasm, under a title such as *gangliocytoma dysplasticum*; against this view is the fact that there is no sign of cellular proliferation. If the cells are what they appear to be – that is, hypertrophic granule cells – their numbers are *reduced*; the expansion of the tissue is due to the enormous increase in size of the individual cells. It is presumably the resulting increased pressure that accounts for the disappearance of the central white matter. Nothing is known of the causes of the disease; but in one instance it affected a mother and her son. In examining a proven case post mortem, we would recom-

Fig. 12.44 Electron micrograph from the tumour shown in Fig. 12.43 showing dense core vesicles in a tumour cell process. Uranyl acetate and lead citrate stain.

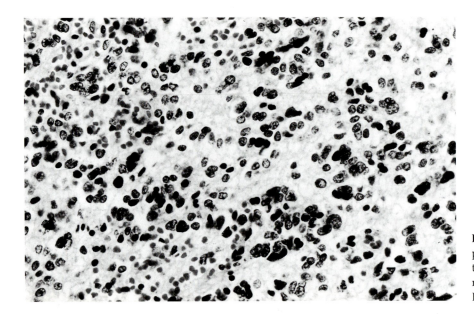

Fig. 12.50 Poorly differentiated pineoblastoma. The cells display little tendency to a radial grouping, show more nuclear pleomorphism and have mitoses. H&E, ×200.

Fig. 12.51 Macroscopic appearance of a medulloblastoma. Some terminal haemorrhage has occurred.

purple, and are friable. They extend into the fourth ventricle, where seedling deposits are frequently released and become transported to the subarachnoid space, there to establish metastases which tend to re-invade the brain or spinal cord.

Microscopically these tumours are densely cellular and composed of diffusely arranged small cells with scanty, ill-defined cytoplasm and dark, hyperchromatic nuclei. Occasional rosette formations may be seen (Fig. 12.52). There are frequently small foci of necrosis, and mitotic figures are plentiful. Most medulloblastomas have a scanty, vascular stroma, but a few extend into the subarachnoid space, where they may provoke a dense, collagenous reaction,

giving rise to an abundant stroma which divides the cells into clusters. This is termed a 'desmoplastic' reaction. Neuroblastic differentiation may be discernible in a small proportion of medulloblastomas in preparations stained with silver, and more frequently if antigenic markers of neural cells (e.g. neurofilaments, neuron-specific enolase) are sought with appropriate antibodies. Evidence of glial differentiation is also sometimes present, as reflected in the expression of GFAP. Rare, related tumours to medulloblastomas are a melanin-containing papillary neuro-ectodermal tumour and a medulloepithelioma, details of which can be found in Russell & Rubinstein (1989) and Becker & Hinton (1986).

Primary CNS lymphomas

Lymphomas are encountered in neuropathological practice at two main sites: in the brain, usually as a primary lymphoma, or as extradural metastases from an extracranial tumour. The primary CNS lymphomas are rare but for reasons that are not clear, are becoming less so. Their increasing incidence is not entirely explained by an increased incidence in immunosuppressed individuals, including those with AIDS. They have a varied naked-eye appearance, which can mimic glioblastoma, metastatic carcinoma, or a brain stem glioma (Fig. 12.53). Those in the cerebrum often form soft, ill-defined grey masses with a granular texture. They occur in any part of the brain, most commonly in the cerebrum or around the lateral and third ventricles. Microscopically they are composed of medium or large, round or polygonal cells, which tend to cluster densely in the Virchow–Robin spaces as well as spilling out in sheets into the brain parenchyma. Wide areas of necrosis occur. Beyond the edge of the main tumour, lymphoid cells

Fig. 12.52 Medulloblastoma composed of small cells with dark-stained nuclei and barely discernible cytoplasm. Cells are arranged in an unusually prominent rosette pattern in this tumour. H&E, ×200.

Table 12.5 Embryonal tumours (WHO 1992).

Medulloepithelioma

Neuroblastoma

Ganglioneuroblastoma

Ependymoblastoma

Primitive neuroectodermal tumours with multipotent differentiation: neuronal, astrocyte, ependymal, muscle, melanotic etc

Medulloblastoma

Medulloblastoma variants:
    desmoplastic medulloblastoma
    medullomyeloblastoma
    melanocytic medulloblastoma

Fig. 12.53 Primary brain lymphoma, situated in the white matter of the left cerebellar hemisphere, causing compression of the brain stem and fourth ventricle. The margins of the tumour are ill-defined, and its texture granular. The naked-eye appearance can be hard to distinguish from that of a malignant glioma, particularly if the tumour is situated in the cerebrum.

Fig. 12.54 Lymphoma cells occupying perivascular spaces above, and surrounding white matter below. H&E, ×100.

Fig. 12.55 Reticulin deposition in infiltrated perivascular spaces in a cerebral lymphoma. ×100.

are found in perivascular spaces in a remarkably wide distribution (Fig. 12.54). The abnormal cells have scanty cytoplasm and large, lobulated nuclei with prominent nucleoli and frequent mitoses (Fig. 4.14). Reticulin is increased in infiltrated perivascular spaces (Fig. 12.55). Investigation of these tumours with antibodies to leucocyte antigens shows that the great majority of them are derived from B-lymphocytes, and very few of them carry antigenic markers specific for macrophages, belying the former term 'microgliomatosis'. However, lymphoma of the brain is accompanied by the widespread occurrence of increased numbers of reactive microglial cells in the surrounding neuropil.

Another rare form of lymphoma involving the CNS is

Fig. 12.56 Macroscopic appearance of the cerebrum in a case of B-cell angiotrophic lymphoma. There was a 6-month history of dementia and focal neurological deficits, which at post mortem seemed to be largely attributable to infarcts and haemorrhages, scattered throughout the cortex and white matter.

Fig. 12.57 Angiotropic B-cell lymphoma. Neoplastic cells occupy the lumen of a small vein. H&E, ×200.

that of a B-cell lymphoma in which the tumour cells are predominantly found in blood vessels, and the symptoms produced are due to ischaemia rather than to space occupation (Figs 12.56 and 12.57). This is referred to as an *angiotropic lymphoma*. Some cases of so-called malignant angioendotheliomatosis now appear to fall into this category.

Further reading and references

Becker LE, Hinton D. 1986. Pathology of neoplasia in children and adolescents. In Finegold M (Ed.) *Major Problems in Pathology.* WB Saunders, Philadelphia. **18**, 397–418.

Burger PC, Scheithauer BW, 1994. Armed Forces Institute of Pathology Atlas of Tumour Pathology, Fascicle 10, third series, Washington.

Burger PC, Vogel FS. 1991. *Surgical Pathology of the Nervous System and its Converings.* John Wiley, New York, 3rd edn.

Daumas-Duport C, Scheithauer BW, Chodkiewicz JP, Laws ER, Vedrenne C. 1988. Dysembryoplastic neuroepithelial tumour of young patients with intractable partial seizures. *Neurosurg* **23**, 545–56.

Kernohan JW, Mabon RF, Svien HJ, Adson AW. 1949. Symposium on a new and simplified classification of gliomas. *Proc Mayo Clin* **24**, 71.

Louis DN. 1994. The p53 gene and protein in human tumours. *J Neuropathol Exp Neurol* **53**, 11–21.

Nishio S, Tashima T, Takeshita I, Fukui M. 1988. Intraventricular neurocytoma: clinicopathological features of six cases. *J Neurosurg* **68**, 665–670.

Rorke LB, Gilles FH, Davis RL, Becker LE. 1985. Revision of the WHO classification of brain tumours for childhood brain tumours. *Cancer* **56** (Suppl), 1869–86.

Rubinstein LJ. 1985. Embryonal central neuroepithelial tumours and their differentiating potential. *J Neurosurg* **62**, 795–805.

Russell DS, Rubinstein LJ. 1989. *Pathology of Tumours of the Nervous System*, 5th edn. Edward Arnold, London.

Kleihues P, Burger PC, Scheithauer BW (Eds.) WHO Histological classification of tumours of the central nervous system. International Histological Classification of Tumours, 2nd edn.

Zulch KJ. 1986. *Brain Tumours, their Pathology and Biology.* Springer, Heidelberg.

13   Other Tumours Affecting the Nervous System

Nerve sheath tumours

In the past there has been impassioned debate about the cells of origin of nerve sheath tumours, and consequently about how they should be named. For our part, we are content to follow Russell & Rubinstein (1989) in recognizing two types: one, derived from Schwann cells, called *schwannoma*, and another derived from perineurial fibroblasts, called *neurofibroma*. The fact that both types of tumour occur in von Recklinghausen's disease, and that both kinds of tissue can sometimes be seen together in a single tumour, suggests that the two are in some way related. Terms now deemed to be objectionable, but still in use, are *neurinoma* and *neurilemmoma*. Tumours of the eighth cranial nerve are commonly referred to by neurosurgeons as *acoustic neuromas*. The objection here is that *neuroma* is also the name of a non-neoplastic tangle of regenerating nerve fibres arising from a severed nerve—a lesion sometimes giving rise to discomfort, or worse, in an amputation stump (Figs 22.7 and 22.8).

Schwannomas

These tumours arise on cranial and spinal nerve roots, and on peripheral nerves. In the cranial cavity, the eighth (vestibulo-acoustic) nerve is by far the commonest site. Schwannomas occurring on both acoustic nerves usually indicate that the patient is suffering from an inherited condition similar to, but distinct from, *von Recklinghausen's disease*. In von Recklinghausen's disease itself, multiple nerve sheath tumours occur in the dermis, attached to deep nerves and on cranial and spinal nerve roots. Both *bilateral acoustic neurofibromatosis* and von Recklinghausen's disease are transmitted by dominant inheritance, whereas solitary nerve sheath tumours are more often sporadic. These tumours are slow growing, encapsulated, firm, discrete masses of variable size (Fig. 11.14). Large acoustic schwannomas may distort and indent the brain stem (Fig. 13.1). Smaller ones occupy the angle between the pons, medulla and cerebellum. The cut surface of the tumour shows a yellow or white, whorled, sometimes partially cystic appearance. There may be evidence of old haemorrhages in the form of foci of rusty discoloration.

Microscopically, schwannomas display intermingled areas containing bundles of compact, interweaving, elongated spindle cells, alternating with areas of looser texture. The former are known as Antoni A and the latter as Antoni B tissues. Overall these tumours show a sparse to moderate degree of cellularity. Antoni A areas show some degree of alignment of nuclei in parallel rows or clusters, referred to as palisading (Fig. 13.2), while in Antoni B areas the cells are haphazardly arranged, have ill-defined boundaries and are set in a microcystic matrix (Fig. 13.3). Mitotic figures are not usually found, though nuclei may show considerable variation in size, shape and staining properties. Blood vessels in schwannomas are notable for the frequent presence of degenerative change with hyaline thickening and fibrin deposition. Haemosiderin deposition is also fairly common in schwannomas. Nerve fibres are not seen coursing through the tumour, but may be seen as a group of compressed fascicles at one margin of the tumour.

(a)

(b)

Fig. 13.1 (a) Schwannoma of the left acoustic nerve, compressing, but not invading, the left cerebellar hemisphere and brain stem. Areas of old and fresh haemorrhage are visible on the cut surface of the tumour. (b) A series of consecutive axial T2W MR images (A–D) through the posterior fossa demonstrate a large extra-axial inhomogeneous solid mass lesion in the left cerebellopontine angle. The mass extends into a widened left IAM. There is distortion of the brain stem and fourth ventricle (D: bottom right: arrow). The appearance is typical of a large schwannoma. The right IAM is normal and the 7th and 8th cranial nerves are well visualized within it (C: bottom left: arrow).

Fig. 13.2 Area of a schwannoma in which the nuclei of the elongated, bipolar tumour cells are aligned in rows ('palisading'). H&E, ×110.

Schwannomas at the cerebellopontine angle may need to be differentiated from meningiomas, which can also occur at this site. Points of distinction in their histology are: the alternating types of tissue (Antoni A and B); palisading of nuclei and degenerative changes in the blood vessel walls in schwannomas; and the presence of psammoma bodies in some meningiomas, which at this site are often of the fibroblastic type (p.234).

Neurofibromas

These rarely occur as single tumours, but are common and

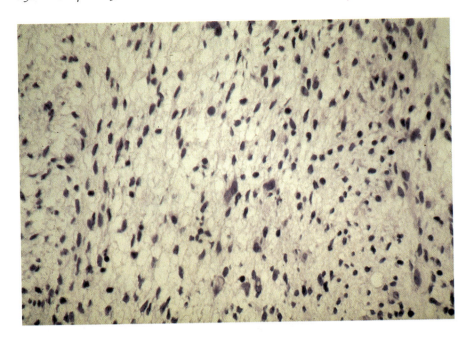

Fig. 13.3 Area of a schwannoma showing the more open, microcystic appearance of Antoni B tissue. This field also shows some nuclear pleomorphism—a feature that does not have sinister implications in these tumours. H&E, ×180.

(a)

(b)

Fig. 13.4 (a) Neurofibromas attached to individual roots of the cauda equina from a case of von Recklinghausen's disease. (b) Small nodules of metastatic carcinoma in the same location. In this case each tumour frequently involves more than one nerve root.

sometimes very numerous in subjects with von Recklinghausen's disease. Most tumours that develop as part of this disease do so in the peripheral nervous system, though paradoxically those subjects who develop the more serious proximal nerve root or CNS tumours often have

little in the way of peripheral disease. Tumours are liable to develop on the cranial and spinal nerve roots (Fig. 13.4). The tumours are schwannomas, neurofibromas or a mixture of the two. Some undergo malignant change. Patients with von Recklinghausen's disease also suffer from an increased incidence of gliomas (especially those involving the optic system), meningiomas, and phaeochromocytomas of the adrenal gland. Neurofibromas usually form an ill-defined expansion of the nerve in which they occur (Fig. 13.5). Microscopically they are sparsely cellular and composed of spindle-shaped cells with narrow, elongated, darkly staining nuclei (Fig. 13.6). Mitotic figures are not usually present. There is an abundance of collagen and reticulin in a structureless matrix which is rich in mucopolysaccharides. Matrix fibres and spindle cells pursue a characteristically wavy course

Fig. 13.5 Macroscopic appearance of a plexiform neurofibroma causing diffuse, irregular expansion of a peripheral nerve and its branches in a patient with von Recklinghausen's disease.

through this matrix. Nerve fibres can be found scattered singly or in small groups throughout the tumour (Fig. 13.7). Over-wrapping of nerve bundles with Schwann cells and fibroblasts may be found in some subjects with von Recklinghausen's disease, even in apparently normal lengths of nerve.

Malignant schwannomas and neurofibromas

Malignant nerve sheath tumours are uncommon, and occur chiefly on the spinal roots, where they often form dumb-bell-shaped tumours expanding inward and outward from an intervertebral foramen. Others occur on deeply situated peripheral nerves. At least half of them occur in subjects with von Recklinghausen's disease. The cell of origin in most cases is thought to be the Schwann cell. The tumours are circumscribed, but may be large—as much as 6 cm across—when first discovered. They are demonstrably related to a peripheral nerve or nerve root. The microscopic appearance is highly cellular, the tumour being composed of interlacing bundles of spindle cells with sausage-shaped nuclei showing pleomorphism and mitotic figures (Fig. 13.8). Foci of necrosis are usually present. Reticulin is widely distributed throughout the tumour. The tumours that occur peripherally can be difficult to distinguish microscopically from other malignant spindle cell tumours of soft tissue. Immunostaining can be helpful, particularly with antibody Leu 7, which can be applied to paraffin sections, and gives a positive reaction with most malignant as well as benign nerve sheath tumours. However, it should be noted that this antibody gives positive reactions with many other CNS tumours. Antibodies to S-100 protein react positively with benign nerve sheath tumours but only rarely do so with their malignant counterparts. They also react with certain other tumours, so again the reaction cannot be regarded as specific for nerve sheath tumours (see Table 4.2).

Meningiomas

Meningiomas arise in the meningeal coverings of the brain and spinal cord. The main cells of origin are thought to be the arachnoid cap cells (p.63; Fig 3.29), particularly those that contribute to the formation of arachnoid villi in the dura. The tumours present chiefly in middle and late adult life. Small ones, often calcified and resembling small stones, are commonly found incidentally at post mortem, usually over the convexities of the cerebral hemispheres. Occasionally meningiomas show evidence of hormone dependency, growing rapidly during pregnancy. Most meningiomas have an attachment to the dura, particularly adjoining the sagittal sinus at the convexity, the sphenoidal ridges, olfactory grooves or tuberculum sellae. Other attachments and locations are well recognized, intracranially

Fig. 13.6 Microscopic appearance of a neurofibroma. The tumour cells are relatively sparse and separated by a pale intercellular matrix. The connective tissue has a wavy profile. H&E, ×250.

Fig. 13.7 Palmgren silver stain on a section of a spinal neurofibroma from a patient with von Recklinghausen's disease. Nerve fibres (arrowed) are scattered within the tumour. ×200.

Fig. 13.8 Malignant nerve sheath tumour. There is a high cell density, and nuclei are pleomorphic. Mitotic figures are present (arrowed). The matrix retains the wavy longitudinal pattern seen in more benign tumours. H&E, ×340.

(a)

(b)

Fig. 13.9 (a) Small meningioma indenting the surface of the right cerebellar hemisphere. Note the clear plane of cleavage between the encapsulated tumour and the brain. (b) Another small meningioma shelled out from the thoracic intrathecal compartment. Spinal meninginomas are almost invariably benign.

Fig. 13.10 Right frontal meningioma displaying an invasive pattern of growth in which there is no clear plane of demarcation between the tumour and brain, or well-defined pia-derived capsule (compare with Fig. 11.2). There is cingulate subfalcine herniation from right to left.

in the leptomeninges or in a lateral ventricle attached to choroid plexus. They also occur in the petrous bone, and rarely extracranially, from presumed ectopic arachnoid cap cells, at sites around the head and neck. The spinal meninges, particularly over thoracic segments of the cord, give origin to spinal meningiomas which occupy the intradural compartment.

Macroscopically, meningiomas appear encapsulated, firm, smooth or slightly lobulated (Fig. 13.9). The majority can be readily shelled out from the tumour bed. Benign meningiomas indent, but do not invade, the underlying brain or spinal cord (Fig. 11.2). However, some meningiomas, particularly those arising around the base of the brain, have a tendency to wrap themselves around neighbouring structures, such as major cerebral arteries or cranial nerves (Fig. 3.32). Meningiomas that display this creeping pattern of growth to a marked extent are sometimes referred to as meningioma 'en plaque'. The adjacent

bone, particularly over the convexities, is occasionally obviously thickened, and nearby venous sinuses may commonly be invaded by tumour, even a benign one. On the cut surface meningiomas usually have a whorled or streaky appearance and feel firm and granular. Frequently they are gritty. They are grey or pink in colour. Those that have undergone xanthomatous degeneration contain yellow areas.

Microscopically there is considerable variation in the appearances of meningiomas. Six basic patterns are recognized among benign forms: syncytial, fibroblastic, transitional, psammomatous, haemangioblastic and angiomatous. Histology of more than one type may be displayed in a single tumour, and the features defining the separate types overlap to some extent, so that the classification is somewhat imprecise. Although most meningiomas displaying features of these subtypes behave as benign tumours, some are more aggressive. Invasion of neigh-

Fig. 13.15 Low-power view of a fibroblastic meningioma to show the swirling, interlacing bundles of strap-like tumour cells. Trichrome, ×100.

Fig. 13.16 Calcified psammoma body at the centre of a whorl in a meningioma. H&E, ×450.

Fig. 13.17 Whorl formations in a transitional meningioma. H&E, ×280.

groups of vacuolated cells lying in pockets of reticulin which separate them from the thin-walled, abundant capillaries. This is sometimes referred to as the haemangioblastic type of meningioma.

Benign forms of meningioma may undergo various forms of secondary degeneration which considerably alter the overall histological appearance of the tumour.

Common forms of degeneration are hyaline, collagenous degeneration and xanthomatous change, in which sudanophilic lipid accumulates focally in groups of cells, giving them a vacuolated appearance in paraffin sections (Fig. 13.18). Less common are myxomatous change and cystic degeneration. Some meningiomas contain hyaline bodies which take the PAS stain.

The final three variants of meningiomas are the least typical in appearance and the most aggressive in their behaviour: the haemangiopericytic, papillary and anaplastic types. They are likely to recur, and occasionally metastasize. *Haemangiopericytic meningiomas*, formerly commonly regarded as variants of angioblastic meningiomas, closely resemble haemangiopericytomas arising in other parts of the body. The tumour cells bear an intimate relation to the lining cells of the sinusoidal blood spaces. The cells are polygonal or angular, rather than spindle shaped (Fig. 13.19). Mitotic figures are invariably present. An intricate reticulin network extends around each of the tumour cells as well as around the closely related blood spaces (Fig. 13.20). Whorls and psammoma bodies are not present.

Papillary meningiomas are rare, malignant tumours. Parts of the tumour may resemble syncytial or transitional forms, but other areas show a distinctly papillary pattern of growth with a striking degree of nuclear pleomorphism and a much less well-differentiated cellular appearance (Fig. 13.21). Most of the cells are large and well defined, with plentiful, eosinophilic cytoplasm and vesicular or hyperchromatic nuclei. Mitoses are frequent. Distinction from metastatic carcinoma may prove difficult in biopsies

Fig. 13.18 Foci of xanthomatous degeneration in a meningioma. The cytoplasm of cells in these areas is paler than that of others. H&E, ×100.

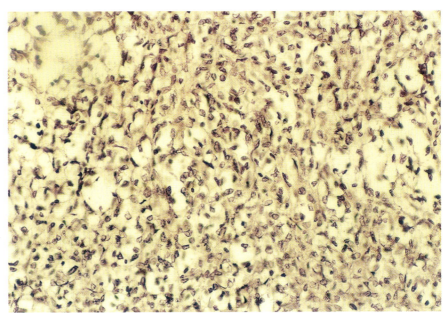

Fig. 13.19 Haemangiopericytic meningioma. Polygonal and spindle cells showing little resemblance to other forms of meningioma. H&E, ×200.

Fig. 13.20 Reticulin pattern of a haemangiopericytic meningioma. There is an intricate network of reticulin around individual tumour cells. ×100.

Fig. 13.21 Meningioma with a papillary growth pattern, rounded cell outlines and nuclear pleomorphism—all features that make differentiation of this tumour from carcinoma difficult. H&E, ×250.

if areas of better-differentiated meningioma are not present.

Anaplastic meningiomas are meningeal tumours in which the histological pattern shows no more than a faint resemblance to one of the better-differentiated forms. There are frequently features suggestive of malignancy, such as invasion of the brain by fingers of tumour (Figs 13.10–13.12), necrosis, and poor cytological differentiation. The tumour cells are spindle shaped, with some tendency to whorl formation (Fig. 13.22). There is a variable collagen and reticulin content. Mitotic figures are numerous. Nuclei are pleomorphic and frequently bizarre, but it should be noted that this feature on its own is not necessarily indicative of malignancy in a meningioma. Anaplastic features can occur focally in a large meningioma. Since their presence influences the prognosis they should be carefully sought by wide sampling of different areas in a large tumour.

With regard to their immunohistological characteristics, meningiomas show variable patterns of reactivity. Most give a positive reaction for vimentin, S-100 protein and epithelial membrane antigen, while some, particularly those that contain PAS-positive hyaline bodies, show focal expression of cytokeratin (Fig. 4.25). These tumours therefore show reactions that are characteristic of both epithelial and mesenchymal tumours.

Meningeal sarcomas

Spindle-celled meningeal tumours with malignant features in which no resemblance to benign meningiomas is apparent in any part of the tumour are regarded as primary meningeal sarcomas, and have a histological pattern closely resembling that of fibrosarcoma.

Fig. 13.22 Malignant meningioma composed of disorderly spindle cells with foci of necrosis (arrowed). H&E, ×200.

Fig. 13.23 Spindle-celled, heavily pigmented melanoma, found at post mortem to have arisen in the leptomeninges. H&E, ×175.

Meningeal melanomas

These are rare tumours with an attachment to the pia mater, though they may burrow deeply into the brain or spinal cord. They usually remain confined to the CNS. They arise more commonly from the leptomeninges overlying the spinal cord than from the brain. Histologically, they resemble the commoner melanomas that are metastatic to the CNS (Fig. 13.23). They are not the only melanin-containing tumours arising in the CNS. Occasional meningiomas, schwannomas, ependymomas, medulloblastomas and choroid plexus papillomas contain melanin.

Haemangioblastomas

These tumours occur usually in the cerebellum, less commonly in the spinal cord, and very rarely elsewhere. In some subjects there is associated angiomatosis of the retina, (von Hippel's disease), non-neoplastic renal or pancreatic cysts, or renal tumours. This constellation of abnormalities is known as Lindau's syndrome. It may be familial, as may be isolated haemangioblastomas. An interesting feature of these tumours is the occurrence in some cases of polycythaemia, which disappears after removal of the tumour. Tumours with an identical appearance to the cerebellar haemangioblastoma also rarely occur around the spinal cord, outside the spinal dura and in the supratentorial meninges, where they are classed as haemangioblastic meningiomas. The classical cerebellar tumours form discrete but unencapsulated masses, frequently cystic, with the tumour appearing as a firm, dark-red nodule in or near the edge of the cyst. The cyst fluid may be rusty-coloured from previous haemorrhage. The tumour has a rich vascular supply, with prominent draining veins.

Microscopically the tumour appears to be composed of two elements, one being endothelial cells forming well-defined capillary channels, and the other intervening stromal cells with pale, foamy, fat-laden cytoplasm (Fig. 13.24). Stromal and capillary elements are irregularly intermixed in varying proportions (Fig. 13.25). The two types of cell appear quite uniform, though there may be nuclear pleomorphism in the stromal cells. Mitotic figures are rarely seen. Abundant reticulin surrounds the capillaries, and may also be seen between the stromal cells. The tumours are slow growing, but recur if incompletely removed, and very occasionally metastasize in the CNS. Multiple cerebellar tumours may occur successively. The origin of the stromal cells in haemangioblastomas is not clear. Some tumours have been shown ultrastructurally to contain neurosecretory granules, suggesting an origin from a neurosecretory cell. In immunohistological reactions most tumours give a focally positive reaction with GFAP antibodies.

Fig. 13.24 Pale, lipid-laden stromal cells of a haemangioblastoma interspersed between capillary endothelial cells. Nuclei are small and regular, without mitoses. H&E, ×300.

Craniopharyngiomas (suprasellar cysts, Rathke's pouch tumours, adamantinomas)

These are cystic, or cystic and solid, lesions occurring in the suprasellar or parasellar region, with a presumed origin from epithelial remnants of the embryonic Rathke's pouch. They present usually in childhood, or early adult life, with symptoms related to compression of the pituitary stalk or gland, or by obstructing the third ventricle, and causing hydrocephalus (Fig. 13.26). The cyst grows slowly, but never undergoes malignant transformation, and does not metastasize. The cyst fluid is usually brown or yellow and contains glistening cholesterol crystals. It has an irritant effect, producing a chemical meningitis if it reaches the subarachnoid space. The wall of the cyst is composed of epithelial cells, and tends to adhere to surrounding struc-

Fig. 13.25 Low-power view of a section of haemangioblastoma showing the abundant capillary spaces that comprise one element of this tumour. H&E, ×70.

tures. When in contact with the brain the lesion excites a dense glial reaction. Microscopically the cyst wall contains stratified epithelium, in some areas flattened and in others focally thickened to form irregular cords or islands (Fig. 13.27). Mitotic figures are not seen. The basal cuboidal layer rests on basement membrane, and elicits a fibrotic and glial reaction where it abuts on the leptomeninges and brain. In the collagenous and glial layers there are frequently cholesterol clefts, calcification, flakes of keratin, multinucleate foreign-body giant cells and other inflammatory cells (Fig. 13.28). Biopsy specimens may contain no epithelial tissue, but the diagnosis can usually be made by exclusion, after discussion of the possibilities with the surgeon.

Dermoid and epidermoid cysts (pearly tumour, 'cholesteatomas')

These are simple cysts, thought to be derived from heterotopic inclusions of epidermal cells. Dermoid cysts are found most frequently in the posterior fossa, particularly in the vermis, or, intraspinally, at the lumbosacral level. Epidermoid cysts occur mainly in the middle and posterior cranial fossae, and occasionally in the cerebral hemispheres and spinal cord. A dermal sinus may be identifiable, connecting a dermoid cyst with an overlying dimple in the skin, and both types of cyst may be associated with local congenital skeletal defects. Macroscopically the cysts are of variable size and are smooth or slightly nodular

Fig. 13.26 Craniopharyngioma occupying and expanding the third ventricle, and causing compression of the right lateral ventricle and obstructive dilatation of the left lateral ventricle. There are cystic and solid, partly calcified, regions in this tumour. Damage to the right temporal lobe was due to previous surgery.

Fig. 13.27 Epithelial cyst wall of a craniopharyngioma. H&E, ×100.

Fig. 13.28 Section of part of the wall of a craniopharyngioma containing numerous cholesterol clefts. H&E, ×100.

and encapsulated. The capsule may be partly calcified. The contents of a dermoid cyst appear thick and yellowish, with some hairs included, while those of an epidermoid cyst are white, waxy or flaky (Fig. 13.29). These cysts give a hyperintense signal on MRI (Fig. 13.30). Microscopically the wall of a dermoid cyst is composed mainly of simple squamous epithelium with variable additional skin ap-

pendages such as hair follicles, sebaceous glands and sweat glands. Epidermoid cysts lack the skin appendages but are otherwise similar. Foreign-body giant cells are commonly found in relation to keratin inclusions in connective tissue deep to the epithelium.

Pituitary adenomas

Most of the tumours removed from the pituitary fossa are adenomas. Many adenomas are received as surgical specimens, and some are found incidentally or unexpectedly at post mortem. With regard to the management of surgical specimens, EM can be helpful in classifying these tumours, and we recommend that small blocks of tissue be fixed and embedded for EM. Ultrathin sections may not need to be examined from the most straightforward cases, but the material is then available, if required. The remainder can be fixed for routine light microscopy. H&E and Orange G/PAS, or a similar stain for distinguishing between eosinophil, basophil and chromophobe cells, are used routinely, and the reticulin stain is useful if there is doubt about whether a sample consists of tumour or pituitary gland. The anterior part of the gland has a distinctive reticulin network which is absent from adenomas (Figs 13.31 and 13.32). A Congo Red stain may show the presence of small amounts of amyloid in some adenomas. Haemosiderin is frequently seen in pituitary adenomas, and occasionally frank haemorrhage and necrosis are found, particularly in tumours from patients with 'pituitary apoplexy'. Simple epithelial-lined cysts may also be encountered in some tumours or occasionally as space-occupying lesions in their own right (Rathke's pouch cyst).

Fig. 13.29 Epidermal cyst in the left frontal lobe of a 24-year-old male. The contents of the cyst are white, flaky and friable. This tumour caused epilepsy, but a decision was made not to operate as the epilepsy was well controlled. The patient died unexpectedly in the bath and was thought to have drowned after suffering a fit.

Fig. 13.30 T2W axial MR image demonstrates the typical appearance of an epidermoid at the left cerebellopontine angle in a young patient with trigeminal neuralgia. It is distorting the pons and displacing the basilar artery (arrow) posteriorly and to the right. The left trigeminal nerve is compressed by the lesion. Note the normal right trigeminal nerve (arrowhead) as it courses from the brain stem towards Meckels cave and the Gasserian ganglion. Epidermoids contain cholestrol and cellular debris and so are typically hyperintense to CSF on MRI.

Fig. 13.31 Reticulin pattern of the anterior pituitary gland, showing epithelial cells in clusters, enclosed by strands shown here by laminin immunocytochemistry. Counterstained with haematoxylin, ×100.

Very small cysts occur as an incidental finding in 'normal' pituitary glands.

Immunohistology using antisera to pituitary hormones is certainly helpful in diagnosis, and can be carried out on paraffin sections. Antisera to the major pituitary hormones are commercially available, those to growth hormone (GH), adenocorticotrophic hormone (ACTH), prolactin (PRL), and the β subunits of thyroid stimulating hormone (TSH), luteinizing hormone (LH) and follicle stimulating hormone (FSH) being probably the most used. As the antisera are expensive and can be used most economically by treating batches of 10–12 tumours at once, our practice is to issue a report on the nature of the tumour based on the light-microscopical appearances in stained sections, and to follow this up with a supplementary report describing the immunohistological findings and EM. In the initial report the traditional classification of adenomas into eosinophil, basophil or chromophobe is used. Although simplistic and largely superseded by classifications based on the hormone content of the tumours, use of this classification does at least assure the surgeon in the initial report that the tumour is indeed a pituitary adenoma and not some other type of tumour. In the supplementary report the tumour is classified according to its hormone content. The main categories of pituitary adenoma are summarized below. A more detailed classification is recommended by some authorities, details of which may be found in the several recent monographs and reviews listed at the end of the chapter.

Fig. 13.32 Reticulin pattern of a pituitary, prolactin-secreting chromophobe adenoma. The amount of reticulin is much reduced compared to that of the anterior pituitary gland. ×100.

Fig. 13.33 Predominantly eosinophil cells in a growth-hormone-secreting pituitary adenoma. Orange G/PAS, ×150.

Growth-hormone-containing adenomas

Acromegaly or gigantism is evident clinically in patients with these tumours. Routine stains on paraffin sections show an eosinophil or mixed chromophobe and eosinophil tumour composed of medium-sized, polygonal epithelial cells usually arranged diffusely (Fig. 13.33). Immunohistology shows some reaction for GH in most or all of the tumour cells, the intensity of the reaction varying from cell to cell (Fig. 13.34). Some PRL-containing cells may be interspersed among those containing GH, but reactions for other hormones are usually negative. EM shows cells with medium- or large-sized granules in the cytoplasm (Fig. 13.35). Another ultrastructural feature present in the cells of some GH tumours is the 'fibrous body'. This occupies perinuclear cytoplasm and is composed of intermingled tubules and filaments (Fig. 13.36).

Occasionally a GH tumour and a ganglioneuroma occur together in the pituitary fossa.

Prolactin-containing adenomas

Symptoms of hyperprolactinaemia are likely to have been detected in premenopausal women with these tumours. Men and elderly women have less overt hormone-related symptoms, and present usually with a space-occupying lesion. The tumours appear chromophobe or weakly

Fig. 13.34 Reaction for growth hormone in a pituitary adenoma associated with acromegaly. A varying intensity of reaction is found in different tumour cells. Immunoperoxidase, counterstained with haematoxylin, ×200.

Fig. 13.35 Heavily-granulated cells of a growth-hormone-secreting pituitary adenoma. Uranyl acetate and lead citrate, ×6630.

Fig. 13.36 Electron micrograph showing perinuclear cytoplasm from a growth-hormone-secreting pituitary adenoma. A fibrous body, consisting of intermingled filaments (11 nm diameter) and microtubules, is present (arrowed) . Uranyl acetate and lead citrate, ×15 440.

Fig. 13.37 Prolactin-secreting chromophobe pituitary adenoma. The section has been treated with a prolacting antiserum, and demonstrates reaction product in all the tumour cells (brown). Immunoperoxidase with haematoxylin counterstain, ×100.

eosinophil with routine stains. The cells are small- or medium-sized, oval or polygonal in shape, and usually arranged diffusely or with a perivascular orientation (Fig. 13.37). Some contain small, scattered calcospherites. PRL-containing tumours which are removed after a prolonged period of bromocriptine treatment are likely to show a reduction in size of the tumour cells and a considerable increase in the collagen and reticulin present between the tumour cells (Fig. 13.38). Immunohistology shows a uniform pattern of PRL-reactivity, often accentuated in the perinuclear cytoplasm, throughout the tumour (Fig. 13.37). There is less positive reaction in tumours that have been

Fig. 13.38 Marked increase in collagen and reticulin content of a prolactin-secreting pituitary adenoma from a patient treated preoperatively with bromocriptine for 36 weeks (compare with Fig. 13.32). ×200.

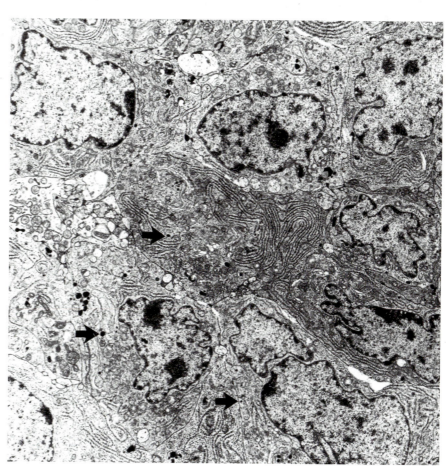

Fig. 13.39 Low-power electron micrograph of a prolactin-secreting pituitary adenoma. Tumour cells contain abundant rough endoplasmic reticulum and sparse, medium-sized secretory granules in the cytoplasm (arrowed). Uranyl acetate and lead citrate, ×4500.

treated with bromocriptine. Occasionally a few GH-containing cells are present. Ultra-structurally the tumour cells contain abundant amounts of rough endoplasmic reticulum and sparse medium-sized secretory granules scattered throughout the cytoplasm (Fig. 13.39). Occasional granules are seen lying between the cell membranes of adjacent cells, a feature referred to as misplaced exocytosis (Fig. 13.40).

Fig. 13.40 Higher power electron micrograph of a prolactin-secreting pituitary adenoma showing a secretory granule (arrowed) situated between the adjacent cytoplasmic boundaries of two tumour cells ('misplaced exocytosis'). Uranyl acetate and lead citrate, ×37 600.

ACTH-containing adenomas

In most cases of Cushing's disease occurring as a consequence of pituitary malfunction, an adenoma can be identified in surgical specimens. The tumour cells are medium- or large-sized, slightly elongated or polygonal and arranged diffusely or in a pseudopapillary pattern (Fig. 13.41). Crooke's hyaline change may be seen in the tumour cells and in basophils of adjacent gland fragments (Fig. 13.42). The tumour cells are basophil or chromophobe. Immunohistology shows uniformly-positive reactions for ACTH in all the tumour cells. Reactions for other pituitary hormones are usually negative. EM shows tumour cells containing medium or large secretory granules scattered throughout the cell cytoplasm or aligned near the cell margins (Fig. 13.43). Fine 7 nm diameter filaments lying in bundles may be seen in perinuclear cytoplasm (Fig. 13.44).

The appearances of tumours removed from cases of Nelson's syndrome show the same features as those described above. In some cases of Cushing's disease, despite evidence of over-production of ACTH by the pituitary gland, there is no identifiable tumour in the surgical specimen. Many ACTH-containing basophils may be found lying adjacent to fragments of neurohypophysis. This is considered by some authorities to represent hyperplasia of ACTH-producing cells. However, the diagnosis of basophil hyperplasia in small surgical fragments of pituitary gland is difficult when it is remembered that normal glands frequently contain sizeable clusters of ACTH-containing basophils in this region.

Non-functioning adenomas

Space-occupying pituitary tumours which produce no clinical evidence of hormone secretion have a variable histological appearance, with cells arranged around sinusoids, or diffusely (Fig. 13.45). Routine staining shows the cells to be chromophobe or eosinophil. Immunohistological reactions may be entirely negative, but in quite a number of the tumours there are found to be scattered groups of cells which react for βFSH, βLH or both. Such tumours and a few others which are negative with these antisera give a positive reaction for the α subunit of the glycoprotein hormones (Fig. 13.46). Some other non-functioning tumours contain small numbers of cells reactive for several different hormones. Ultrastructurally these tumours contain small secretory granules which may be aligned close to the cell membranes or scattered more diffusely in the cytoplasm (Fig. 13.47). Some also contain many mitochondria (oncocytic change; Fig. 13.48) or multivesicular bodies.

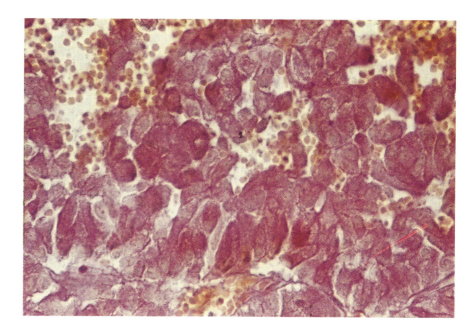

Fig. 13.41 Basophil tumour cells in an ACTH-secreting pituitary adenoma. Orange G/PAS, ×500.

Fig. 13.42 A basophil cell showing Crooke's hyaline change in the anterior pituitary gland from a subject with Cushing's disease. Granules are displaced to the margin of the cell where they give a positive reaction for ACTH (arrowed), and the perinuclear cytoplasm is pale. Counterstained with haematoxylin, ×400.

Other pituitary adenomas

Rare examples occur of TSH-containing and other pituitary adenomas, details of which can be found in Robert & Martinez (1986).

Malignant or invasive pituitary adenomas

A few pituitary tumours, among both hormonally active and inactive ones, show an invasive local growth pattern and even metastasize. Such tumours are generally not distinguishable histologically from their benign counterparts.

Cytological features of nuclear pleomorphism and high mitotic activity are seen in a minority of pituitary adenomas, and are certainly worth noting in reports, but have not been clearly shown to relate to clinical behaviour of the tumours.

Post mortem examination on cases of pituitary tumour

At post mortem it is not uncommon to find incidental adenomas of the pituitary gland. Most of these are no more than a few millimetres across, but a few are larger and

Fig. 13.50 Pituitary tumour arising in the posterior part of the gland and composed of bipolar cells orientated around blood vessels, showing histological appearances closely resembling those of pituicytes (modified astrocytes). H&E, ×100.

Fig. 13.51 Granular cell myoblastoma of the posterior pituitary. The tumour cells have pale, granular cytoplasm and regular, dark-staining nuclei. Cell margins are outlined in this immunocytochemical preparation for laminin. Counterstained with haematoxylin, ×220.

Fig. 13.52 Germinoma, showing intermingled large tumour cells and small stromal lymphocytes. H&E, ×220.

Mitotic figures are plentiful in the large, polygonal cells. These tumours are malignant and have a capacity to metastasize in the subarachnoid space.

Tumours extending locally to involve the CNS

There are many tumours which arise in and around the skull and vertebral column and involve the CNS by direct extension. Some of those arising in the eye are, indeed, derived from the CNS itself. Apart from pituitary adenomas, which have already been described, most of these tumours will be familiar to the general pathologist and the following will not be described here.

1 Carcinomas arising in the paranasal sinuses, the ear, upper nasopharynx, skin of the face and parotid gland.
2 Orbital tumours.
3 Skull and vertebral column tumours: osteogenic sarcomas (especially arising in association with Paget's disease), osteomas, osteochondromas, chondromas, chondrosarcomas, chordomas, fibromyxosarcomas, fibrosarcomas and malignant giant cell tumours of bone, and myelomas.
4 Tumours invading the spinal extradural space from the retroperitoneum, especially lymphomas and soft-tissue sarcomas.
5 Glomus jugulare tumours, which can arise from chemoreceptor cells in the jugular bulb and invade the posterior fossa or compress the lower cranial nerves.
6 Olfactory neuroblastomas.
One practical point is that the neuropathologist may be required to become familiar with the appearances of these tumours in smear preparations or frozen sections, since they may be biopsied by the neurosurgeon under circumstances that demand rapid diagnosis. Illustrations of some of these tumours as they appear in smears can be found in Chapter 4.

Metastatic tumours

Malignant tumours metastatic to the CNS are fairly common. They are blood-borne and frequently multiple. Their size varies from microscopic to 6 cm or more across. Carcinomas are the commonest tumours to metastasize to the CNS. They usually produce spherical masses in the brain, and much less commonly in the spinal cord. Nerve roots may also be affected (Fig. 13.4b). They may occupy or project into a ventricle and cause hydrocephalus (Fig. 13.53). Uncommonly adenocarcinomas spread as a thin layer, barely discernible by the naked eye, in the subarachnoid space (Fig. 13.54). The solid tumours appear relatively well circumscribed, firm and white or yellowish (Fig. 11.4). Areas of necrosis are usually obvious to inspection and there may also be haemorrhages. In some cases there is severe surrounding oedema (Figs 11.3 and 11.4a). Primary tumours particularly liable to metastasize to the CNS include oat cell and other lung carcinomas (by far the commonest source), breast, stomach, colon, kidney, thyroid, chorio- and testicular carcinomas, and melanomas. Metastatic lymphoma may produce a mass lesion in the CNS or diffuse infiltration in the subarachnoid space and around nerve roots. One rare form of lymphoma occupies small cerebral blood vessels and causes ischaemic lesions in the brain. This was formerly known as malignant angio-endotheliomatosis (p.227). Metastatic lymphoma or carcinoma also commonly invades the spinal extradural

Fig. 13.53 Multiple carcinoma deposits in the cerebellum, fourth ventricle and pons from a primary gastric carcinoma. The tumours appear deceptively well demarcated from surrounding brain, but they are not encapsulated, and are very difficult to remove entire.

These variants of MS are not always totally distinct pathologically from the more classical lesions and do not therefore warrant consideration as distinct diseases, as they have sometimes been considered in the past.

In severe, long-standing MS with extensive cerebral lesions there is usually a degree of cerebral atrophy, with compensatory enlargement of the lateral ventricles. In cases with severe involvement of the optic nerves the optic tracts show shrinkage and discoloration (Fig. 14.12). A severely affected spinal cord appears shrunken and grey. Extensive lesions in which there has been severe oedema may show a post-oedematous cystic state (Fig. 11.9). At the other end of the spectrum of severity that MS displays are cases in which a few small, chronic plaques are found incidentally at post mortem examination in a patient who had no history of neurological disease. Such incidental plaques are most likely to be found at the lateral angles of the lateral ventricles (Fig. 14.13). Very occasionally gliomas have been found in brains of subjects with MS and some appear to have arisen in a plaque.

In any individual case of MS, correlation of the siting of plaques with clinical symptomatology is often possible, for example when the lesions are situated in the optic nerves, brain stem or spinal cord. Cerebral plaques tend to be harder to correlate with clinical features, but are often extensive in patients with prominent mental changes. In every case note should be taken of the particular clinical features that were present and an attempt made to discover lesions that account for them.

Microscopy of MS: dating of lesions

Many patients with MS eventually die several decades after the onset of their disease. There is often little evidence of disease progression clinically in the latter years, and death may be due to a disease quite unrelated to MS, or to complications resulting from a static neurological deficit, as for example when a patient dies from renal failure secondary to repeated urinary tract infections precipitated by loss of bladder control, or from pneumonia consequent on immobility. The MS lesions in such patients are mainly of a type regarded as inactive, or showing no evidence of recent demyelination. Microscopically these lesions appear less cellular than the surrounding tissue (Fig. 14.14), and in general the chronicity of the lesions is inversely related to cellularity. There is abrupt loss of myelin as one moves into the plaque (Fig. 14.15), and oligodendrocyte nuclei are reduced in numbers or abolished in the plaque (Fig. 14.14). Axons are for the most part preserved, and there is a dense felt-work of glial fibres forming scar tissue. This is clearly seen with a Holzer stain (Figs 3.20, 14.16 and 14.17). Inflammation is sparse, and macrophages few or absent in the lesion. Neutral fat cannot be demonstrated in more than an occasional cell (Fig. 14.18). Partially myelinated axons, lying in groups, are frequently found inside or just beyond the margins of chronic plaques, and as these regions stain palely with myelin stains they are termed areas of 'shadow' plaque (Fig. 3.20). Many of these areas probably represent areas of remyelination, though in other

Fig. 14.13 Incidental finding of small, chronic demyelinated plaques in a patient dying of carcinoma of the colon. These are situated at the margin of the inferior horn of the right lateral ventricle, and in the right thalamus (arrowed).

(a)

(b)

Fig. 14.14 Comparison of nuclei in a chronic MS plaque (a), and normal white matter (b). In the plaque nuclei are fewer in number, less regularly distributed, and most clearly belong to astrocytes. In normal white matter most of the nuclei are smaller, more uniform and rounded, with appearances of oligodendrocyte nuclei. This population of cells is severely depleted in chronic MS plaques. H&E, ×250.

Fig. 14.15 Low-power view of myelin stained section of a lateral column chronic MS plaque in the spinal cord. The border of the plaque is sharply defined. LBCV, ×18.

contexts, for example in acute plaques, areas of myelin pallor may in contrast be due to incomplete demyelination, or to oedema (Fig. 14.19). Extensive chronic plaques are often associated with some wallerian degeneration due to loss of chronically demyelinated axons. The site at which such secondary degeneration can be demonstrated will vary according to the site of the plaques. For example, chronic plaques in the cervical spinal cord may be associated with wallerian degeneration in the lateral corticospinal tracts at lower levels of the cord.

Intermingled with the inactive plaques described above there may be other plaques whose centres appear inactive, but whose edges are hypercellular (Fig. 14.20). These

Fig. 14.16 Adjacent section to that shown in Fig. 14.10, stained by the Holzer technique to show glial fibres. The whole demyelinated area is densely gliotic.

Fig. 14.18 Inactive, gliotic periventricular plaque stained to show neutral fat (red). Only small amounts are present in scattered macrophages.

Fig. 14.17 Adjacent sections of midbrain containing inactive paques. (*Above*) Myelin stain. (*Below*) Holzer stain showing gliosis within the plaques.

Fig. 14.19 Low-power view of myelin-stained section from a case of acute MS. Margins of the irregular, demyelinated zone appear blurred on account of oedema. Note also some residual myelin remaining adjacent to, and within the corpus callosum.

Fig. 14.20 Margin of MS plaque (right), showing increased numbers of microglial cells at and beyond the margin (left). The plaque itself contains plump-bodied macrophages (right). Ricin communis agglutinin-1 lectin. Counterstained with Mayer's haemalum, ×200. (Slide prepared by Dr CS Morris.)

Fig. 14.21 A small, acute plaque showing intense cellularity. H&E, ×150.

are thought to be plaques at the margins of which demyelination is intermittently continuing. The increased cells at the margins consist of macrophages, a few lymphocytes, astrocytes and possibly increased numbers of oligodendrocytes. Some of the macrophages may contain neutral fat, representing breakdown products of degenerate myelin (Fig. 3.37). Areas of shadow plaque may also be present in the vicinity. These marginal zones probably represent areas where demyelination and partial remyelination alternately occur.

Patients occasionally die with a relatively short history of MS, or during a relapse. The brain and spinal cord of such patients contain lesions that show evidence of active demyelination. Many of them are small and intensely cellular (Fig. 14.21). They show loss of myelin, though this may not be complete, and contain many macrophages, some of which have ingested fragments of myelin which still react with myelin stains. Oligodendrocytes are also increased in density (Fig. 14.22). Reactive astrocytes with enlarged cell bodies may be present, but glial fibres are

Table 15.1 The main clinical and pathological features of five relatively common degenerative conditions.

Disease	Main clinical features	Naked-eye changes	Histological changes
Motor neuron disease 'Classical' form	Usual onset in sixth and seventh decades. Rarely familial. Progressive weakness and wasting of skeletal muscles, excluding ocular muscles	Muscle wasting and pallor. Wasting of anterior spinal roots. Medullary pyramids may be wasted	Loss of motor cells from anterior grey horns, and from cranial motor nuclei V, VII, (X), XI, XII. Denervation changes in muscles. Pyramidal tract degeneration
Werdnig–Hoffmann disease	Onset in late fetal life onwards. Recessive inheritance. 'Floppy baby'	Muscle wasting and pallor. Wasting of anterior spinal roots	Loss of motor cells. Denervated muscles. Pyramidal tracts not affected
Paralysis agitans (Parkinson's disease, idiopathic parkinsonism)	Usual onset in seventh and eighth decades. Not familial. Bradykinesia, resting tremor, 'cogwheel' rigidity, festination, mask-like facies, etc. Autonomic failure in some cases	Loss of pigment from substantia nigra and locus ceruleus. Basal ganglia appear normal	Loss of pigmented cells from substantia nigra and locus ceruleus; intracytoplasmic inclusions (Lewy bodies) in cells of these nuclei, nucleus basalis (substantia innominata) and elsewhere. No striatal cell loss. Intermediolateral column cell loss in some cases
Multiple system atrophy	Usual onset in fifth to seventh decades		
Striatonigral type*	Parkinsonism (not responding to (L-dopa). Autonomic failure (Shy–Drager syndrome) in some cases	Atrophy and discoloration of putamen. Loss of pigment from substantia nigra and locus ceruleus	Cell loss and gliosis in putamen, substantia nigra, locus ceruleus, intermediolateral columns
Pontocerebellar type*	Progressive ataxia and dysarthria	Atrophy of pons, olives, cerebellar cortex and white matter, middle and inferior cerebellar peduncles	Cell loss and gliosis in pontine nuclei, olives, Purkinje cells. (Different selection of lesions in different cases. Motor cells and sensory ganglia occasionally affected, but mildly. Likewise pyramidal tracts)
Friedreich's ataxia	Onset in first and second decades. Progressive ataxia, beginning in lower limbs. Mild sensory changes. Signs of cardiomyopathy, with abnormal ECG. Death commonly from heart failure	Atrophy of posterior spinal roots, spinal cord, brain stem, superior cerebellar peduncles; in some cases atrophy of globus pallidus, subthalamic nuclei, optic nerves. Cerebral infarcts rather common. Hypertrophy and fibrosis of heart	Cell loss from sensory ganglia (lower cord segments), dorsal and accessory cuneate nuclei, and dentate nuclei. Loss of axons in sensory nerves, posterior columns, pyramidal and spinocerebellar tracts, superior cerebellar peduncles, etc. Chronic myocarditis

ECG, electrocardiogram.
*These two types are often combined.

ataxia, for example, the *heart* is affected; thus in any case of progressive ataxia coming on in early life, a careful examination of several regions of the heart should be carried out.

In any case of suspected neuronal degeneration, samples of peripheral nerve, sensory and autonomic ganglia, and muscles from neck and upper and lower limbs should be taken. In selecting muscles, it should be borne in mind that the final state of muscles which have undergone severe neurogenic atrophy is practically indistinguishable from that of muscles affected by dystrophy or other myopathies. For this reason, it is advisable to take samples of mildly affected, and of apparently unaffected, muscles. In any denervating condition pallor of the muscle, due to loss of myoglobin, is a rough naked-eye indication of the degree of denervation. Samples of muscles supplied by cranial nerves should be taken in any case suspected of motor neuron disease. A procedure for obtaining these is described on pp.5–6.

The choice of blocks for histological examination should depend on a careful reading of the clinical notes.

Motor neuron diseases

A small to moderate degree of motor cell loss occurs in a variety of degenerative conditions, including multiple system atrophy. To make a diagnosis of 'classical' motor neuron disease (*amyotrophic lateral sclerosis*) one must not only demonstrate motor cell loss in the anterior horns of the cervical and lumbar enlargements, and in the hypoglossal nuclei, but also show that there is no obvious degeneration in other parts of the CNS—in particular, the basal ganglia, the cerebellar system and the sensory pathways. In most cases of motor neuron disease a certain amount of degeneration is also seen in the corticospinal (pyramidal) tracts. This may be apparent, in myelin preparations, over the full extent of the tracts, from Rolandic cortex to the sacral segments of the cord. In other cases, it may be detectable only in the lowest cord segments. It was Charcot's (1874) observation of greyness of the crossed pyramidal tracts in sections of the cord that gave rise to the term 'lateral sclerosis'. Strictly speaking, the diagnosis of 'amyotrophic lateral sclerosis' is inappropriate for cases of motor neuron disease not showing this feature. The process is one of 'dying back'; that is, it begins at the distal ends of the axons, and works its way back to the cells of origin. As the axon dies, its myelin sheath breaks down, and the fatty degradation products can be selectively stained by the Marchi method (p.67), which gives positive evidence of tract degeneration when the negative evidence provided by the myelin stain is inconclusive (see Figs 3.38 and 3.39).

When the process has reached up to midbrain level, myelin and Marchi preparations show it to be confined to the middle thirds of the cerebral peduncles (Fig. 2.30).

Fig. 15.1 Camera lucida tracings from Marchi preparations on horizontal sections of a case of motor neuron disease.
(a) Upper midbrain. (b) Basal ganglia. (c) Centrum ovale and corpus callosum. (d) Superior frontoparietal region. The stippled areas indicate positive Marchi degeneration. C = caudate nucleus; cc = corpus callosum; cg = cingulate gyrus; Cl = claustrum; cs = central sulcus; GP = globus pallidus; Hyp = hypothalamus; I = insula; L = lateral ventricle; ot = optic tract; P = putamen; R = red nucleus; T = thalamus; III = third ventricle.

(a)

(b)

(c)

Fig. 15.5 (a) Normal lentiform nucleus. Coronal section, level P1. Klüver–Barrera stain. (b) Same area, same stain. Woman, aged 58, with multiple system atrophy. Note the pallor and shrinkage of the putamen. The minor degree of pallor and shrinkage in the globus pallidus is mainly due to loss of myelinated axons coming from the putamen. (c) Same area, same stain. Woman, aged 71, with progressive supranuclear palsy. The putamen, and its myelinated bundles, appear normal, but the globus pallidus is grossly atrophic, and the subthalamic nucleus (arrowed) is shrunken and pale.

Pontocerebellar (olivopontocerebellar) atrophy

This is a relatively common type of degeneration causing ataxia. In spite of heroic attempts to sort out the various forms of this condition, it is still not clear whether it is one disease or several. Most cases are sporadic, but some show dominant, others recessive, inheritance. Some, at least, belong to the group referred to above (p.275) under the heading *multiple system atrophy*, and are liable to show major or minor lesions in the putamen, pigmented nuclei

and/or intermediolateral columns. Parts of the cerebellar system involved—sometimes severely—are the pontine nuclei and their efferent tracts in the middle cerebellar peduncles, the inferior olives and their efferents in the inferior cerebellar peduncles, and the Purkinje cells (all areas of cerebellar cortex may be affected). In consequence the cerebellar white matter is shrunken and gliotic, leaving an enlarged fourth ventricle (Figs 8.11 and 15.9); and the dentate nuclei, although there is no appreciable cell loss, are gliotic because of loss of incoming Purkinje axons. Ad-

(a)   (b)

Fig. 15.6 (a) Anterior and lateral horns, at mid-thoracic level. 20 μm section, Klüver–Barrera stain. There is a normal number of cells in the intermediolateral column (arrowed). (b) Same area and stain, in a man aged 58, suffering from multiple system atrophy, with autonomic failure. Only one nerve cell is visible in the intermediolateral column.

(a)   (b)

Fig. 15.7 (a) Surface view of normal pons and medulla. (b) Same view, in a case of multiple system atrophy. The leptomeninges have been stripped away. The pons and olives are greatly shrunken. Woman aged 76, suffering from parkinsonism and ataxia.

Fig. 15.8 Multiple system atrophy. Section of pons, stained for myelin, showing atrophy of the basis pontis and middle cerebellar peduncles, with normal-looking tegmentum, superior cerebellar peduncles and corticospinal tracts. The entering roots of the trigeminal nerves are conspicuously preserved. Woman of 54 with parkinsonism, ataxia and autonomic failure.

ditional lesions – not usually severe – may be found in sensory ganglia, anterior horn cells, dorsal (Clarke's) nuclei, and in spinocerebellar and/or corticospinal tracts.

Friedreich's ataxia

Some clinicians apply this term indiscriminately to any form of progressive familial ataxia; but since the 'classical' type of Friedreich's disease is exceptionally constant in its clinical and pathological manifestations, it is better to confine the eponymic title to more or less typical cases.

The onset of the disease is at some time in the first two decades of life, with a peak at ten years of age. The first symptom is ataxia of the lower limbs; later, the arms become ataxic, and finally the bulbar musculature is involved, and the patient's speech becomes dysarthric. A further symptom, not giving rise to much distress, is loss of common sensation, again affecting the legs before the arms, and rarely involving the face. A few patients suffer progressive visual or auditory loss. Outside the nervous system, the *heart* is almost always affected. The ECG is abnormal, the heart enlarges, and heart failure is the commonest immediate cause of death. Cerebrovascular accidents, attributable to emboli from the heart, are fairly common.

The most striking naked-eye changes include atrophy of the posterior roots in the lumbosacral region and cauda equina, and of the spinal cord and brain stem. Histological

(a)

(b)

Fig. 15.9 Multiple system atrophy. Sections of upper medulla stained (a) for myelin and (b) for fibrous gliosis (Holzer). The fourth ventricle is enlarged because of cerebellar atrophy. The inferior olives are shrunken and densely gliotic, and there is

myelin pallor and heavy gliosis of the cerebellar white matter, seen in top left and right hand corners, but not of the superior cerebellar peduncles above the roof of the fourth ventricle. Man, aged 62. Main complaint, ataxia. Familial case.

sections of lower spinal posterior roots and their ganglia show loss of ganglion cells and of their axons. In the cord there is well-marked degeneration of the posterior columns, affecting the gracile more than the cuneate funiculus, and of the pyramidal and spinocerebellar tracts, accounting in large measure for the overall shrinkage of the cord (Figs 15.11 and 15.12). Anterior and lateral horn cells are preserved, but there is severe loss of cells in the dorsal (Clarke's column) nuclei. In the brain stem, cell loss is seen in the accessory cuneate nuclei (the cephalic homologues of

the dorsal nuclei) and in the gracile nuclei in long-standing cases – presumably due to transneuronal degeneration. In the cerebellum, the dentate nuclei are nearly always severely affected, and the superior cerebellar peduncles correspondingly shrivelled (Figs 15.13 and 15.14). Purkinje cells and inferior olives are generally unaffected; when they are involved, it is probably as a result of ischaemia sustained in episodes of heart failure. At higher levels, some cases show symmetrical cell loss in the globus pallidus and subthalamic nucleus, and in some there is shrinkage and loss of fibres in the optic nerves and tracts. The usual findings in the heart are of chronic myocarditis, with fibrosis.

Ataxia–telangiectasia

Progressive ataxia, starting in childhood, is not always due to Friedreich's disease. An alternative cause is ataxia–telangiectasis (Louis–Bar syndrome). This is a familial condition, probably with autosomal recessive inheritance. Ataxia develops in early childhoold, and is followed by the appearance of telangiectatic areas in the conjunctivae and elsewhere. The victims are unduly prone to respiratory infections. Bodily growth is retarded, and mental deterioration may occur in the later stages of the disease. There is an enhanced liability to develop malignant growths, particularly lymphomas; these, along with recurrent infections, account for most of the patients' deaths. Laboratory findings include low levels of IgA in serum and other

Fig. 15.10 Oligodendrocyte inclusions in multiple system atrophy stained golden brown by methenamine silver. Counterstained with cresyl violet, ×200.

Fig. 15.11 Friedreich's ataxia. Boy, aged 10 years at death. Onset of ataxia at age 6. Lower lumbar cord and surrounding nerve roots, stained for myelin. The posterior roots, and the posterior columns, are pale and shrunken.

Fig. 15.12 Friedreich's ataxia. Man, aged 31. Onset of ataxia at age 10. 8th cervical segment, stained for myelin. Posterior roots are less affected than in Fig. 15.11. The gracile funiculi are more affected than the cuneate. Both dorsal and ventral spinocerebellar tracts, and the corticospinal tracts, are severely affected. (Note that there is no uncrossed pyramidal tract on the right side of the picture: and that the areas of the crossed pyramidal tract on the right and the uncrossed tract on the left add up to the area of the crossed tract on the left. This type of asymmetry, due to partial decussation at the lower end of the medulla, is very common.)

Fig. 15.13 Friedreich's ataxia. Upper medulla and cerebellum, stained for myelin. There is severe shrinkage and pallor of the pyramids, and of the hila of the dentate nuclei. The solitary tracts are almost invisible. In contrast with the cases of multiple system atrophy illustrated above, the cerebellar white matter and inferior olives appear normal.

Fig. 15.14 Same case as in Fig. 15.13. The basis pontis and tegmentum appear normal; but there is shrinkage and pallor of the superior cerebellar peduncles (arrowed), due to cell loss in the dentate nuclei.

fluids, defective responses of blood lymphocytes to phytohaemagglutinin and, in many cases, lymphopenia. Post mortem findings include hypoplasia, or even absence, of the thymus, general reduction of lymphoid tissue, hypoplastic gonads and widespread infiltration of viscera by large cells with bizarre nuclei. The telangiectases consist of dilated, tortuous venules. In the CNS, there is atrophy of the cerebellar cortex, with extensive loss of both Purkinje and granule cells, and retrograde cell loss in the inferior olives. Some cases show degeneration of the posterior columns, especially of the gracile funiculus. Posterior root ganglia show a deficiency of satellite cells, and of the larger ganglion cells; and in some cases there is drop-out of motor neurons, with consequent atrophy of muscles.

Correlation of clinical and anatomical changes

There is at present no body of knowledge connecting particular types of ataxic disturbance with lesions in particular components of the cerebellar system. This is aside from the general rule that midline lesions affecting the vermis are responsible for truncal ataxia and lesions of hemispheres for limb ataxia. The same can be said of the state of knowledge connecting particular kinds of abnormal movement, such as chorea or athetosis, with focal lesions in the basal ganglia. An exception is the frequent, but not invariable, association of *hemiballism* with lesions of a *subthalamic nucleus*.

Huntington's chorea

This is the best-known example of a dominantly-transmitted neuronal degeneration. It presents, usually during the third to fifth decades of life, with a combination of movement disorders and mental disturbances. Of these two, either may precede the other; occasionally, one does not occur at all. The movement disorder progresses from a slightly fidgety behaviour to frank chorea. The mental disorders are variable, and include dementia and schizophrenia. Some patients spend years in a psychiatric hospital before neurological signs develop. Since the threat posed by the disease is usually known to the whole family before it shows itself, it is not surprising that anxiety and depression are listed among the mental disturbances suffered by patients; and as it is common knowledge that there is no effective treatment, it is not surprising that many sufferers fail to consult a doctor. An uncommon variant of the disease, with onset in the second decade, is characterized by muscular rigidity rather than chorea, with epilepsy as an additional feature.

The characteristic naked-eye change is a severe symmetrical shrinkage of the *corpus striatum* (lentiform and caudate nuclei), with compensatory dilatation of the anterior horns of the lateral ventricles (Figs 8.9 and 15.15). A similar striatal atrophy occurs in some cases of Pick's disease, but in these there is a concomitant atrophy of the temporal lobes (Figs 8.10 and 15.16). There may also be a slight generalized thinning of the cortical ribbon. Under the low power of the microscope, one finds a devastating loss of small neurons in the caudate nucleus and putamen, with relative sparing of the large cells, and loss of the myelinated fibre bundles passing through the pallidum. The atrophied regions are densely gliotic. Apart from the corpus striatum, cell loss of varying severity may be found in the cerebral cortex, thalamus, hypothalamus, substantia nigra, cerebellar cortex, dentate nuclei, olives, and other brain stem nuclei. Further details, including electron microscopic and neurochemical abnormalities, are given by Oppenheimer & Esiri (1992).

Fascinating enlightenment about the genetics of this disorder has come recently with the demonstration that the defect responsible, on chromosome 4, is an expansion of a repeat sequence of 3 nucleotides (CAG), coding for a polyglutamine tract which varies in length in normal individuals between 11 and 34 and is expanded to 37–121 in Huntington's disease. This type of trinucleotide expansion

Fig. 15.16 Pick's disease. Man, aged 57. As in Fig. 15.15, the caudate nucleus is atrophic: the obvious difference lies in the extreme atrophy of the temporal lobe in this case, with compensatory dilatation of the inferior horn of the lateral ventricle.

Fig. 15.15 Huntington's disease. Man, aged 52. Myelin-stained section at level A1. The dilatation of the anterior horn of the lateral ventricle is due mainly to shrinkage of the caudate nucleus, and to a lesser extent of the lentiform nucleus. Note the normal size of the inferior (temporal) horn of the lateral ventricle.

is responsible for other inherited neurological diseases in addition to Huntington's disease (La Spada *et al.* 1994).

Progressive supranuclear palsy

This rare condition was first reported by Steele, Richardson and Olszewski in 1964. The onset is in the fifth to seventh decades of life, and men are twice as often affected as women. The disease is not familial. Clinical disturbances include paralysis of upward gaze, dysarthria, and muscular rigidity, which is most marked in the muscles of the neck. The most striking naked-eye change is a symmetrical atrophy of the globus pallidus and subthalamic nucleus (Fig. 15.5c). Microscopically, there is cell loss and gliosis in these nuclei, and in the red nuclei, substantia nigra, tectum of the upper brain stem, and the dentate nuclei of the cerebellum. A further peculiarity is the presence of neurofibrillary tangles in neurons in many areas, including some where cell loss is not apparent (Fig. 15.17). These tangles differ from those of Alzheimer's disease, Down's syndrome, the parkinsonism–dementia of Guam and post-encephalitic parkinsonism, which are very similar to each other, in their electron microscopic features (for references, see Oppenheimer and Esiri 1992).

Dentato-rubro-pallido-luysian atrophy (DRPLA)

Another rare disease, reported mainly but not exclusively from Japan, is dentato-rubro-pallido-luysian atrophy (DRPLA). In this condition (or group of conditions) the clinical features are very variable, even when the pathological findings are closely similar. The main disturbances consist of involuntary movements, variously described as ataxic, athetotic, choreic, ballistic or myoclonic. The condition is reviewed by Iizuka *et al.* (1984). The genetic defect in this disease, as in Huntington's disease, is a triplet repeat expansion.

Peroneal muscular atrophy (Charcot–Marie–Tooth disease)

This condition is generally classed as a progressive neuropathy, along with a number of other familial neuromuscular disorders. It does not appear to differ in any important respect from the CNS degenerations discussed above. There is loss of anterior horn cells and their axons, as in motor neuron disease, and of sensory ganglion cells and their processes, similar to that occurring in Friedreich's ataxia. In practice, the neuropathologist has the task of examining both the central and the peripheral nervous systems.

Fig. 15.17 Progressive supranuclear palsy. Same case as in Fig. 15.3c. Neurofibrillary tangle in brain stem. H&E, ×1200.

(a)

(b)

Fig. 15.18 Strümpell's disease (familial spastic paraplegia). Man aged 67. Onset of weakness in legs during adolescence: little change since then. (a) Section of cervical cord, stained for myelin, showing diffuse pallor in the lateral white columns, and specific fibre loss in the crossed and uncrossed pyramidal tracts and gracile funiculi. (b) Thoracic cord from the same case. Degeneration of the crossed pyramidal tracts is more marked, but the posterior columns at this level appear intact.

(a)

(b)

Fig. 15.19 Pontobulbar palsy with deafness. Boy aged 23 months. Sections of the junction of pons and medulla, stained (a) for myelin and (b) for fibroglia. The cut is slightly asymmetrical, with a higher level on the right side of the picture. Severe loss of myelin is seen in both acoustic nerves and ventral cochlear nuclei (arrowed), with corresponding gliosis.

Table 15.2 Sites of selective cell loss in various conditions.

Site	'Degenerative'	Metabolic, etc.	Toxic
Hippocampus	AD	Hypoxia Epilepsy	
Sensory, visual and auditory cortex			Organic mercury (p.356)
Motor cortex (Betz cells)	MND FA		
Striatum	Hunt MSA CJD	Wilson's disease (p.335) Hepatic failure (p.345)	Methyl alcohol (p.358) Manganese (p.356)
Pallidum	DRPLA PSP FA	Hallervorden–Spatz disease (p.338)	Manganese (p.356)
Subthalamic nuclei	DRPLA PSP FA	Wilson's disease (p.335)	Manganese (p.356)
Substantia nigra	PA MSA		MPTP (p.358)
Locus ceruleus	MSA AD PA		
Pontine nuclei	MSA		
Inferior olives	MSA CCD Hunt		Clioquinol (p.353)
V, VII and XII motor nuclei	MND PBP		

continued

Table 15.2 *continued.*

Site	'Degenerative'	Metabolic, etc.	Toxic
Dorsal nucleus X	MSA PA		
Dentate nuclei	FA PSP DRPLA	Wilson's disease (p.335)	
Purkinje cells	MSA CCD AT	Hypoxia Epilepsy Carcinoma	Ethyl alcohol (p.352) Methyl alcohol (p.358)
Cerebellar granule cells	CJD AT		Ethyl alcohol (p.352) Methyl alcohol (p.358) Organic mercury (p.356)
Spinal cord Motor cells	MND, WHD CMTD, CJD	Poliomyelitis	
Autonomic (intermedio-lateral)	MSA PA		
Dorsal (Clarke's column) nuclei	FA		
Sensory ganglia	FA	Avitaminoses Tabes dorsalis Carcinoma	
	CMTD	Hereditary sensory neuropathy	

AD, Alzheimer's disease; AT, Ataxia–telangiectasia (p.279); CCD, Cerebellar cortical degeneration (p.275); CJD, Creutzfeldt–Jakob disease (p.311); CMTD, Charcot–Marie–Tooth disease (p.283); DRPLA, Dentato-rubro-pallido-luysian atrophy (p.283); FA, Friedreich's ataxia (p.278); Huntington's disease (p.281); MND, Motor neuron disease (p.271); MSA, Multiple system atrophy (p.278); PA, Paralysis agitans (Parkinson's disease) (p.273); PBP, Pontobulbar palsy (p.285); PSP, Progressive supranuclear palsy (p.254); WHD, Werdnig–Hoffmann disease (p.273).

Doubtfully degenerative conditions

There are at least two conditions generally classed as progressive degenerations, though once they have developed their course are relatively stable. One is Strümpell's *familial spastic paraplegia*. This has its onset in the second decade of life, but normally remains static after bodily growth ceases. It does not shorten life. In most cases, paraparesis is a fairer description than paraplegia. The lesions are found in the spinal cord. In the cervical region, the posterior columns and spinocerebellar tracts are thinned; in the lumbosacral segments the pyramidal tracts are affected (Fig. 15.18). The other is the Brown–Vialetto–van Laere disease (*pontobulbar palsy with deafness*). The condition is often familial. It presents at any age, but most commonly in early life. The onset is sudden, with total hearing loss developing over a period of a few hours, accompanied or followed by paral-

ysis of some or most of the muscles supplied by the lower cranial nerves. After this, the patient's condition may remain static for some years, or for the rest of her life (most of the patients are female); or another episode of rapid deterioration may follow. This is not the pattern of relentless progression seen in most cases of primary neuronal degeneration. Histological features include loss of cells from the lower cranial motor nuclei, and of acoustic nerve fibres, with degeneration of the ventral cochlear nuclei (Fig. 15.19).

'Abiotrophy'

The idea that the neuronal degenerations represent a premature ageing of nervous tissue ('abiotrophy'), proposed by Gowers in 1902, is still current. It would, in any case, be difficult to disprove. It is also difficult to see how this idea, even if true, helps with our understanding of these diseases. Certain changes do undoubtedly take place in the CNS with advancing years. One such, which is easily confirmed by cell counting, is a tendency to thinning-out of the Purkinje cells in the cerebellum. They are also thinned out in several of the diseases discussed above; but in other conditions they survive, while other cell types disappear. It is often stated in print that after the age of 15 (or perhaps 25, or 35) the brain loses cells at the rate of 1000 (or 30000, or 100000) a day. These statements, we believe, belong to the realm of scientific journalism rather than of scientific research.

Sites of selective cell loss in various 'degenerative', toxic and metabolic diseases are shown in Table 15.2.

Further reading and references

Daniel S. 1992. The neuropathology and neurochemistry of multiple system atrophy. In Bannister R, Mathias C (Eds) *Autonomic failure: a textbook of diseases of the autonomic nervous system*, 3rd edn. Oxford University Press, pp.564–85.

Iizuka R, Hirayama K, Maebara K. 1984. Dentato-rubropallido-luysian atrophy. *J Neurol Neurosurg Psychiat* **47**, 1288–98.

La Spada AR, Palmson HL, Fischbeck KH. 1994. Trinucleotide repeat expansion in neurological disease. *Ann Neurol* **36**, 814–22.

Oppenheimer DR, Esiri MM. 1992. Diseases of the basal ganglia, cerebellum and motor neurons. In Adams JH, Duchen LW (Eds) *Greenfield's Neuropathology*, 5th edn. Edward Arnold, London, Chapter 15.

Rosen DR. Siddique T, Patterson D *et al*. 1993. Mutations of copper/zinc superoxide dismutase gene are associated with familial lateral sclerosis. *Nature* **362**, 52–62.

16 Malformations of the Central Nervous System

Causes of malformations

Knowledge of the causes of CNS malformations is at present rather sketchy. There has been a good deal of experimental work on teratogenesis in animals, and a little is known about factors affecting human embryos. These include genetic traits, intoxications, nutritional defects, maternal infections and irradiation. In this chapter we shall confine ourselves to the description of some of the commoner developmental anomalies. The conditions mentioned here are without doubt heterogeneous, since we know of no sure means of distinguishing between malformations due to genetic or 'idiopathic' causes and those due to toxic or metabolic disturbances. Further information on these matters is to be found in Keeling (1993) and Harding (1992).

Malformations of the spinal cord

The most commonly encountered of these are associated with *spina bifida*, i.e. failure of the spines and laminae of certain vertebrae to fuse in the midline, leaving a gap through which the spinal meninges may protrude. The lumbar vertebrae are the ones most often affected. In a *meningocele* the dura and arachnoid are ballooned backwards, and lie immediately beneath a layer of thinned-out skin; underneath, there is a sac containing CSF and nerve roots. In a *meningomyelocele* part of the spinal cord is included, and nerve roots are found stuck to the walls of the sac. The cord itself is usually malformed in this region. Muscles of the lower limbs, normally supplied by the affected nerve roots, are more or less denervated, wasted and useless. The sac is present at birth. If it is not treated surgi-

cally, the thin overlying skin is apt to become ulcerated, and infection sets in. Purulent meningitis is a common, and commonly fatal, outcome. At post mortem a sample of the contained fluid should be withdrawn for bacteriological examination. In *spina bifida occulta* there is a less capacious sac, with similar involvement of nerve roots, but no obvious protrusion on the surface. In some cases there is a dimple in the skin over the affected vertebra, marking the position of a dermal track, which leads to the spinal meninges. In all cases of spina bifida, it is best to take the entire vertebral column at post mortem. If this is not done, a careful dissection of the region should be carried out when the spinal cord is removed.

Other malformations, sometimes but not always associated with a spina bifida, are *diastematomyelia*, in which the left and right sides of the cord are separated by a space, or by a layer of connective tissue, and *diplomyelia*, in which two more or less complete cords lie side by side. Some degree of *hydromyelia* (expanded central canal) is a common finding in all these types of malformation.

Malformations of the brain stem and cerebellum

Chiari malformations, types 1 and 2

In Chiari's type 1 malformation there is elongation of one or both cerebellar tonsils, which dangle through the foramen magnum into the upper part of the spinal canal (Fig. 16.1). This deformity may cause no symptoms until, for one reason or another, intracranial pressure is increased. Since the capacity of the cisterna magna is reduced, the risk of foraminal herniation, with impaction, is

(a)

(b)

Fig. 16.1 (a) Chiari malformation, type 1. Incidental finding in a man aged 62. No other malformations present. The lower end of the medulla has been cut away to display the elongated right cerebellar tonsil (on the left of the picture). (b) T1W parasagittal MR image demonstrates extension of the cerebellar tonsils through the foramen magnum into the upper cervical canal. There is also associated syringohydromyelia (occurs in up to 25% of Chiari 1) and moderate hydrocephalus which also occurs in up to 25% of Chiari 1.

enhanced. The patient may, for example, die suddenly in the course of an acute feverish illness. In a case of this kind examined in our department, the patient had suffered a series of episodes, with signs and symptoms referable to the lower brain stem, which were very reasonably ascribed to MS.

Chiari's type 2 malformation (commonly referred to as the *Arnold–Chiari malformation*) is unfortunately far commoner, and is the commonest cause of congenital hydrocephalus. The principal features of this condition are listed below (see Figs 16.2 and 16.3).

1 The vault of the skull varies in size from large to enormous. The fontanelles are very wide, and do not close. The posterior fossa is small and shallow.

2 Enlargement of the skull is caused by, and corresponds with, enlargement of the lateral and third ventricles. The aqueduct is usually patent, but the fourth ventricle is not enlarged.

3 The outer surfaces of the cerebral hemispheres are flattened, with virtual obliteration of the cerebral sulci and disappearance of the subarachnoid space. The cortex and underlying white matter are thinned; in a severe case, the distance between the pia and lateral ventricle may be less than a centimetre throughout.

4 The tentorium and falx cerebri are paper-thin, and often fenestrated.

5 The anatomy of the thalamus, basal ganglia and upper brain stem is more or less normal.

6 The cerebellum, lower brain stem and fourth ventricle are grossly deformed. The cerebellar tonsils are prolonged for a distance of 10 cm or so into the spinal canal, and are accompanied by an irregularly folded medulla oblongata and an elongated fourth ventricle.

7 There is a lumbar spina bifida, with a protruding meningomyelocele. The lower end of the spinal cord is splayed open, and its emergent nerve roots are embedded in the wall of the sac.

8 Lower limb muscles supplied by these nerve roots show varying degrees of denervation atrophy.

One or more of these features may be lacking in individual cases. How many of them are causally linked, and whether they can all be traced to a single mishap in early development, are still subjects of debate, which we shall not attempt to pursue here.

To display the features of either type of Chiari malformation, one should avoid the conventional method of removing the brain at post mortem, as this entails cutting through the herniated cerebellar tonsils when the brain stem is separated from the spinal cord. For the type 2 malformation, the technique described on p.8 gives a good display (see Figs 16.2 and 16.3). Unless it is intended to carry out a detailed study of the disordered brain stem anatomy, the whole specimen can be divided in the midline, and mounted as a museum specimen. For the type 1 malformation, a transverse cut can be made through the upper cervical cord from behind, before extracting the brain from the skull (the diagnosis has often been made radiologically before death).

(a)

(b)

Fig. 16.2 Chiari malformation, type 2. The brain and spinal column have been removed by the method described on p.8. Infant, aged 4 months, with congenital hydrocephalus and meningomyelocele. (a) A midline cut shows an enormous lateral ventricle, a paper-thin falx cerebri, and a malformed hindbrain, with the cerebellar tonsils extending far down into the spinal canal, accompanied by a downward extension of the fourth ventricle. (b) A midline cut shows a misshapen spinal column, with a lumbar kyphus instead of lordosis, and deficient lumbar and sacral bony arches. Above (arrowed), the downward extension of the medulla oblongata appears to be folded over the spinal cord. Below, the roots of the cauda equina are attached to the walls of a large meningocele.

Cerebellar hypoplasia

The cerebellum as a whole may be abnormally small, or parts of it may be hypoplastic, or even missing. When one cerebellar hemisphere is hypoplastic, the inferior olive and pontine nuclei on the opposite side also tend to be under-developed. In *pontoneocerebellar hypoplasia* the lateral lobes of the cerebellum, pontine nuclei and middle cerebellar peduncles are reduced in size (Fig. 16.4), whereas the vermis and flocculi are of more or less normal size. In other cases, the lateral lobes may be normal, while the vermis is hypoplastic or absent. In the *Dandy–Walker malformation* the vermis is partially or completely replaced by a large ependyma-lined cyst (Fig. 16.5); and there is often an as-sociated hydrocephalus, and agenesis of the corpus callosum.

Disorderly development of patches of cerebellar cortex gives rise to a condition variously known as *pachygyria* or *microgyria* (the same two terms are used for two quite dis-tinct types of malformation of cerebral cortex). In the cere-bellar condition, the cellular elements—Purkinje cells, granule cells and the rest—in a number of adjacent folia are jumbled up, and divisions between folia are lost. The con-dition is said to be rare, but tiny areas of similar cellular disorder are quite commonly seen in the neighbourhood of the foramina of Luschka as incidental findings. Less com-monly, areas of ectopic cortical cells are found within the cerebellar white matter.

In *cerebrocerebellar* (*crossed cerebellar*) *atrophy* smallness of one cerebellar hemisphere is associated with smallness of the opposite cerebral hemisphere (Figs 16.6 and 16.7). The primary lesion in such cases, which may be one of a great variety of prenatal or postnatal mishaps, is to be found in the cerebrum. The affected cerebellar hemisphere may be histologically more or less normal. More often, there is loss of cells and glial scarring, which in many cases can be plausibly attributed to the effects of repeated epileptic attacks.

Fig. 16.3 View from behind of a cord with the Chiari type 2 malformation. As in the last example, the medulla extends far down into the spinal canal. The posterior spinal nerve roots, which normally slope downward from the cord, here slope upward, and undergo a sharp bend downward at the points where they penetrate the dura. The patient was a boy aged 18 years, with spina bifida and a lumbar meningomyelocele. He was mentally normal. He died of a purulent meningitis.

Malformations of the cerebral hemispheres

In this, as in the preceding sections, we wish to make it clear that most of the italicized words/headings are not the names of diseases, but merely labels attached, for convenience, to certain naked-eye and microscopic appearances. The diseases causing them remain for the most part unknown. We hope, and indeed expect, that a more satisfactory nomenclature will emerge in the course of the next ten or twenty years. An analogous process has taken place in the naming of the lipidoses. At first they were known by the names of their original describers. Next, they were subdivided according to their clinical and histological characteristics. Now, they are generally referred to in terms of missing enzymes (Table 19.1).

Microencephaly and megalencephaly

Microencephaly and megalencephaly do not seem to us to be very useful terms. The weights of normally-functioning brains vary within wide limits; they may even weigh less than 1 kg or more than 2 kg without causing trouble. Very large and very small brains often show abnormalities, gross or histological, apart from size; and it is these abnormalities which determine the diagnosis.

Fig. 16.4 Pontoneocerebellar hypoplasia in a 14-month-old infant. Total brain weight 658 g; hindbrain alone, 21 g. Cerebrum, pyramidal tracts and cerebellar vermis more or less normal. Pontine nuclei, middle cerebellar peduncles and hemispheres tiny. Incomplete cell loss in dentate nuclei and olives.

(a)

(b)

Fig. 16.5 (a) Dandy–Walker malformation in a week-old infant with patent ductus arteriosus. The cerebellar vermis is replaced by a large cavity. (b) T1W sagittal (A) and T2W axial (B) MR images elegantly demonstrate features of the Dandy–Walker malformation. The posterior fossa is large with elevation of the tentorium, dysgenesis of the cerebellar vermis, hypoplasia of the cerebellar hemispheres and cystic dilatation of the fourth ventricle. There is hydrocephalus which occurs in approximately 75% of cases by 3 months of age. The skull vault is grossly thickened as a result of chronic hydrocephalus. The exact aetiology is not known but theories include failure of development of the embryonic roof of the fourth ventricle, atresia of outlet foramina and an insult to the developing cerebellar hemispheres and fourth ventricle.

Down's syndrome

In Down's syndrome (mongolism) the brain is usually of below average size, with relative smallness of the hindbrain. The cerebrum appears short from front to back, with a small parietal lobe; and there is often a hypoplasia of the superior temporal gyri (Fig. 16.8). Various histological ab-normalities have been described, but none peculiar to Down's syndrome, with the possible exception of a minor malformation of the thoracic cord, described by Benda (1947), consisting of fusion across the midline of the dorsal (Clarke's) nuclei. It has also been observed that patients reaching middle age tend to show numerous cortical plaques and neurofibrillary tangles, resembling those seen in Alzheimer's disease, in cortical nerve cells.

Fig. 16.7 Cerebellar degeneration in a man of 25 with Sturge–Weber disease (see p.298) affecting mainly the left cerebral hemisphere. Epilepsy, mental defect and right hemiplegia from infancy. Left hemispherectomy at age 16, with good results. Deterioration for 1 year before death, due to intracranial bleeding. Post mortem: superficial haemosiderosis, and gross atrophy of left side of brain stem and right side of cerebellum, with extensive loss of cortical neurons and dense gliosis. Dilated veins in the left cerebellar hemisphere are part of the original disease.

Fig. 16.6 Cerebrocerebellar degeneration in a woman aged 62. Left spastic hemiparesis, epilepsy and mental defect since infancy. Cause not known. Right cerebral hemisphere shrunken: areas of ulegyria. Shrinkage and scarring of right side of brain stem and left cerebellar hemisphere.

Fig. 16.8 Down's syndrome. Man, aged 43. The brain is generally small (weight 1035 g) and short from back to front. The superior temporal gyrus is relatively narrow.

Fig. 16.9 Holoprosencephaly. Brain of neonate, seen from behind. There is a single forebrain cavity, covered partly with a rudimentary cortex and partly with a thin membrane. Here the membrane has been torn, giving an indecent exposure of the thalamus and basal ganglia, which have a relatively normal structure.

Other trisomies

Down's syndrome is usually associated with trisomy 21. There is also a wide range of malformations associated with trisomy of the 13–15 group. The simplest of these is *arrhinencephaly*, i.e. absence of the olfactory parts of the forebrain. This may be combined with the rather common major malformation of *holoprosencephaly*. In this, the hemispheres are not separated, and there is a single large cavity replacing the lateral ventricles (Fig. 16.9). The skull and facial bones are malformed, and in some cases there is *cyclopia*, i.e. a single, malformed, centrally-placed eye. Trisomy 18 is found in some cases of this type. For a fuller discussion see Laurence (1987).

Disorders of cell migration

In fetal life these are held responsible for two types of malformation: *heterotopias* and *lissencephaly* (Fig. 16.10). In the former, heterotopic (or ectopic) masses of grey matter are found in unexpected places, such as the centrum ovale,

or the cerebellar white matter. In the latter, there seems to be a generalized failure of outward migration of cells from the mantle layer to the cerebral cortex. As a result of this, the normal pattern of cortical gyri and sulci, and the normal six-layered cortex, fail to develop. Externally, the hemispheres show either a grossly simplified convolutional pattern, with a few broad gyri (*pachygyria*), or a lack of sulci other than a shallow depression representing the lateral fissure (*agyria, lissencephaly*). On slicing, the hemispheres are separate, with normally-placed, but dilated, lateral and third ventricles; the centrum ovale, though normally myelinated, is much reduced in bulk; and outside this is a layer, 2 cm or so thick, of grey matter in which the cells, though showing lamination of a kind, are not readily equated with the six layers of normal cortex. Passing through the abnormal cortex are radial bundles of myelinated fibres. Associated abnormalities in the CNS include defective development of the corpus callosum, heterotopic grey matter in the cerebellum, and malformations of the inferior olives. Malformations may also be present in viscera such as heart and kidneys. Some cases are familial.

Agenesis of the corpus callosum

Partial or total absence of the corpus callosum may be part of a complex of cerebral anomalies, or it may occur in isolation, in the absence of clinically-observed defects (Fig. 16.11). The pattern of sulci on the medial aspects of the hemispheres is commonly abnormal, lacking a cingulate sulcus.

Schizencephaly

In this condition there is a cleft, extending from the lateral surface of one hemisphere (or more commonly both) to the ependyma of the lateral ventricle (Fig. 16.12). The lips of the cleft may be apposed, or separated by a subarachnoid space. The cortex lining the cleft is commonly malformed, and there may be heterotopic masses of grey matter. In some cases the Rolandic cortex and corticospinal tracts are lacking. These clefts are distinguished from so-called *porencephalic cysts* by the fact that there is no sign of tissue destruction during the prenatal or perinatal periods.

Encephaloceles

These are protrusions of cerebral tissue through defects in the cranium. They occur most commonly through an occipital defect, or, more rarely, through a gap between the frontal and ethmoid bones (anterior meningocele or encephalomeningocele). The latter condition is said to be rare in Europe, but relatively common in South East Asia. Posterior encephaloceles can become very large, and may

(a)

(b)   (c)

Fig. 16.10 Pachygyria (lissencephaly) in a 5-month-old girl with multiple congenital defects. (a) Coronal slice at the level of the optic chiasm, showing a somewhat simplified convolutional pattern, with an abnormally wide cortical ribbon and a corresponding paucity of central white matter. The corpus callosum is present, but thin. The lateral ventricles are large, and there is a conspicuous cavum septi pellucidi. (b) A myelin-stained section at anterior thalamic level shows relatively normal thalamus and corpus striatum, and normal myelination of the deeper white matter. Between this and the cortex proper there is a zone within which bundles of myelinated fibres are mixed with cells which have failed to migrate outward. Sulci between convolutions are very shallow. (c) Posteriorly, ectopic islands of grey matter lie in the periventricular white matter.

(a)

(b)

Fig. 16.11 (a) Agenesis of the corpus callosum in a 2-year-old child with polymicrogyria and aqueduct stenosis. (b) Agenesis of the corpus callosum is elegantly demonstrated by MRI particularly on a T1W sagittal image. This T2W coronal MR image, however also demonstrates many features associated with callosal agenesis, in particular, the third ventricle is widened and extends superiorly between the bodies of the lateral ventricles. The frontal horns appear concave because of eversion of the cingulate gyrus (small arrow) and Probst bundles (larger arrow). (Axons that usually cross in corpus callosum instead run medial to the medial walls of the lateral ventricles parallel to the interhemispheric fissure. These are known as the longitudinal callosal bundles or bundles of Probst.)

contain an extension of the posterior horn of the lateral ventricle.

Cavum septi pellucidi

This, on its own, barely qualifies as a malformation, though it may be combined with more serious deformities, as in Fig. 16.10. It is normally present in fetal life, and may persist. A cavum septi is also said to be a characteristic acquired feature in the brains of professional boxers.

Polymicrogyria

This is a condition affecting large or small, generally asymmetrical, areas of cerebral cortex. The pathogenesis is still uncertain, but there is often a history suggesting a toxic, infective or hypoxic episode occurring at some time before the sixth month of fetal life. The external appearance has been compared to the surface of a cauliflower or of a peeled chestnut. Slicing (Figs 16.12 and 16.13) shows a much-wrinkled cortical ribbon, with pia mater covering multiple tiny wrinkles, not dipping between them. Within the ribbon, it is usually possible to distinguish four layers, of which the first (outer) and third are sparsely populated, while the second and fourth are richly supplied with neurons. A detailed description, with discussion of the theoretical aspects of the condition, is given by Harding (1992).

The condition is not uncommon. Mental defect and epilepsy are common in affected patients; but small lesions may be clinically silent.

Ulegyria

This is a type of cortical scarring dating from early life. It is not, as is sometimes suggested, confined to lesions acquired before or at the time of birth; it has been seen, for instance, in material removed in the operation of hemispherectomy for epilepsy consequent upon infantile hemiplegia, when the original vascular mishap occurred at the age of 12 months or more. On the surface of the hemisphere there may be little sign of damage. On section, the affected gyri show cell loss, shrinkage and gliosis in the depths of sulci, whereas the crowns of the gyri appear intact (Fig. 16.14). The condition is discussed on pp.125 and 370.

Anencephaly

This is a relatively common fetal malformation of the head. The skull is grossly abnormal, and the brain is replaced by a mass of vascular connective tissue. The causes are not known. *Hydranencephaly*, in spite of the name, is a totally different condition, attributed to perinatal cerebral ischaemia. It is discussed by Harding (1992).

General recommendation

In any case of CNS malformation, the pathologist should search the clinical notes for clues to the aetiology: in particular, one should look for records of maternal infections (such as rubella), intoxications, or episodes of hypoxia or hypotension.

Vascular malformations

These are classified according to the predominant structural component. The commonest and least clinically important are *capillary telangiectases*, which may be found incidentally at post mortem, particularly in the pons or cerebral cortex and subjacent white matter. These are usually solitary lesions composed of a cluster of dilated, congested capillary channels. They rarely bleed spontaneously.

Cavernous angiomas

These occur at similar sites, are usually solitary but occasionally multiple, and are rather larger than capillary telangiectases, measuring up to 4 cm across. They appear dark red, resembling a mulberry, and may show evidence of having bled. They are composed of thin-walled, blood-filled spaces of variable size, some very large in comparison with the thinness of their walls (Fig. 6.16). The walls contain a single endothelial layer and a thin rim of collagen. Gliotic brain parenchyma lies between these blood-filled spaces, and may contain haemosiderin-laden macrophages, testifying to former leakage of red blood cells. Occasionally cavernous angiomas give rise to haemorrhage, and those in or close to the cerebral cortex may be associated with epilepsy.

Arteriovenous malformations

These types of vascular malformation are of greatest clinical importance (Figs 16.15 and 16.16). They may give rise to symptoms (i) by bleeding, (ii) by provoking epileptic attacks, (iii) by enlarging and so acting as compressing lesions, or (iv) by diverting blood from neighbouring structures, which are thereby rendered ischaemic. In the brain they are commonest in the cerebrum, and are usually related to a leptomeningeal or ependymal surface. They form a more or less circumscribed tangle of vessels, some of which, on microscopic examination, are found to be arteries, and others veins. In the arteries there is frequently reduplication of elastic tissue and irregularity in width of the media. Aneurysmal dilatation, with gross thinning of the wall, may be seen. The veins show collagenous thickening of their walls, with some admixed smooth muscle. The veins are particularly prominent in spinal arteriovenous malformations, which are discussed on p.35.

Sturge–Weber disease (encephalofacial angiomatosis)

In this rare condition there is an extensive, diffuse capillary and venous malformation in the leptomeninges of one cerebral hemisphere, and an associated cutaneous 'port wine' naevus in the ipsilateral trigeminal distribution.

Fig. 16.15 Arteriovenous malformation. Operation specimen from temporal lobectomy of a boy aged 12, who presented with psychomotor epilepsy.

Fig. 16.16 Arteriovenous malformation. Coronal slice, at level P3, from a 70-year-old woman with a 43-year history of uncontrollable epilepsy. There is a massive tangle of blood vessels in the left cerebral hemisphere.

Fig. 16.17 Hemispherectomy specimen from a case of Sturge–Weber disease illustrating the thickened and abnormally vascular leptomeninges. (Courtesy of Dr B McDonald.)

Over the affected cerebral hemisphere the leptomeninges are thickened and contain a multitude of fine-calibre blood vessels (Fig. 16.17). The underlying cortex is frequently atrophic and contains numerous calcified fine vessels. The parenchyma is usually gliotic, with variable neuronal loss.

There is an interesting twilight zone in which the category of congenital (sometimes hereditary) malformations merges into that of neoplasia. Two of the better-known conditions in this area are the syndromes of Lindau and Bourneville.

Lindau's syndrome

This comprises haemangioblastoma of the cerebellum (more rarely of the cord), haemangioblastoma of the retina (von Hippel's disease), a relatively benign tumour of the kidney ('benign hypernephroma') and cysts, thought to be congenital, in pancreas and kidneys. The syndrome affects only a minority of patients with a cerebellar haemangioblastoma, but is commoner in patients with (i) a family history of such tumours, and (ii) multiple tumours in the cerebellum. In making a post mortem examination on *any* case of cerebellar haemangioblastoma, the pathologist should look carefully at the *spinal cord*, both *kidneys*, and *pancreas*. For histological details of the tumour, see p.239.

Tuberous sclerosis complex (Bourneville's disease)

Clinically, this disorder comprises epilepsy, mental defect, adenoma sebaceum of the face, other skin lesions, and haematuria. The associated structural lesions include 'tubers' in the brain, rhabdomyomas of the heart muscle, and angiomyolipomas of the kidney. The condition, when familial, is said to be transmitted by an autosomal dominant gene. Within an affected family, its expression is very variable, with one member exhibiting the full disease, while another merely shows a benign kidney tumour.

The brain lesions occur in two main sites: cerebral cortex

Fig. 16.18 Tuberous sclerosis. Axial T2W MR images of a child with seizures demonstrates hamartomas (tubers) involving the cortical and adjacent subcortical white matter causing flattening of the gyri giving them an almost pachygyric appearance. Subependymal hamartomas or tubers (arrowheads) within the walls of the lateral ventricles are better seen on the axial image.

and the ependyma of the lateral ventricles (Fig. 16.18). On the surface, the cortical tubers are firm to the touch (more noticeably so before fixation), pale in colour, and appear as focal expansions of the gyri in which they occur (Fig. 16.19). Under the microscope they show a disorderly arrangement of cells, with loss of the normal lamination, dense gliosis, and numerous bizarre giant cells (Fig. 16.20), which are not easily classified as neurons or glial cells. The paraventricular lesions, described as 'candle-gutterings' by a generation familiar with the behaviour of candles, are elongated nodules, projecting into the ventricular cavity, composed of a variety of glial cells, among which large gemistocytic types of astrocyte are conspicuous. It is these lesions that on occasion give rise to expanding neoplasms, which are described on p.203. As a rule, neither the cortical nor the paraventricular lesions become neoplastic. As specimens from both types of lesion may turn up unexpectedly as biopsies, or even smears, it is important not to confuse them with malignant gliomas—a mistake facilitated by the presence of bizarre giant cells.

(a)

(b)

Fig. 16.19 Tuberous sclerosis. Girl, aged 10 months. Epileptic, with malformed heart and polycythaemia. Brain weight 900 g. (a) Right lateral view, showing cortical tubers (arrowed). (b) Coronal slice at level A2, showing cortical tubers (arrow heads) and 'candle-gutterings' (arrowed) in the walls of the lateral ventricles. (Courtesy of Dr Betty Brownell.)

General comments

In many places antenatal monitoring by ultrasound has greatly reduced the prevalence of major malformations since these are now detected at an earlier stage of pregnancy and the pregnancy terminated.

Malformations of the CNS vary greatly in their consequences. Some, such as anencephaly and holo-

(a)   (b)

Fig. 16.20 Same case as in Fig. 16.19. (a) Section through a cortical tuber. Pial surface at top-right corner. Abnormal lamination of nerve cells. In a deeper layer, there is a group of bizarre giant cells. Cajal's gold sublimate, ×100. (b) Higher power view of abnormal cells in tuber. Cajal's gold sublimate, ×250.

prosencephaly, are fatal shortly after birth. Others, including encephaloceles and meningoceles, may be successfully patched up by the surgeon. Here, the main risk to life is a purulent meningitis. Minor malformations, such as polymicrogyria or agenesis of the corpus callosum, may give rise to epilepsy, 'cerebral palsy', and/or varying degrees of mental defect in childhood and after. As a general rule, minor malformations cause inconvenience or distress to the patient, whereas major ones, if they are compatible with continued life, are responsible for years of misery suffered by members of patients' families. They also constitute a drain on the resources of the social services. Research into the causes of malformations is well worth while, both for the light it may throw on embryological processes, and in the hope that better understanding may, in at least some of these conditions, suggest preventive measures.

Further reading and references

Benda CE. 1947. *Mongolism and Cretinism*. Grune and Stratton, New York.

Keeling JW (Ed.). 1993. *Fetal and Neonatal Pathology*, 2nd edn. Springer, Berlin, Chapter 23.

Harding BN. 1992. Malformations of the nervous system. In Adams JH, Duchen LW (Eds) *Greenfield's Neuropathology*, 5th edn. Edward Arnold, London, Chapter 10.

17 Dementia

In this chapter we discuss the pathological diagnosis in cases of progressive dementia with onset in adult life. Dementia, in which there is loss of previously intact mental faculties, needs to be distinguished from mental defect, in which these faculties may never have developed normally. Dementia in childhood is due to a different range of diseases from those found in adults. However, it should be noted that rare adult cases of inherited metabolic disease, more commonly presenting in childhood, may present with dementia. There are many diseases in which dementia may occur in adults as part of the clinical picture, for example in cases of MS, diffuse cerebral tumour or PML. These cases are not our primary concern here, though they may be expected to turn up as occasional causes of unexplained progressive dementia. So too may conditions giving rise to confusion, memory loss or aphasia (Chapter 25), which may be mistakenly diagnosed clinically as dementia. Progressive supranuclear palsy (p.282) is sometimes regarded as a dementing condition, but the cognitive impairment in that disease is due more to slowed reactions than to a true dementia. A fixed, rather than progressive, dementia dating from an acute onset may occur following severe head injury or a hypoxic insult to the brain. Most adult cases in which the clinical disease is dominated by progressive mental deterioration will be found to be suffering from one of the conditions dealt with in this chapter. Further information on these conditions may be found in Tomlinson (1992) and Esiri & Morris (1996).

The pathologist usually becomes involved with the diagnosis of cases of dementia after patients have died, but there are some medical centres that undertake cerebral biopsy as part of the investigation of cases of dementia. If a biopsy is taken, it is desirable that part of it be submitted for biochemical assay of choline acetyltransferase activity, which is selectively reduced in the cerebral cortex in Alzheimer's disease. The remainder is examined by light and electron microscopy (p. 94). It is recommended that the sample for biochemistry is snap-frozen in liquid nitrogen or at $-70°C$ and stored until microscopy has been carried out on the remainder of the sample. In this way a diagnosis of Creutzfeldt–Jakob disease (CJD) can usually be excluded before any biochemical investigation is undertaken.

Precautions regarding the agent responsible for Creutzfeldt–Jakob disease (CJD)

Cases of progressive dementia on which a post mortem examination has been carried out may occasionally be found (when sections for microscopy become available), contrary to expectation, to be cases of CJD. CJD is a horrible, and at present untreatable, disease. It is also the subject of unsettled controversy. It is certain that transmission has been effected inadvertently, via penetrating electro-encephalogram (EEG) electrodes, a corneal graft and most recently by injections of pituitary extract administered to growth-hormone-deficient children. There is also strong evidence for occurrence of a closely related condition, the Gerstmann–Sträussler syndrome, as an autosomal dominant disease, and there have been transmissions from such familial cases to experimental animals. Strict precautions have been recommended by the Committee on Health Care Issues of the American Neurological Association (1986) and others (HMSO 1991, 1994; Bell & Ironside 1993), for the post mortem handling of tissues

Table 17.1 Guide to the examination of the brain in cases of adult progressive dementia.

Macroscopic appearance	Probable significance	Blocks recommended
Foci of softening	MID (but AD may also be present)	Softened foci, temp/hippo to exclude AD
Normal, or mild, generalized atrophy	Probably AD; other possibilities CJD (especially if illness <1 yr), MID (micro-infarcts), schizophrenia, paraneoplastic encephalitis (see p.184)	AD blocks (see text); CJD blocks (see text); cortex/white matter for MID
Marked atrophy of cortex (focal/generalized) and comp. vent. dil.	Possible AD; Pick's disease (post 2/3 of sup. temp. gyrus spared); CJD with long survival; syphilis (meninges thick); frontal lobe dementia	Pick's disease blocks (see text); AD blocks (see text); CJD blocks (see text); frontal lobe/ventricular surface for syphilis frontal/temp lobe for frontal lobe dementia
Atrophy of caudate with normal or atrophic cortex and comp. vent. dil.	Huntington's chorea; milder caudate atrophy−Pick's disease; AD	See p.281 for Huntington's chorea; Pick's disease blocks (see text); AD blocks (see text)
Enlarged ventricles without atrophy	'Normal pressure' or obstructive hydrocephalus	Leptomeninges and outlet of 4th ventricle; temp/hippo to exclude AD
Cerebral white matter discoloration/softening; cortex preserved	Binswanger's disease; also consider AIDS (see p.174)	Foci of softening/discoloration; temp/hippo to exclude AD; for AIDS see p.174
Pale SN	PD with dementia; prog. supranuc. palsy with dementia cortico basal degeneration	Midbrain, pons, cingulate gyrus, AD blocks (see text); basal ganglia; for prog. supranuc. palsy see p.282
Chronic subdural haematoma	If small, probably secondary to atrophy; if large may be cause of dementia	If small, look for disease causing atrophy (see above)
Cerebellar atrophy	If mainly vermis, alcoholism; CJD	For alcoholism see p.352; CJD blocks (see text)

AD, Alzheimer's disease; CJD, Creutzfeldt–Jakob disease; MID, multi-infarct dementia; SN, substantia nigra; temp/hippo, temporal lobe and hippocampus; comp. vent. dil., compensatory ventricular dilatation; prog. supranuc. palsy, progressive supranuclear palsy; sup. temp. gyrus, superior temporal gyrus.

from suspected cases; but the actual risks involved are quite unknown. Over 50 years elapsed between Jakob's description of the disease and the demonstration that it could be transmitted to animals. During this time cases were examined without precautions, yet there are still no recorded cases of CJD in pathologists or mortuary attendants, though two cases have recently been reported in laboratory technicians. It is impossible to say whether these anecdotal cases are coincidental or related to occupational exposure. As the incubation period can last for decades, the connection between infection and the development of symptoms would be easy to miss. It should be remembered that formalin fixation is insufficient to destroy the transmissible agent. However, the procedures recommended in Appendix C will sterilize tissue and other materials so there is no good reason to avoid examination of biopsy or post mortem material on safety grounds, provided these recommendations are followed. Confimed cases of CJD in

the UK should be notified to the CJD Surveillence Office (see Appendix B).

Provision of post mortem material for research purposes

It has been realized during the last 20 years that brain samples obtained post mortem from cases of dementia provide a valuable source of research material. Many enzymes retain activity after death provided the body is refrigerated rapidly. Arrangements are made by some laboratories to collect deep-frozen material from pathologists able to supply it. Relatives of the deceased must be consulted, and usually give ready consent. As with biopsy samples, it is essential on safety grounds that the diagnosis of CJD should have been excluded by the pathologists for any case from which material is supplied for such purposes. The exact manner in which the specimens are taken from the

Table 17.2 Causes of progressive dementia seen in a series of over 500 adults autopsied cases in Oxford 1980–94.

Alzheimers disease – alone or with additional CHS pathology

Cerebrovascular disease – alone or with additional pathology

Parkinson's disease – with or without cortical Lewy bodies and with or without Alzheimer's disease and/or cerebrovascular disease

Cerebral tumour

Creutzfeldt–Jakob disease

Wernicke's encephalopathy and alcoholic cerebellar degeneration

Paraneoplastic encephalitis

Huntington's chorea

Pick's disease

Frontal lobe dementia – with or without pathology of motor neuron disease

Normal pressure' hydrocephalus

Metachromatic leucodystrophy

Adreno leukodystrophy

Chronic subdural haematoma

Schizophrenia

AIDS encephalitis

Familial cerebral amyloid angiopathy

Progressive supranuclear palsy

Progressive multifocal leucoencephalopathy

---

fresh brain to be deep frozen is a matter for agreement between the pathologist and research worker, but one practical, convenient and usually acceptable procedure is to divide the brain into right and left halves by cutting through the corpus callosum, thalamic connection, floor of the third ventricle and hindbrain. One-half of the brain is deep frozen whole or sliced while the other half can be fixed by suspension if the basilar artery is retained with it. As the diseases that are likely to be responsible for progressive dementia virtually always involve both sides of the brain, there is very little danger of missing the diagnosis by adopting this procedure.

Naked-eye examination of the brain
(Table 17.1)

Although the list of pathological diagnoses in cases of dementia is very long (Table 17.2), in practice most cases are accounted for by a small number of conditions, and it is only when such conditions have been excluded, or one is confronted with the macroscopic evidence, that one needs to consider the rare alternatives. Most of the responsible conditions require only that the brain, and not other parts of the nervous system, be examined in detail. But if motor neuron disease with dementia is suspected, it is essential to examine the spinal cord as well.

The macroscopic appearance of the brain is of considerable help in distinguishing between likely causes of dementia. Findings in other parts of the body may also be important, particularly the state of the heart and blood vessels, the possible presence of tumours in viscera, and the state of the reticuloendothelial system. In multi-infarct dementia the brain is likely to show multiple areas of softening due to infarction (Fig. 17.1), and the cardiovascular system is likely to show advanced atheromatous disease. Occasionally, however, multi-infarct dementia occurs in the absence of gross lesions, there being innumerable tiny infarcts, barely visible to the naked eye, or an extensive cribriform state of the white matter. In most such cases, and in those in which there is more diffuse damage to white matter associated with a predominantly dementing illness, as occurs in Binswanger's disease, there is usually evidence of long-standing hypertension. In Alzheimer's disease, which is much the commonest cause of progressive dementia in adults, the naked-eye appearances of the brain are variable; occasionally it appears grossly atrophic, with narrowed cortical gyri, gaping sulci and enlarged subarachnoid spaces (Fig. 17.2), but more often it is only mildly atrophic, or within normal limits for the age of the patient. The MRI appearances in Alzheimer's disease are shown in Fig. 17.3. Cortical atrophy is more readily seen if the leptomeninges are stripped from the surface of the brain. In brain slices, cases of Alzheimer's disease show variable dilatation of the lateral ventricles, with narrowing of the corpus callosum. Some cases show mild atrophy of the caudate nuclei and others, particularly very elderly cases, focal atrophy of the hippocampus, amygdala, and temporal lobe, with compensatory dilatation of the inferior horns of the lateral ventricles (Figs 17.3 and 17.4). In Pick's disease there is focal, quite often asymmetrical, or generalized cerebral cortical atrophy, often of severe degree (Figs 8.10, 15.16, 17.5 and 17.6). The posterior two-thirds of the superior temporal gyri are characteristically spared. In slices, the brain may show atrophy of the caudate nuclei, and marked dilatation of the lateral ventricles (Fig. 8.10). Some cases of dementia have atrophy of the frontal lobes and in this respect resemble Pick's disease, but lack definitive microscopic features of the disease. Such cases have come to be known as cases of *frontal lobe dementia*. In Parkinson's disease with dementia, pallor of the substantia nigra is usually evident (Fig. 2.17), and in 'normal pressure hydrocephalus' there is marked ventricular dilatation, particularly of the lateral ventricles (see p.145). Evidence of obstruction to CSF flow should be sought, but cannot always be found. Most commonly it occurs in the subarachnoid space as a consequence of leptomeningeal thickening. In Huntington's chorea there is severe atrophy of the caudate nuclei and putamen (p.282; Figs 8.9 and 15.15), and in Binswanger's disease grey discoloration, possibly with foci of softening, in white matter of the

Fig. 17.1 Cerebral hemisphere slices from a case of multi-infarct dementia. Old infarcts (arrowed) are present in the left inferior frontal gyrus, insula, superior temporal gyrus and basal ganglia bilaterally, right parieto-temporal white matter and left calcarine region.

Fig. 17.2 Unusually severe, generalized, cortical atrophy in Alzheimer's disease. The leptomeninges have been stripped to show the narrowing of cortical gyri and widening of sulci (compare with Fig. 2.2).

centrum ovale (Figs 7.23 and 7.24). In CJD the brain usually appears normal to naked-eye examination, but in cases with exceptionally long survival, there may be marked atrophy of the cerebrum and/or cerebellar cortex (Fig. 17.7). In dementia associated with alcoholism the lesions of Wernicke's encephalopathy, or of cerebellar degeneration, may be visible to the naked eye (p.359).

Microscopic examination of the brain

The choice of blocks for microscopy depends on the clinical diagnosis and the range of possible pathological diagnoses that present themselves once the brain has been examined with the naked eye. Table 17.1 provides a guide to procedures, taking as the starting point the macroscopic appearance of the brain. Summarized alphabetically below

(a)

(b)

Fig. 17.3 Consecutive axial (a) and temporal lobe orientated (b) cranial CT scans in a 67-year-old female patient with progressive memory loss for recent events demonstrates moderate generalized changes of cerebral atrophy with enlargement of the sulci, ventricles and Sylvian fissures. In addition there is atrophy of the mesial temporal structures with enlargement of the choroidal fissures and temporal horns of the lateral ventricles. At autopsy the diagnosis of Alzheimer's disease was confirmed.

are the specific microscopic findings which should be identified in order to diagnose the most important diseases causing dementia. These represent minimum diagnostic requirements. Obviously in the context of many research projects there may be an indication to examine more widespread sites.

AIDS encephalopathy

This is a recently encountered cause of dementia in adults who may or may not be known to be suffering from AIDS at the time that psychiatric or neurological symptoms appear. The features found in the brain in AIDS encephalopathy, and the blocks recommended for examination if this is suspected, are described on p.174.

Alzheimer's disease

The characteristic microscopic findings are listed below.
1 The presence of numerous argyrophilic plaques in the hippocampus, neocortex (cortex outside the hippocampus and its immediate surroundings) and some subcortical nuclei, particularly the amygdala.
2 The presence of numerous neurofibrillary tangles in hippocampal pyramidal neurons and neurons of the subiculum, entorhinal region and parahippocampal gyrus,

Fig. 17.4 Comparison of normal temporal lobe and amygdala (left) with the same area from an elderly case of Alzheimer's disease (right). The latter shows atrophy of the amygdala (arrowed), with compensatory dilatation of the inferior horn of the lateral ventricle. In addition, the temporal lobe cortex and white matter are reduced in volume in Alzheimer's disease. (Compare with Fig. 2.4, level A1.)

Fig. 17.5 Lateral view of the cerebrum in Pick's disease. The lateral aspect of the temporal lobe is severely atrophied. Note relative sparing of the posterior part of the superior temporal gyrus (arrowed).

and of some neurofibrillary tangles in neurons of the neocortex, amygdala, nucleus basalis, raphé nuclei of the midbrain and certain other subcortical nuclei. The neocortex is not uniformly affected by tangle formation in Alzheimer's disease; for example, areas of association cortex tend to be severely affected, whereas primary sensory areas, apart from the olfactory cortex, are relatively spared, as is the primary motor cortex. Figures 2.26d and 2.32 show where the structures affected by tangle formation in Alzheimer's disease can be found.

3 The presence of neuropil threads, thread-like argyrophilic neuritic processes in grey matter, usually in association with neurofibrillary tangles (Fig. 17.8).

4 The presence of granulovacuolar degeneration (Fig. 17.14) in hippocampal pyramidal neurons. The same neurons may also contain Hirano bodies (Fig. 17.9).

5 Amyloid deposits in small leptomeningeal and cortical blood vessels (Fig. 3.35).

Fig. 17.6 Six consecutive axial cranial scans in a 61-year-old male patient suffering from memory loss, loss of concentration, disorientation and gait disturbance demonstrate atrophy involving the frontal lobes, anterior temporal lobes and caudate nuclei, consistent with a diagnosis of Pick's disease. Note the disproportionate enlargement of the sulci in these areas, enlargement of the Sylvian fissures and frontal horns of the lateral ventricles. The temporal horns were also dilated (not shown).

Fig. 17.7 Coronal slice through the left cerebellar hemisphere, vermis and medulla from a case of CJD. There is marked atrophy of the cerebellar folia.

Fig. 17.9 Hirano body (pink) lying adjacent to a hippocampal pyramidal neuron. H&E, ×800.

Fig. 17.8 Neurofibrillary tangles shown in a paraffin section stained by Cross' modification of the Palmgren stain (Appendix A). Many neuropil threads can be seen in the background. ×200.

6 Some neuron cell loss, not usually very conspicuous, at many of the sites that contain neurofibrillary tangles. Argyrophilic plaques are foci of degeneration in neural parenchyma containing abnormal neuritic processes and sometimes having at their centre a core of amyloid. Some silver stains (e.g. the methenamine silver stain shown in Fig. 3.16, see Appendix A) show up additional, diffuse, plaques which lack neuritic processes. Diffuse plaques can also be demonstrated by antibodies to A4/β amyloid protein (Fig. 3.44) and a number of other antibodies e.g. to

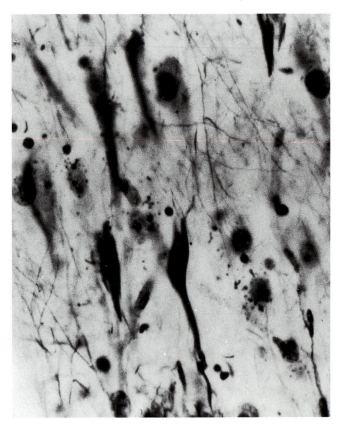

Fig. 17.10 Neurofibrillary tangles in a frozen section of the hippocampus in Alzheimer's disease. von Braunmühl, ×700.

complement components and apolipoprotein E. A4/β protein is thought to be the main component and the significance of these additional proteins for pathogenesis of the lesions is uncertain, but genetic evidence indicates that a

Fig. 17.11 Electron micrograph of a cortical pyramidal neuron containing a neurofibrillary tangle in a biopsy sample from a case of Alzheimer's disease. The bundles of paired helical filaments occupy the centre of the cell, where they are admixed with some lipofuscin. Uranyl acetate and lead citrate, ×6250. Inset top right: high-power view of the paired helical filaments. ×47 000. (Courtesy of Dr JJ Sloper.)

particular genotype coding for apolipoprotein E4 is a clear risk factor for Alzheimer's disease. The abnormal neurites are argyrophilic, and are more or less condensed into discrete, shrubby masses 20–200 μm across (Fig. 3.16). Neurofibrillary tangles are abnormal collections of argyrophilic, congophilic fibrillary material in neuron cell bodies (Figs 3.14, 17.8 and 17.10). Ultrastructurally, tangles are composed of bundles of helically wound, paired filaments (Fig. 17.11). A few filaments of the same type can also be found in the neurites in argyrophilic plaques and in neuropil threads (Fig. 17.12). Neuritic plaques and tangles, occurring together, are the most diagnostically useful pathological features of Alzheimer's disease. Plaques are not generally visible in H&E-stained sections, but can be seen with the PAS stain and are best shown with an appropriate silver method, such as that of Bielschowosky or methenamine silver (p.441), or with a stain for amyloid which shows up the core. Neurofibrillary tangles can be seen with H&E but are much easier to detect with silver stains, of which the best, in our hands, is Cross' modification of the Palmgren stain (see Appendix A). An amyloid stain demonstrates tangles quite well, and tangles also react with some neurofilament and tau antibodies (Fig. 17.13). Granulovacuolar degeneration is the accumulation

Fig. 17.12 Low-power electron micrograph of a cortical plaque in a biopsy sample from a case of Alzheimer's disease. The area occupied by the plaque is outlined by the dotted line. Details of the plaque structure cannot be displayed at this magnification, but clearly recognizable are expanded, dystrophic nerve endings containing dense bodies (D) and neuritic processes containing paired helical filaments (N). Uranyl acetate and lead citrate, ×3200. (Courtesy of Dr JJ Sloper.)

of abnormal argyrophilic granules in small, cytoplasmic spaces in neuron cell bodies (Fig. 17.14), and Hirano bodies are rod-shaped eosinophilic structures, composed principally of actin, lying adjacent to neuron cell bodies (Fig. 17.9). Both these structures are well seen with the H&E stain.

Cases of Alzheimer's disease occurring before the age of 65 years are easy to confirm pathologically because all the structures described above are usually present in profusion, whereas in normal brains of the same age they are present in no more than trivial numbers. In elderly cases of Alzheimer's disease, particularly those over 80 years, the microscopic changes of the disease are not so clearly distin-

guished from those found in 'normal' ageing, because all the features described above may occur to some extent in aged, undemented individuals. We do not intend to imply by this statement that the pathological features of Alzheimer's disease are an inevitable consequence of ageing; rather that very mild, locally restricted, clinically trivial, Alzheimer's lesions are exceedingly common in the very old. The pathologist needs to beware of attributing clinically evident dementia to the presence of some plaques in the cerebral cortex and some tangles in the hippocampal and related regions of the brain shown in Figs 2.26d and 2.32. A definition of Alzheimer's disease in the very old becomes a matter of quantitative distinction

Fig. 17.13 Cortical pyramidal neurons showing an abnormal reaction with neurofilament monoclonal antibody RT97. An adjacent section stained with silver showed reactive neurons contained neurofibrillary tangles. Counterstained with haematoxylin, ×200.

Fig. 17.14 Granulovacuolar degeneration in hippocampal pyramidal neurons from a case of Alzheimer's disease. Multiple, small cytoplasmic vacuoles contain basophilic granules (arrowed). H&E, ×670.

(Khachaturian 1985; Mirra *et al.* 1991). However, there is one feature which almost never occurs in 'normal' ageing, and that is the presence of tangles in the neocortex—that is, cortex outside the hippocampus and related entorhinal and parahippocampal regions. This we regard as the most useful single distinguishing feature of Alzheimer's disease in old age. Tangles are also greatly increased in number in the hippocampus and para-hippocampal/subicular regions in Alzheimer's disease, but detection of this increase above that found in normal ageing requires experience of tangle numbers that the pathologist may not have had the oppor-

tunity to acquire. In Alzheimer's disease in the very elderly, cortical tangles are not as widespread as in younger cases and are largely confined to temporal lobe neocortex. For this reason a block of temporal lobe cortex is the best place in which to search for the features of Alzheimer's disease in the very old. One or two additional areas of cortex should also be examined, e.g. frontal and parietal cortex, and the hippocampus should be examined for tangles, granulovacuolar degeneration and Hirano bodies. Sections of the mid brain (for substantia nigra and raphé) and pons (for locus ceruleus) should also be examined for tangles and to exclude additional features of Parkinson's disease which may co-exist with Alzheimer's disease. If substantial numbers of cases of Alzheimer's disease are likely to need diagnosis, or if a systematic study of elderly brains is being undertaken, we recommend use of the CERAD protocol (Mirra *et al.* 1991). Plaques tend to be most numerous in the outer three layers of the cortex, while tangles tend preferentially to occur in pyramidal cells of cortical layers 3 and 5. It is important to realize that most of the microscopic features that occur in Alzheimer's disease (albeit with slight modifications in the case of plaques) also occur in other diseases (Table 17.3), and it is the combination of all or most of them together in the same brain, and in the characteristic locations, that is diagnostic of Alzheimer's disease.

Chronic subdural haematoma

This condition may arise following a head injury or develop apparently spontaneously in the elderly. Usually there is some headache or clouding of consciousness, but occasionally dementia is the main presenting feature. Fluctuation in clinical state is usually obvious. There may be a chronic subdural haematoma membrane over one or both cerebral hemispheres (Fig. 11.1) (see also p.113). The underlying brain is frequently mildly oedematous, or may show evidence of recent or earlier ischaemic/hypoxic damage.

Creutzfeldt–Jakob disease

This is a rare disease associated with the presence in the brain of an, as yet, incompletely characterized transmissible agent. The agent, and the pathology it produces, closely resemble those found in another even rarer human disease, 'kuru', and in three animal diseases: scrapie in sheep, bovine spongiform encephalopathy in cows and mink encephalopathy. The agents responsible for CJD and scrapie, on which most work has been done, have unusual biological and chemical properties; the diseases they produce have unusually long incubation periods, measured in months or years, the agents themselves are resistant to most (but not all) physical and chemical agents that inacti-

Table 17.3 Other diseases showing one of the microscopic features of Alzheimer's disease.

Argyrophilic plaques
Normal ageing*
Down's syndrome (from early middle age)
Familial cerebral amyloid angiopathy (p.123)
Gerstmann–Sträussler syndrome

Neurofibrillary tangles
Normal ageing†
Postencephalitic parkinsonism (p.273)
Post-traumatic brain injury in boxers (p.108)
Parkinson–dementia complex of Guam
Subacute sclerosing panencephalitis (p.173)
Progressive supranuclear palsy (p.282)
Down's syndrome (from early middle age)
Familial cerebral amyloid angiopathy (p.123)
Gerstmann-Straussler syndrome

Granulovacuolar degeneration
Normal ageing*
Pick's disease
Parkinson–dementia complex of Guam
Down's syndrome

Hirano bodies
Normal ageing*
Parkinson–dementia complex of Guam
Down's syndrome
Many other conditions (see Tomlinson 1992)

---

*Small to moderate numbers compatible with normal mental state in old age.
†Limited to hippocampus and parahippocampal gyrus/subiculum in normal old age.

vate pathogens, and their infectivity is closely associated with the presence of a glycoprotein, prion protein, which tends to accumulate after extraction as amyloid-like fibrils. This associated protein is host derived—a fact that may explain another odd feature of these diseases, the lack of any agent-specific immune reaction.

When selecting blocks for microscopy from cases of suspected CJD it is preferable on safety grounds to avoid the use of formalin-frozen sections and to rely instead solely on paraffin sections. Three or four blocks of cerebral cortex, two or three of deep grey matter, and one or two of the cerebellar cortex should provide sufficient evidence with which to confirm or refute the diagnosis of CJD. For safety reasons the blocks should be immersed in formic acid for five minutes before being further processed (Appendix C). The characteristic microscopic features of the disease are spongy change (status spongiosus), neuron loss, and reactive gliosis (Figs 17.15 and 17.16). A few cases also show

amyloid plaques, which differ from Alzheimer plaques in their lack of peripheral neuritic processes, in their common location in the cerebellar cortex (Fig. 17.17), and their immunoreactivity for prion protein (Fig. 17.18). The spongy change is the most useful diagnostic feature, as the others are entirely non-specific. Spongy change is readily seen with the H&E stain, but is more impressive in a PTAH-stained section, which also shows the astrocytic reaction clearly. In most cases of CJD, spongy change, cell loss and gliosis are all quite widespread in the cerebral cortex, though they vary in severity from lobe to lobe, and the hippocampus tends to be relatively spared. Cerebellar cortex is also regularly affected, and shows mainly loss of the granule cells and spongy change in the molecular layer (Fig. 17.19). Deep grey matter involvement is variable, with the putamen liable to be affected and brain stem nuclei usually spared. In some cases there is loss of anterior horn motor neurons in the spinal cord. Reactive gliosis in CJD occurs not only at sites that have lost neurons, but also at sites whose afferent innervation has been destroyed (Fig. 17.20). Neuron loss is usually, but not always, severe enough to be appreciated by inspection of sections. Care must be taken to distinguish the spongy state of CJD from artefactual vacuole formation which may occur following dehydration during processing, particularly of oedematous brain. A useful point of distinction is that artefactual vacuoles surround neurons or small blood vessels, whereas the spongy state of CJD consists of empty vacuoles 5–50 μm across, located mainly in grey matter parenchyma. A condition known to be closely related to CJD, and capable of being transmitted to animals, is the Gerstmann–Sträussler syndrome, an inherited disease characterized by progressive dementia and ataxia. Spinocerebellar tracts show degeneration in this disease, and there are amyloid plaques in cerebral and cerebellar cortex, together with neuron loss and gliosis in the same areas. Spongy change is, however, not a feature of this disease, but some cases show β/A4 as well as prion protein plaques and some neurofibrillary tangles.

Frontal lobe dementia and dementia associated with motor neuron disease

Cases that conform clinically and pathologically to Pick's disease, but lack Pick cells and Pick bodies are now often referred to as cases of frontal lobe dementia. The pathology of this condition was recently reviewed (Mann *et al.* 1993). Macroscopically these cases show a variable degree of frontal lobe atrophy. Microscopically the feature of particular note is spongy change in layer two of the cortex in parts of the frontal and temporal lobes (Fig. 17.21). This is not a specific change but it is highly characteristic. There is also variable loss of neurons from the same areas and gliosis of cortex and underlying white matter. Certain subcortical

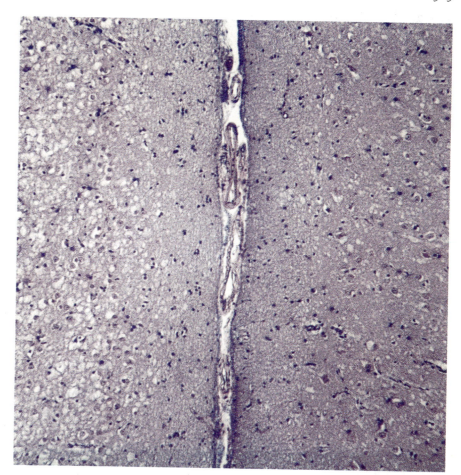

Fig. 17.15 Foci of spongy change (left) in the cerebral cortex from a case of CJD. The gyrus on the right is not affected. PTAH, ×100.

Fig. 17.16 Cerebral cortex from a case of CJD showing depletion of neurons and a marked excess of reactive astrocytes. PTAH, ×295.

Fig. 17.17 Amyloid plaques in the granule cell layer of the cerebellum in CJD (arrowed). PAS, ×560. (Courtesy of Prof. JH Adams.)

Fig. 17.18 Reaction for prion protein (brown) in cerebral cortex of a case of CJD. Conterstained with haematoxylin, ×400. (Section courtesy of Dr J Bell.)

Fig. 17.19 CJD. Spongy change in the molecular layer of the cerebellum. H&E, ×150.

nuclei are liable to show neuron loss, including the substantia nigra. There are no characteristic intraneuronal inclusions.

Case of dementia with motor neuron disease usually show pathological features of frontal lobe dementia with, in addition, pathological features of motor neuron disease (p.274). The latter may be confined to the anterior horns and hypoglossal nuclei in the medulla and not involve upper motor neurons.

General paralysis of the insane

This formerly common dementing disease, due to infection of the brain by *Treponema pallidum*, and a manifestation of tertiary syphilis, has fortunately become rare with the widespread availability of penicillin. It produces marked atrophy of the brain, particularly of the frontal lobes, with thickening of the overlying leptomeninges. The ventricles are moderately dilated, and their surfaces covered with tiny warts composed of glial fibres (Fig. 9.10). Microscopically, the affected parts of the cortex in untreated cases show an overall increase in cellularity and diffuse neuron loss. The extra cells are microglial cells, perivascular inflammatory cells and reactive astrocytes. Small blood vessels are also unusually prominent and endothelial cells hypertrophied. Iron deposits are found in microglial and endothelial cells. *Treponema* is found in untreated cases using appropriate stains, in groups or scattered singly in

(a)

(b)

Fig. 17.20 Adjacent sections from the hippocampus from a case of CJD showing the marked gliosis (a) that may occur despite preservation of the neurons (b). The gliosis in this case was attributable to loss of afferent fibres to the region. (a) Cajal, (b) Nissl, ×140.

Fig. 17.21 Frontal cortex from a case of frontal lobe dementia in which features of Pick's disease were absent but there was loss of cortical neurons and spongy change confined to layer 2, as shown here. H&E, ×100.

the neuropil of the cerebral cortex, in endothelial cells, and ingested in microglia. The overlying meninges in chronic cases show fibrosis and mild inflammation.

Multi-infarct (vascular) dementia

Cases of dementia due to cerebrovascular disease, the second most common cause of dementia in old age, are usually distinguishable clinically from those due to Alzheimer's disease. At post mortem examination the brains of such cases contain infarcts of various sizes ranging from grossly visible extensive areas of softening to numerous microscopic infarcts, or areas of white matter rarefaction around hyalinized cerebral arterioles. Binswanger's disease, in which the latter changes are accompanied by more diffuse damage to cerebral white matter (Fig. 17.22), is also thought to be due to an attenuated blood supply in patients with long-standing hypertension. Occasionally there are numerous small cortical infarcts and tiny haemorrhages associated with extensive amyloid

Fig. 17.22 Horizontal section of posterior parietal and occipital lobe from a patient with vascular dementia, stained for myelin (blue). There is diffuse pallor of myelin staining in subcortical parietal white matter. The cortex also showed small foci of infarction.

deposition in leptomeningeal and cortical blood vessels (Fig. 3.35). This may be associated with evidence of occlusion of some of the affected vessels, sometimes with recanalization, or with an inflammatory reaction around them. Such cases are almost always associated with some plaque and tangle formation, though this may not be sufficiently extensive to warrant a diagnosis of Alzheimer's disease. Conversely, although cerebrovascular amyloid deposition is a characteristic feature of Alzheimer's dis-

ease, it is not, in most cases, associated with cortical infarction of the type described above. However, it is not uncommon for the features of Alzheimer's disease to coexist along with cerebral infarction due to atheroma or embolism in elderly subjects, and it is therefore necessary, in cases of possible multi-infarct dementia, to exclude coexisting Alzheimer's disease by examining a temporal lobe/hippocampal section for the features of this disease as well as examining sections of softened areas to confirm the presence of infarction and to try to identify the pathology of the underlying vascular disease (see Chapter 7). Arteritis or lymphomatous blockage of small vessels are among the rarer causes of multi-infarct dementia.

Parkinson's disease with dementia

The lesions responsible for the development of dementia in a minority of cases of Parkinson's disease are not clearly established. The lesions of Parkinson's disease, neuron loss and Lewy body formation (p.273), though principally located in the pigmented nuclei of the brain stem, are not confined to these sites, but are also found in the nucleus basalis and in the cerebral cortex. It is possible that damage to these structures provides an explanation of the dementia in some cases of Parkinson's disease, and these sites should be examined microscopically in such cases (see Fig. 2.26c and d for the location of the nucleus basalis). Lewy bodies in the cortex are most abundant in the parahippocampal gyrus, cingulate gyrus and insula. The appearance of the bodies here is less distinctive than in the substantia nigra. They may be more readily detectable with an antibody to ubiquitin than in haematoxylin and eosin preparations (Fig. 17.23). Features of Alzheimer's disease should also be sought, as some cases show pathological features of both

(a)

(b)

Fig. 17.23 Appearance of cortical Lewy bodies (arrows) in the cerebral cortex (a) with haematoxylin and eosin (b) ubiquitin immunostaining. ×400.

(a)

(b)

Fig. 17.24 Low-power view of cerebral cortex from a severely affected temporal lobe in Pick's disease (above), with control (below). The width of the cortex in Pick's disease is approximately halved, and larger neurons, which are just detectable at this power in the control, are almost entirely absent in Pick's disease. LBCV, ×25.

Parkinson's disease and Alzheimer's disease. It is possible that dementia in Parkinson's disease is attributable to damage to structures such as the nucleus basalis by the process responsible for Parkinson's disease, summating with plaque and tangle formation which is of a degree that would, on its own, be insufficient to produce clinical dementia.

Other conditions to consider in cases of dementia with nigral cell loss but no Lewy bodies are progressive supranuclear palsy (p.282) corticobasal degeneration and frontal lobe dementia. Corticobasal degeneration is a rare form of neurodegeneration characterized clinically by pro-gressive weakness, apraxia and rigidity with, in the late stages, memory impairment and dysphasia. Neuropathologically there is atrophy of the pre- and post-central gyri with loss of neurons and gliosis. Large, pale ballooned neurons resembling those seen in Pick's disease are also found.

Parkinsonism–dementia complex of Guam

Symptoms of progressive dementia, parkinsonism and motor neuron disease occurring in combination in the same subject or in different members of one community are

Fig. 17.25 Swollen neuron cell body with pale cytoplasm (Pick cell) in the temporal lobe cortex from a case of Pick's disease. Nissl, ×800.

(a)

(b)

Fig. 17.26 Pick bodies; rounded cytoplasmic, argyrophilic inclusions (a) in hippocampal pyramidal neurons (arrowed); (b) in the dentate fascia granule cells in Pick's disease (black). (a) H&E, ×250. (b) Cross' modification of Palmgren, ×100.

remarkably common among the Chamorro tribe of the Mariana Islands in the Pacific. The pathology of this condition is reviewed by Hirano & Llena (1986).

Pick's disease

This rare autosomal dominant (occasionally sporadic) disease produces distinctive appearances in the brain, with severe focal cerebral atrophy most commonly confined to the frontal and temporal poles (Figs 8.10, 15.16 and 17.5), but sometimes occurring in a more widespread distribution (Fig. 8.10). A characteristic feature is sparing of the posterior two-thirds of the superior temporal gyrus. The cortex displays the most marked atrophy, but there may also be atrophy of the caudate nuclei and loss of cerebral white matter. Microscopy should be performed on sections of atrophic cortex, less severely affected cortex, hippocampus and brain stem. The worst affected areas show severe neuron loss (Fig. 17.24), with reactive astrocytosis and fibrillary gliosis of underlying white matter. Some neuron cell bodies are greatly expanded by argyrophilic collections of neurofilaments (Pick cells) (Fig. 17.25). Others contain collections of neurofilaments (Pick bodies) that do not actually expand the cell body (Fig. 17.26). Pick cells may be focally plentiful, but can be difficult to find in cortex that has been largely depleted of neurons. Pick bodies can usually be found in the dentate granule cell and pyramidal cell layers of the hippocampus (Fig. 17.26). Granulovacuolar degeneration also occurs in the hippocampus, and occasional cases show other features of Alzheimer's disease, including plaques and tangles.

Cases of dementia without specific pathology

In around 5–8% of cases in published series of elderly subjects with well-documented histories of dementia, no specific pathology has been found within the brain. Particular groups of such patients are recognized.

1 Those with dementia and symptoms of motor neuron disease: such cases show the pathology of motor neuron disease (p.271), but no more than slight spongy change in layer 2 of the cortex (precentral motor cortex and elsewhere) to account for their dementia.

2 Chronic alcoholics who were demented may show lesions of Wernicke's encephalopathy (p.359), or those of repeated head injury (p.108), but some show none of these lesions, and in these cases the cause of dementia may remain undefined.

3 Chronic schizophrenics who become demented (see p.427).

4 Those with 'toxic' dementia (e.g. dialysis dementia).

5 Very old subjects who may show a mild degree of plaque and tangle formation that is insufficient to justify a diagnosis of Alzheimer's disease. Such cases may also have small areas of vascular or hypoxic damage to the brain, which may precipitate development of symptoms of dementia in people who would otherwise remain asymptomatic.

6 Some cases of prion disease—for example, familial dementia in which other family members have shown well-developed features of CJD—have shown no specific brain pathology.

Further reading and references

Bell JE, Ironside JW. 1993. How to tackle a possible Creutzfeldt–Jakob disease necropsy. *J Clin Pathol* **46**, 193–7.

Committee on Health Care Issues of the American Neurological Association 1986. Precautions in handling tissues, fluids and other contaminating materials from patients with documented or suspected Creutzfeldt–Jakob disease. *Ann Neurol* **19**, 75–7.

Esiri MM, Morris JH (Eds) 1996. *Neuropathology of dementia.* Cambridge University Press, (in press).

Hirano A, Llena J. 1986. Neuropathological features of Parkinsonism–Dementia complex of Guam: reappraisal and comparative study with Alzheimer's disease and Parkinson's disease. In Zimmerman HM (Ed) *Progress in Neuropathology* **6**. Raven Press, New York, 17–31.

HMSO. 1991. Health Services Advisory Committee. *Safety in Health Service Laboratories.* HMSO, London.

HMSO. 1994. Health Services Advisory Committee. *Precautions for work with human and animal transmissible spongiform encephalopathies.* HMSO, London.

Khachaturian ZS. 1985. Diagnosis of Alzheimer's disease (Conference Report). *Arch Neurol* **42**, 1097–104.

Mann DMA, South PW, Snowden JS, Neary D. 1993. Dementia of frontal lobe type; Neuropathology and immunohistochemistry. *J Neurol Neurosurg Psychiat* **56**, 605–14.

Mirra SS, Heyman A, McKeel D, *et al.* 1991. A consortium to establish a registry for Alzheimer's disease (CERAD). Part II. Standardisation of the neuropathologic assessment of Alzheimer's disease. *Neurology* **41**, 479–86.

Roth M, Iversen LL (Eds) 1986. Alzheimer's disease, and related disorders. *Br Med Bull* **42**, No. 1. Churchill Livingstone, Edinburgh.

Tomlinson BE. 1992. Ageing and the dementias. In Adams JH, Duchen LW (Eds) *Greenfield's Neuropathology*, 5th edn. Edward Arnold, London, 951–1025.

18   Epilespy

Epilepsy is an episodic disorder due to excessive synchronous electrical discharges by groups of neurons. Isolated epileptic fits occurring in the context of a generalized metabolic disorder are not included in the definition, and do not give rise to specific cerebral pathology in most cases. It is the task of the pathologist to attempt to identify pathological changes occurring in the brain of an epileptic subject in material examined either after surgical removal or at post mortem. The pathological changes associated with epilepsy range from gross lesions such as large tumours to minute or even microscopic irregularities, the significance of which is often doubtful. In some instances there may be dispute as to whether the lesions are the cause or the effect of the patient's fits. In about two-thirds of cases in published series an acceptable cause for epilepsy can be identified, though the exact proportion varies with age and with duration of epilepsy. In the remaining third of the cases no structural lesion can be identified. It should be pointed out that most of the literature on the pathology associated with epilepsy is concerned with severe cases, and the proportion of mild cases in which lesions can be identified is probably much lower.

In those cases in which a structural lesion is present, the mechanism that allows the excessive electrical discharge which generates the fit to occur is obscure. It is thought likely that interference with normal inhibitory influences acting upon pyramidal cortical neurons, particularly those mediated by the neurotransmitter gamma-aminobutyric acid (GABA), is involved. In those cases of epilepsy in which no structural lesion can be identified there may be an important genetic predisposition to epilepsy (McKusick 1983), but the structural basis for such a predisposition, if any, is unknown.

The commonest brain lesions thought to play a causative role in epilepsy are, in children, birth and neonatal injuries (Chapter 21), a preceding febrile convulsion (especially if prolonged), vascular accidents, head injuries (Chapter 5) and malformations (Chapter 16). The ultrastructural observation that in young monkeys an episode of hypoxia results in degeneration of predominantly symmetrical, inhibitory synapses in the cerebral cortex may be relevant to the pathogenesis of epilepsy in infants suffering perinatal brain damage (Sloper, Johnson & Powell 1980). In adults the commonest related conditions are cerebral tumours (Chapters 11 and 12) or head injury (Chapter 5), followed by infections of the brain and its coverings – bacterial, viral or parasitic (Chapters 9 and 10) – and in later life, degenerative diseases such as Alzheimer's disease (Chapter 17) or cerebrovascular disease (Chapter 7). Table 18.1 lists a number of conditions giving rise to epileptic fits.

Post mortem examination of the body of a known epileptic is sometimes required in circumstances that make it unclear whether epilepsy was responsible for the terminal event. For example, the subject may have been found dead at home unexpectedly. In these cases it is necessary to search for evidence of a recent fit, such as incontinence or tongue-biting. Not infrequently there is evidence of inhalation of vomit while unconscious. Clues of this sort are more likely to establish a cause of death in such cases than an examination of the brain.

When examining the brain of an epileptic patient post mortem the areas of special interest are the cerebral cortex, hippocampus and cerebellum. It is factors acting on the cerebral cortex that tend to initiate epilepsy, and these factors are most likely to be epileptogenic if they are situated near the central sulcus. The two most characteristic lesions in the brains of epileptics are cell loss and gliosis in the hippocampus and cerebellar cortex. These are now generally regarded as effects rather than causes of fits. These two areas are well known to be vulnerable to hypoxia, however caused; similar lesions can be produced in animals subjected to experimental seizures. There is increasing support for the view that the hippocampal lesion may result from the toxic effect of excess excitatory neurotransmitter. Cerebral hypoxia during prolonged fitting may also contribute. According to one view, the hippocampal lesion (commonly referred to as Ammon's horn sclerosis) may itself act as an epileptic focus, and a sequence has been suggested in which febrile convulsions in childhood lead to Ammon's horn sclerosis, which leads to temporal lobe epilepsy in later life.

Table 18.1 Some major causes of epilepsy.

Focal intracranial lesions
Tumour
Abscess
Angioma

Inflammatory conditions
Meningitis
Encephalitis

Trauma
Perinatal brain injury
Head injury
Operative neurosurgery

Congenital abnormalities and malformations

Degenerations and inborn errors of metabolism
Neuronal storage disorders
Leucodystrophies
Pick's disease
Alzheimer's disease
Creutzfeldt–Jakob disease

Vascular disorders
Infarction
Haemorrhage
Hypertensive encephalopathy
Eclampsia
Autoimmune disorders (e.g. systemic lupus erythematosus)
Intracranial aneurysm

Intoxications

No apparent cause (idiopathic)

Naked-eye appearance of the brain

Appearances of the brain in epileptics will obviously differ, depending on the cause. The external surface should be carefully inspected for focal cortical lesions such as a tumour (Fig. 18.1), or malformation, such as polymicrogyria (Fig. 16.13) or tuberous sclerosis (Figs 16.19 and 16.20). There may be evidence of acute or chronic meningitis, subdural empyema, old contusions due to head injury, or venous thrombosis.

Caution is needed in attributing epilepsy to contusions, as they may also be a consequence of falls suffered during fits (Fig. 18.2). Convincing evidence linking head injury causally to epilepsy has however come from follow-up studies during life of head injury victims. They have shown a particularly high risk of epilepsy developing if there has been an open head injury, i.e. one in which the skull was fractured and the dura breached. The prevalence in these conditions reaches 40% by 5 years after injury, whereas after a closed injury the equivalent figure is 10%. The important pathological lesion would appear to be a pial tear and mechanical damage to the underlying cortex (contusion). Slightly more than half of those developing epilepsy after a head injury do so after an interval of months or years, and there may be a similar delay before epilepsy develops following an infection such as a brain abscess. The reason for this delay is said to be the gradual evolution of an epileptogenic scar at the site of the lesion.

Tumours causing epilepsy can be fully assessed and described after the brain has been fixed and sliced. They are variable in size. Large tumours are almost certain to have been detected clinically (Fig. 18.3), but small ones sometimes escape clinical detection (Fig. 18.4). Slowly growing tumours are particularly liable to cause epilepsy. They are usually situated above the tentorium, and frequently impinge directly on the cortex. Common tumour types responsible for epilepsy are gliomas, metastases, meningiomas, angiomas, hamartomatous lesions and tuberous sclerosis (Chapter 16).

Of infective causes of epilepsy, abscesses and granulomas are likely to be evident macroscopically, as is herpes simplex encephalitis and meningitis. Other infections may require microscopy for identification.

Vascular causes of epilepsy include cerebral arterial and venous infarction, subarachnoid and intracerebral (especially lobar) haemorrhage, and perinatal vascular in-

Fig. 18.1 Temporal lobectomy specimen illustrating the external appearance of a small, superficial oligodendroglioma (arrowed).

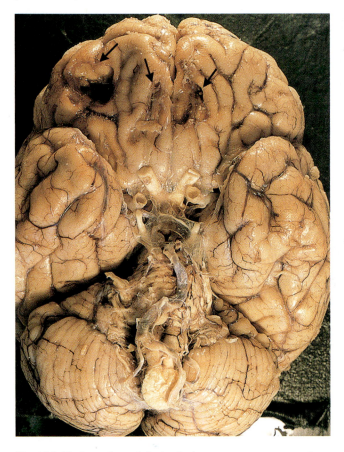

Fig. 18.2 Undersurface of the brain from a young woman who had suffered from epilepsy since early childhood. She had no history of trauma preceding the onset of epilepsy, but had suffered frequent falls during her fits. There are old, cortical scars attributable to these (arrowed).

sults. They are usually readily visible externally or when the brain is sliced.

Some of the lesions that result from epilepsy can be detected by careful naked-eye inspection of the brain. They include cerebral hemiatrophy (Fig. 16.6) in which the whole or most of one cerebral hemisphere, the ipsilateral thalamus and contralateral cerebellar hemisphere are smaller than on the other side. Also detectable by inspection are laminar cortical necrosis (Fig. 7.5), and atrophy of the hippocampus on one or, rarely, both sides (Fig. 7.7), which may be accompanied by atrophy of the ipsilateral fimbria and mamillary body.

Microscopic examination of the brain

In selecting blocks any lesions visible macroscopically should be included in the samples. It is also recommended that bilateral hippocampal blocks and a block of cerebellar cortex should be examined microscopically whether or not they show macroscopic lesions. Whether to take more blocks, if the brain appears normal macroscopically, is more problematic. We favour taking at least one additional block from the amygdala and another to include neocortex from an arterial boundary-zone territory, as damage to the neocortex, if present, tends to be maximal in such regions. It is also worth examining any parts of the neocortex which were known to have exhibited abnormal electrical activity on EEG recording, and in cases of Jacksonian epilepsy the appropriate part of the motor cortex should be examined.

Surgical specimens removed from subjects with epilepsy are likely to be either a tumour resection, which should be treated as discussed in Chapter 4, or an anterior temporal

Fig. 18.3 Right temporo-occipital astrocytoma from a case in which epilepsy, including psychomotor fits, dominated the clinical course.

Fig. 18.4 A small, superficial oligodendroglioma from a patient with psychomotor epilepsy. This is the cut surface appearance of the tumour shown in Fig. 18.1.

Fig. 18.5 Cortical dysplasia. Low power view of Nissl-stained section of cortex from a temporal lobectomy specimen showing a focus of disorganized neuronal architecture. There are abnormally large neurons scattered haphazardly through the cortical layers.

lobe resection or amygdalo-hippocampectomy performed for the relief of temporal lobe epilepsy. The latter is best sliced coronally, blocks for microscopy being taken to include any macroscopic lesions and, even in their absence, from each slice. If well-preserved temporal lobectomy specimens are regularly received in a department, it is likely that special investigations will be undertaken on them, since they are a scarce and valuable source of material that can be studied to advance understanding of human cortical organization in general and epilepsy in particular. Golgi studies, histochemistry and EM are all techniques of value for use on such material, but their choice depends on local interest and expertise, and they are not essential for routine diagnostic purposes.

Occasionally a hemispherectomy operation is performed for severe and intractable epilepsy. The surgical specimen received from this resection includes the cerebral cortex and white matter of all the main lobes from one cerebral hemisphere, together with variable portions of the amygdala and hippocampus. The specimen is usually sliced coronally after fixation and blocks for microscopy prepared from macroscopically abnormal areas from each slice, or from representative samples from each slice if no naked-eye lesions are visible. Small samples of tissue for special investigations, such as those outlined above for temporal lobe specimens, can be taken immediately after arrival of the specimen in the laboratory. Hemispherectomy specimens commonly show gross

(a)

(b)

Fig. 18.6 (a) Loss of neurons in the end folium in a case of long-standing epilepsy. (b) Normal end folium for comparison. (a) and (b) ×200.

lesions such as ulegyria (p.295; Fig. 16.14). The operation is sometimes complicated by postoperative bleeding and the development of superficial siderosis (p.124; Fig. 6.16), which may be found in patients dying after an interval of years.

In the absence of a macroscopic lesion in an epileptic brain, Nissl-stained sections are useful in searching for abnormalities in neuron populations or abnormal cyto-architecture in the cerebral cortex as occurs, not infrequently, in a focus of cortical dysplasia (Fig. 18.5). A glial

Fig. 18.7 Dentate fascia in epilepsy with Ammoni's horn sclerosis. Note how some of the cells are displaced to form a double layer. Nissl stain, ×100.

Fig. 18.8 Coronal SPGR MR image through the body of the hippocampal formations in an 18-year-old female patient with long standing left temporal lobe epilepsy, refractory to medical treatment. Compare the normal right hippocampal formation (arrow) with the atrophied left hippocampal formation indicating left hippocampal sclerosis. (High signal is often seen on T2W MRI within the atrophied hippocampal formation in hippocampal sclerosis due to gliosis.)

stain, particularly the Holzer stain, is also useful to detect areas of focal gliosis. Loss of neurons and gliosis should be searched for in the hippocampus, neocortex and cerebellum. Small degrees of cell loss will be missed unless quantitative studies are undertaken, but this is more appropriate for research than for routine investigation. The

sites most likely to show cell loss and gliosis in the hippocampus are the Sommer sector of the pyramidal cell layer (H1) (Fig. 7.8). and the end folium (H4) (Fig. 18.6). The granule cells for the dentate fascia are also reduced in some cases and a proportion of remaining cells may be displaced (Fig. 18.7). The H2 region is characteristically preserved. The hippocampal atrophy that results from the loss of these neurons and their fibres causes focal dilatation of the neighbouring inferior horn of the lateral ventricle. There may also be cell loss in the amygdala and temporal cortex, particularly in the fusiform, inferior and middle temporal gyri. The cell loss in the temporal lobe cortex is often accentuated at the depths of sulci, and it is usually laminar in distribution, affecting principally layers 2 and 3. It may extend outside the temporal lobe to arterial boundary zones in frontal, parietal and occipital lobes, or may involve the entire hemisphere and produce hemiatrophy. *Mesial temporal sclerosis* is a term used for the hippocampal and related pathology. It is interesting that in the great majority of cases it is a unilateral lesion (Fig. 18.8). Similar lesions can be induced in experimental animals by focal injection of kainic acid, and investigations of these lesions suggest that the hippocampal damage may be produced by neurotoxic effects of excess release of the excitatory neurotransmitter glutamate.

The cerebellar Purkinje cells, and to a lesser extent the granule cells, are susceptible to damage in epilepsy (Fig. 18.9). They may be affected together with, or independently of, the neocortical and hippocampal pathology. Prolonged seizures appear to cause physiological changes that are sufficient to reproduce similar experimental damage in animals. Although phenytoin, used extensively in the treatment of epilepsy, gives rise to cerebellar malfunction as a

Fig. 18.9 Low-power view of the cerebellar cortex from a case of long-standing epilepsy. Very few Purkinje cells remain, and the granule cell layer is somewhat reduced in width. The patient had received high doses of phenytoin for many years. H&E, ×35.

toxic side-effect, it is not certain whether it can give rise to cell loss of the type and extent seen in the cerebellum in some long-term epileptics.

Temporal lobe (psychomotor) epilepsy

The commonest lesion found in temporal lobe specimens surgically resected for the relief of temporal lobe epilepsy is mesial temporal sclerosis, which is present in 50–60% of cases (Meldrum & Corsellis 1984). Small glial or vascular tumours, scars due to previous head injury, old vascular lesions, inflammatory lesions and cortical dysplasia are also described, and in about 20% of cases no lesion is identifiable. Prognosis for cessation of fits following surgery is best if the lesion identified is mesial temporal sclerosis or a benign, completely resected tumour. The fact that removal of the focus of damage, which mesial temporal sclerosis constitutes, can frequently lead to cessation of temporal lobe (psychomotor) fits supports the view that this lesion, or one closely related to it, can itself act as an initiator or perpetuator of temporal lobe fits.

Status epilepticus

Epileptic fits lasting longer than an hour carry an appreciable mortality. Deaths in acute cases, particularly in adults, may be accompanied by no specific neuropathological changes. In most cases the brain appears swollen and congested and there may be a few petechial haemorrhages. Histological examination of the brain should include sampling the hippocampus on both sides, neocortex, thalamus and cerebellum. Quite frequently there is ischaemic cell change in a patchy or laminar distribution in the cortex, in the Sommer sector of the hippocampus, and in the thalamus and cerebellum. After several days' survival,

neuron loss and a microglial and astrocytic reaction are likely to be found at the same sites.

Myoclonic epilepsy

Myoclonus may occur as a symptom in a number of different diseases (Fahn *et al.* 1986). As a principal feature it occurs together with epilepsy in a rare, familial, metabolic condition, *Lafora body disease*. In this disease, which can be diagnosed during life on the basis of appearances in a liver or muscle biopsy, there is an abundance of concentric microscopic inclusions occurring in neuronal cytoplasm, axons and dendrites, and lying free in the neuropil of the brain. The Lafora bodies are most numerous in the thalamus, globus pallidus, substantia nigra, superior olives, brain stem reticular formation, lateral geniculate bodies, dentate nuclei and pre- and post-central gyri. Blocks for microscopic examination, if this condition is suspected, should be prepared from these sites. The inclusions are intensely stained by PAS and stains for acid mucopolysaccharides. They appear basophilic with haematoxylin, a point of distinction from Lewy bodies, which they otherwise resemble. They closely resemble corpora amylacea (see p.73; Fig. 3.47).

Occasionally severe myoclonus occurs in the absence of Lafora bodies. Such cases may show features of a system degeneration, such as dentatorubral atrophy, or there may be predominantly cerebellar pathology. Myoclonus may occur as one of a number of features in other diseases, such as SSPE (Chapter 10), sialidosis type 1, Creutzfeldt–Jakob disease, or Alzheimer's disease (Chapter 17).

Further reading and references

Corsellis JAN, Bruton CJ. 1983. Neuropathology of status

epilepticus in humans. In Delgado-Escueta AV, Wasterlain CG, Treimen D, Porter RJ (Eds) *Status Epilepticus: Mechanisms of Brain Damage and Treatment*. Raven Press, New York, pp. 129–39.

Dam AM. 1980. Epilepsy and neuron loss in the hippocampus. *Epilepsia* **21**, 617–29.

Fahn S, Marsden CD, van Woert MH (Eds). 1986. Myoclonus. *Advs in Neurology* **43**. Raven Press, New York.

Jennett WB. 1965. Predicting epilepsy after blunt head injury. *Br Med J* **1**, 1215–16.

Jennett WB, Lewin W. 1960. Traumatic epilepsy after closed head injury. *J Neurol Neurosurg Psychiat* **23**, 295–301.

McKusick VA *et al*. 1983. *Mendelian Inheritance in Man*, 10th edn. William Heinemann, London.

Meldrum BS, Corsellis JAN. 1992. Epilepsy. In Adams JH, Duchen LW (Eds) *Greenfield's Neuropathology*, 5th edn. Edward Arnold, London, pp. 921–50.

Russell WR, Whitty CWM. 1952. Studies in traumatic epilepsy. 1 Factors influencing the incidence of epilepsy after brain wounds. *J Neurol Neurosurg Psychiat* **15**, 93–8.

Sloper JJ, Johnson P, Powell TPS. 1980. Selective degeneration of interneurons in the motor cortex of infant monkeys following controlled hypoxia: a possible cause of epilepsy. *Brain Res* **198**, 204–9.

Table 19.2 Diagnostic procedures for metabolic CNS diseases.

Condition	Useful investigations outside CNS	Definitive biochemical investigation	Tissues
GM$_2$ gangliosidosis	HCh + EM on suction rectal bx	Assay hexosaminidases A and B	WBC, CF, AFC
GM$_1$ gangliosidosis	HCh + EM on suction rectal bx	Assay β-galactosidase	WBC, CF, AFC
Neuronal ceroid lipofuscinosis	HCh + EM on skin, conjunctiva, blood	None	
Niemann–Pick disease (A, B)	HCh + EM on suction rectal bx, conjunctiva, bone marrow	Assay sphingomyelinase	WBC, CF, AFC
Gaucher's disease	HCh + EM on bone marrow	Assay β-glucocerebrosidase	WBC, CF, AFC
Mucopolysaccharidoses	HCh + EM on bone marrow	Mucopolysaccharide analysis; assay for suspected enzyme defect in light of findings in urine	WBC, CF, AFC
Mannosidosis	HCh + EM on bone marrow, blood, suction rectal bx	Assay α-mannosidase	WBC, CF, AFC
Fucosidosis	HCh + EM on bone marrow, blood, suction rectal bx	Assay α-fucosidase	WBC, CF, AFC
Aspartylglycosaminuria		Assay aspartylglycosylamine amidohydrolase, urinary metabolites	WBC, urine, CF, AFC
Fabry's disease	HCh + EM on skin biopsy	Examine urine for excess ceramide hexosides; assay lysosomal α-galactosidase A	Plasma, tears, urine, CF, AFC
Leigh's encephalopathy	Some cases show mitochondrial abnormalities in EM of muscle bx	Pyruvate metabolism and respiratory chain enzymes; blood lactate usually elevated	Variable; e.g. muscle, liver, cultured fibroblasts
Metachromatic leucodystrophy	HCh + EM on skin and nerve biopsies	Examine urine sediment for metachromatic granules, assay arylsulphatase A	Urine, serum, WBC, CF, AFC
Krabbe's leucodystrophy	–	Assay lysosomal galactocerebroside β-galactosidase	Serum, WBC, CF, AFC
Adrenoleucodystrophy	EM on adrenal cortex	Assay very-long-chain fatty acids	Serum, CF, AFC

AFC, cultured amniotic fluid cells (for prenatal diagnosis); EM, electron microscopy; CF, cultured fibroblasts; HCh, histochemistry; WBC, white blood cells; bx, biopsy.

into two main groups according to whether the grey or the white matter of the CNS is predominantly involved. We believe such a division can be helpful in the initial stages of the neuropathological diagnosis of difficult cases (Table 19.3). Detailed description of the individual diseases is not given here, but may be obtained from current textbooks of neuropathology such as *Greenfield's Neuropathology* (1992). In examining cases of inherited metabolic disease it is very important to reserve some fresh tissue for biochemical and histochemical study before fixing the remainder of the tissue. Tissues should also be taken for EM.

Inherited metabolic diseases chiefly affecting grey matter

Lysosomal disorders

The gangliosidoses

These are a group of disorders with autosomal recessive inheritance in which excess amounts of gangliosides of normal chemical structure are present in the brain, and, in some cases, in other organs as well. Two main groups are recognized:

Table 19.3 Guide to neuropathological diagnosis of diseases in which there is abnormal stored material in the CNS. (See Table 19.2 for confirmatory biochemical investigations.)

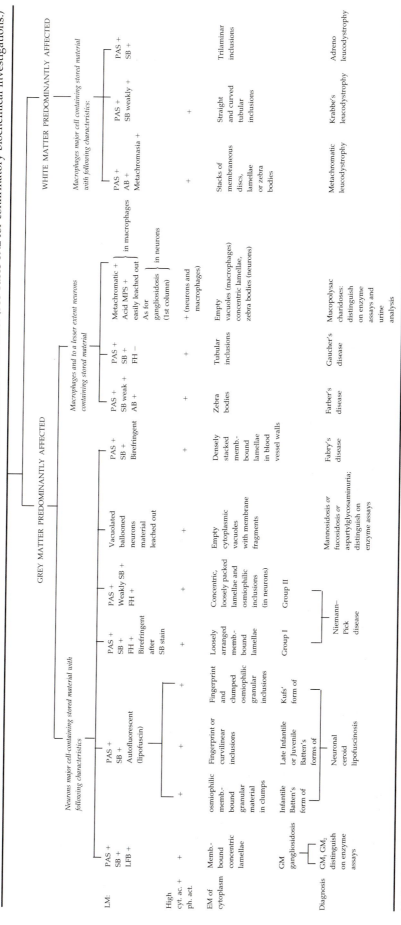

GREY MATTER PREDOMINANTLY AFFECTED

Neurons major cell-containing stored material with following characteristics:

	LM	High cyt. ac. + ph. act.	EM of cytoplasm	Diagnosis
	PAS +, SB +, LFB +	+	Memb.-bound concentric lamellae	GM gangliosidosis (GM₁, GM₂ distinguish on enzyme assays)
	PAS +, SB +, Autofluorescent (lipofuscin)	+	osmiophilic memb.-bound granular material in clumps; Fingerprint or curvilinear inclusions; Fingerprint and clumped osmiophilic granular inclusions	Neuronal ceroid lipofuscinosis — Infantile Batten's form of; Late Infantile or Juvenile Batten's forms of; Kufs' form of
	PAS +, SB +, FH +, Birefringent after SB stain	+	Concentric, loosely packed lamellae and osmiophilic inclusions (in neurons) — Group II	Niemann–Pick disease
	PAS +, Weakly SB +, FH +	+	Loosely arranged memb.-bound lamellae — Group I	Niemann–Pick disease
	Vacuolated ballooned neurons material leached out	+	Empty cytoplasmic vacuoles with membrane fragments	Mannosidosis or fucosidosis or aspartylglycosaminuria; distinguish on enzyme assays

Macrophages and to a lesser extent neurons containing stored material

	LM	High cyt. ac. + ph. act.	EM of cytoplasm	Diagnosis
	PAS +, SB +, Birefringent	+	Densely stacked memb.-bound lamellae in blood vessel walls	Fabry's disease
	PAS +, SB weak +, AB +	+	Zebra bodies	Farber's disease
	PAS +, SB +, FH −	+	Tubular inclusions	Gaucher's disease
	Metachromatic +, Acid MPS + easily leached out } in macrophages; As for gangliosidosis (1st column) } in neurons	+ (neurons and macrophages)	Empty vacuoles (macrophages); concentric lamellae, zebra bodies (neurons)	Mucopolysaccharidoses: distinguish on enzyme assays and urine analysis

WHITE MATTER PREDOMINANTLY AFFECTED

Macrophages major cell containing stored material with following characteristics:

	LM	High cyt. ac. + ph. act.	EM of cytoplasm	Diagnosis
	PAS +, AB +, Metachromasia +	+	Stacks of membraneous discs, lamellae or zebra bodies	Metachromatic leucodystrophy
	PAS +, SB weakly +		Straight and curved tubular inclusions	Krabbe's leucodystrophy
	PAS +, SB +		Trilaminar inclusions	Adreno leucodystrophy

AB, Alcian blue; EM, electron microscopical appearance; FH, ferric haematoxylin; LFB, Luxol-fast blue; LM, light microscopical appearance; MPS, mucopolysaccharide; PAS, periodic acid schiff; SB, Sudan black; cyt. ac. ph. act., cytoplasmic acid phosphatase activity.

The GM$_2$ gangliosidoses. These include infantile, juvenile and adult forms. Affected individuals are usually normal at birth but, in the infantile form, fail to achieve developmental milestones from a few months of age and develop blindness and progressive neurological abnormalities. A cherry-red spot is present at the macula on ophthalmological examination. At post mortem examination the brain may be normal in size, enlarged or atrophic. There is loss of a clear distinction between grey and white matter, and the cortical ribbon may be narrowed. All parts of the brain show microscopic abnormalities, the most striking being ballooning of neuronal cytoplasm, with compression of the nucleus to one margin of the cell. Large neurons are affected more than small ones, and neurons of sensory and autonomic ganglia are not exempt. In microscopic sections, in addition to the ballooning of neurons and a foamy appearance to their cytoplasm, there is an increase in number and size of microglial cells, which contain excess PAS-positive material. Stored material in neurons stains positively with Sudan black and Luxol fast blue. The ganglioside is found in increased numbers of large lysosomes, which can be demonstrated histochemically using the acid phosphatase reaction. EM of the stored material shows membrane-bound lysosomal structures filled with concentric lamellae. The enzyme which is deficient is hexosaminidase A, or, in Sandhoff's disease, hexosaminidase A and B.

GM$_1$ gangliosidosis. This presents in infants, young children or, rarely, in adults. In the infantile form there is hypotonia at birth, developmental delay, skeletal deformities, failure to thrive and hepatosplenomegaly. The brain at post mortem may be macroscopically normal or may show cor-

tical atrophy. Microscopically it shows ballooned neurons alongside normal ones in all areas (Fig. 19.1), and similar changes are present in the myenteric and submucosal plexuses of the gut. Appearances resemble those seen in GM$_2$ gangliosidosis, but the enzyme that is deficient is the lysosomal enzyme, β-galactosidase.

Neuronal ceroid lipofuscinosis

There are various forms of this condition, which differ in clinical features, age of onset and pathology, particularly at the ultrastructural level. The infantile form of Batten's disease presents from about 8 months with rapidly progressive motor and mental retardation, visual loss, ataxia and hypotonia. Death occurs at 3–10 years. Late infantile Batten's disease has its onset between 18 months and 4 years. Progressive mental and motor retardation with visual disturbance occur, with death eventually supervening at 4–10 years. In juvenile Batten's disease the initial presentation is with visual impairment in later childhood, followed by fits, gait disturbance and weakness, leading to death in the second or third decade. In the adult form (Kufs' disease) onset of symptoms may occur in childhood or adult life, with progressive dementia, ataxia, epilepsy and extrapyramidal movement disturbance. Most forms are recessively inherited.

In all forms of the disease the brain is found post mortem to be very atrophic and covered by thickened leptomeninges, and the skull is also thickened. The cerebral and cerebellar cortex are greatly narrowed and the white matter firm and gliotic. In general the changes are most severe in the infantile form. Microscopic sections show neuron loss, reactive gliosis and macrophage infiltration in

Fig. 19.1 GM$_1$ gangliosidosis. Appearance of swollen neurons in pontine nuclei. The cytoplasm is pale, and many of the nuclei are displaced from the centre of the cell. PAS. ×170.

many areas. All surviving neurons in infantile Batten's disease, and most in the other forms, contain prominent granular material with the histochemical characteristics of lipofuscin (PAS and Sudan black positivity and strong autofluorescence). Excess acid phosphatase activity can be demonstrated histochemically. Ultrastructural examination shows inclusions of differing type in the different forms of the disease. In infantile Batten's disease they consist of osmiophilic, granular, clumped material surrounded by a unit membrane. In late infantile Batten's disease they are curvilinear in form, in the juvenile disease fingerprint bodies are described and in Kufs' disease there are fingerprint and clumped osmiophilic inclusions. Outside the CNS stored material is present in neurons in peripheral ganglia, and in viscera, endothelium and muscle. The chemical nature of the stored material has not been identified, nor an enzyme defect uncovered.

Niemann–Pick (and related) disease

Two major subgroups of this disease are recognized: group 1, with sphingomyelinase deficiency, in which clinical forms with and without CNS involvement, in addition to visceral involvement, are distinguishable; and group 2, with normal sphingomyelinase activity, in which, again, there may or may not be early neurological involvement. All forms show enlargement of liver and spleen, and, in infants, failure to thrive. Infants in group 2 may also suffer severe neonatal jaundice. Childhood and adult cases, as well as infantile ones, occur in both groups. In group 1

cases with neurological involvement, the brain is slightly atrophic and the white matter firm. Neurons and glial cells are ballooned (Fig. 19.2), and white matter demyelinated, gliotic and infiltrated with foamy macrophages containing stored material. Similar macrophages, 20–90 μm across, infiltrate lymphoreticular tissue, and can be found also in most organs. These cells contain sphingomyelin and give a positive reaction in cryostat or frozen sections with Sudan black and ferric haematoxylin. The cytoplasmic deposits are also PAS-positive and show red birefringence under polarized light after Sudan black staining. The acid phosphatase reaction is strongly positive around the foamy vacuoles. By EM the neuronal inclusions contain loosely arranged lipid lamellae in membrane-bound vacuoles. There is a demonstrable deficiency of lysosomal sphingomyelinase in many tissues, including white blood cells and cultured fibroblasts. In group 2 cases with CNS involvement there may be slight cerebral atrophy and the white matter is gliotic, but not demyelinated. Ballooning of neuronal cytoplasm is present in all regions, and is accompanied by some axonal swelling. The stored material in neurons is not sphingomyelin, and in frozen sections is only weakly sudanophilic and stains positively with ferric haematoxylin and PAS. Spleen foam cells, however, do contain sphingomyelin, with the histochemical properties described above for group 1 cases. The neuronal stored material consists at the EM level of concentric, membrane-bound, loosely packed lamellae accompanied by dense osmiophilic inclusions. The enzymatic basis of the group 2 defect is not known.

Fig. 19.2 Appearance of ballooned neuronal cytoplasm in Niemann–Pick disease. Holmes/Luxol fast blue, ×530.

abnormal mitochondrial structure in some cases in skeletal muscle and, in a few cases, in the brain.

Hallervorden–Spatz disease

This is a rare, familial, slowly progressive disorder in which one noteworthy macroscopic change is found in the brain at post mortem: rusty-brown discoloration of the globus pallidus and reticular zone of the substantia nigra. In microscopic sections this can be seen to be due to deposition of brownish-yellow pigment in the cytoplasm of nerve cells, microglia and astrocytes. Extracellular pigment deposits are also present, particularly around blood vessels in the same areas. These deposits give a strong reaction for iron and are PAS-positive and Sudan-black-positive. Neurons are depleted in the globus pallidus and reticular zone of the substantia nigra and in some cases in the subthalamic nuclei and cerebellum (Purkinje cell layer and dentate nuclei), and reactive gliosis occurs at the same sites. A characteristic finding is of axonal swellings, appearing as round or oval bodies in a widespread distribution. The spinal cord may show pyramidal tract and posterior column fibre loss.

Neuro-axonal dystrophies are rare degenerative diseases in which axonal swellings similar to those seen in Hallervorden–Spatz disease are found widely distributed in the central and peripheral nervous system. These cases lack the pigment deposition characteristic of Hallervoden–Spatz disease.

Zellweger's cerebrohepatorenal syndrome

This is an uncommon autosomal recessive disorder of infancy in which there is a characteristic facial appearance and hepatomegaly progressing to cirrhosis, renal cysts and severe neurological abnormalities. The brain may show developmental abnormalities such as polymicrogyria, pachygyria or grey matter heterotopias (Chapter 16). There is also accumulation of neutral fat in astrocytes. EM studies

Fig. 19.8 Proliferated capillaries from a case of Leigh's encephalopathy. PAS, ×150.

Fig. 19.9 Microscopic appearance of the lesion shown in Fig. 19.7. This is a long-standing lesion in which pericapillary fibrosis is prominent, and there is some rarefaction of the neuropil (left). In more recent lesions the nerve cells tend to be fairly well preserved. Holzer, ×100.

Fig. 19.10 Metachromatic leucodystrophy. Myelin-stained section of occipital cortex and white matter. The pale streak coincides with the 6th cortical layer. Most of the white matter myelin is lost, though some is preserved in the immediately subcortical layer.

Inherited metabolic diseases chiefly affecting white matter

In inherited white matter disorders there is diffuse and widespread, though not universal, degeneration of myelin. Fibres lying just below the cortex tend to be spared, and elsewhere the damage is seldom uniform. The cerebral white matter is usually the most severely affected, with cerebellar and brain stem white matter better preserved. In some disorders peripheral myelin as well as central white matter is affected. Sampling of tissues at post mortem should therefore include peripheral nerves as well as spinal cord and brain. Fresh frozen cryostat blocks should be prepared from cerebral white matter and peripheral nerves, and further frozen samples need to be stored if biochemical analyses are to be carried out. Clinical suspicion of a disorder of white matter is likely to be present at the time of death, and a CT scan may have added weight to that suspicion. However, occasional cases present post mortem, and the pathologist should suspect the presence of one of these diseases from the peculiar feel of the brain after removal. The surface looks and feels normal, but a curious sensation is imparted of woody hardness inside, which is produced by the intense white matter gliosis. In occasional cases, in contrast, the white matter is unduly soft.

Lysosomal disorders

Metachromatic leucodystrophy

There are three forms of metachromatic leucodystrophy, all autosomal recessive disorders, but differing in the age

of the liver in this condition show a deficiency of peroxisomes, and there is absence of certain peroxisomal enzymes, such as acyl CoA dihydroxyacetone phosphate acyltransferase in cultured fibroblasts.

Fig. 19.11 Pontine bundles, showing partially preserved myelin sheaths, from a case of metachromatic leucodystrophy. The small, dark bodies are masses of metachromatic material. There are very few glial nuclei remaining. LBCV, ×130.

of onset and rate of progression. In the commonest, late infantile, variety there is progressive motor disability and later dementia. Some adult cases have a clinical diagnosis of schizophrenia.

Post mortem the brain appears normal or only slightly atrophic externally, but feels very abnormal. On slicing it after fixation there is found to be undue firmness and discoloration of the cerebral white matter. Cavitation is sometimes seen in the region of the lentiform nuclei and internal capsules. Microscopic sections show loss of myelin, with relative sparing of axons, diffuse gliosis (Fig. 19.10) and infiltration by macrophages, which in routine paraffin sections appear PAS-positive, and in cryostat sections can be shown to contain metachromatic, Alcian-blue-positive granules (Fig. 19.11), but no neutral fat. Although there is fibrillary gliosis, many neuroglial cell bodies disappear, imparting an air of desolation to the tissue. Metachromatic material (sulphatide) also accumulates in peripheral nerves and to some extent in the liver, gall bladder wall, and especially in the kidney. Deposits similar in nature to those found in the brain macrophages are also found in neurons in basal ganglia, brain stem and cerebellum, but not usually in cerebral cortex or peripheral ganglionic neurons. The ultrastructure of the stored cytoplasmic material is variable, but includes stacks of membranous discs, concentric or radial lamellae, paired membranes or zebra bodies. It consists chemically of sulphatide (cerebroside sulphate), and its accumulation is due to deficiency of arylsulphatase A. The diagnosis can be made by assaying the enzyme in blood leucocytes or cultured fibroblasts. A useful initial pointer to the diagnosis during life is provided by finding metachromatic granules in the urinary sediment.

Krabbe's leucodystrophy

This is a rare autosomal recessive disease with onset usually in early infancy, after normal development in the first few postnatal months. Neurological deficits are progressive, and epilepsy may occur. At post mortem the brain is usually small, and the white matter abnormally firm and discoloured (Fig. 19.12). Microscopically there is severe myelin loss, with astrocytic gliosis and prominent collections of enlarged macrophages, including epithelioid and multinucleated globoid cells (Fig. 19.13), but little or no neutral fat. Axons are relatively spared, but some are even-

Fig. 19.12 Krabbe's leucodystrophy. Cerebral slice showing discoloration and central spongy degeneration of the white matter.

Fig. 19.13 Krabbe's leucodystrophy. Globoid cells in perivascular spaces and brain parenchyma. LFB/PAS, ×400.

tually lost, and oligodendrocytes disappear from the most severely affected parts of the white matter. Globoid cells are found chiefly in perivascular spaces. They are derived from macrophages and measure up to 50 μm across. Some are multinucleate. They contain PAS-positive cytoplasm, and in fresh-frozen sections are weakly sudanophilic, show no metachromasia and react strongly for acid phosphatase. EM of the stored material shows straight or curved tubular inclusions scattered or aggregated in globoid cell cytoplasm. Neurons do not contain obvious stored material, but there may be some neuron loss in dentate nuclei and among Purkinje cells of the cerebellum, and in some brain stem nuclei, including the inferior olives. Peripheral nerves show segmental demyelination and increased acid phosphatase activity in Schwann cells but no collections of globoid cells. The enzyme which is deficient is lysosomal galactocerebroside-β-galactosidase. This can be assayed in blood leucocytes or cultured fibroblasts.

X-linked recessive leucodystrophies

Adrenoleucodystrophy

This is probably the most common form of sudanophilic leucodystrophy. Associated leucodystrophy and adrenal insufficiency in boys was its first recognized manifestation. There are now known to be infantile and adult varieties, not all sex-linked, as well as the juvenile form. Expression of the adrenal insufficiency is variable, and may occur only late in the course of the disease. Adult cases occur with cerebral disease or with a chronic myeloneuropathy, and females in affected families occasionally develop symptoms. In cases with cerebral disease the brain appears externally normal at post mortem, but on slicing shows diffuse white matter discoloration and firmness (Fig. 19.14). The most severe changes commonly occur in parieto-occipital and posterior temporal lobe white matter. Microscopically there is diffuse demyelination with relative, but far from complete, sparing of axons, and gliosis (Fig. 19.15). Macrophages containing sudanophilic material and reactive astrocytes are found in the affected white matter. There is also a prominent perivascular lymphocytic infiltrate, particularly at the sites of active myelin breakdown (Fig. 19.16). In the spinal cord there may be loss of distal axons in pyramidal tracts and posterior columns, and these changes may be the only abnormality found in the nervous system in adrenomyeloneuropathy (Fig. 19.17). Peripheral nerves show mild axonal loss. Macrophages in affected cerebral white matter and lymphoreticular tissue, Schwann cells in peripheral nerves, adrenal cortical cells and interstitial cells in the testis show typical ultrastructural cytoplasmic trilaminar inclusions (Fig. 19.18). The adrenal cortex is usually atrophic, and cortical cells have a fibrillary, or striated

cytoplasmic appearance on microscopy. There is known to be an excess of very-long-chain fatty acids in serum and cultured fibroblasts, and assays of these allow a diagnosis to be made and heterozygotes to be identified. The disease appears to be a peroxisomal disorder, with deficiency of the peroxisomal enzyme lignocerocyl Co A synthetase, which is required for β-oxidation of very long chain fatty acids (Naidu & Moser 1990).

Pelizaeus–Merzbacher disease

There are several recognized varieties of this rare disease, varying in age of onset and rate of progression. At post mortem examination the brain is frequently atrophic and the lateral ventricles dilated. White matter is discoloured and firm. Microscopically the white matter shows loss of myelin with some preservation of axons, reactive gliosis, but only rare macrophages which contain sparse

Fig. 19.14 Adrenoleucodystrophy. Granular discoloration of the parieto-occipital white matter.

(a)

(b)

Fig. 19.15 Adrenoleucodystrophy. (a) Parieto-occipital white matter, extensively demyelinated. (b) Adjacent section, showing diffuse gliosis in the demyelinated white matter. (a) Myelin stain, (b) Holzer stain.

Fig. 19.16 Adrenoleucodystrophy. Prominent lymphocytic cuffing around a vein in the demyelinated white matter. Reactive astrocytes are seen bottom right. H&E, ×160.

sudanophilic material. The loss of myelin is not uniform, but shows characteristic preservation of myelin around blood vessels. Oligodendrocytes disappear from the demyelinated zones. Absence of proteolipid apoprotein has recently been demonstrated in the CNS in this disease. The peripheral myelin, which normally lacks this protein, is unaffected.

Other forms of sudanophilic leucodystrophy

Cases of diffuse and widespread myelin loss, apparently sporadic or familial, are seen from time to time in which no distinguishing features of diagnostic significance are present. Macrophages in areas of myelin breakdown contain neutral fat. Most such cases show no consistent abnormalities outside the CNS. Better characterization of these cases awaits biochemical analysis. The diagnosis is made largely by exclusion of other, better-defined diseases causing sudanophilic breakdown of CNS myelin, including the Schilder type of MS (Chapter 14).

Fig. 19.17 Adrenoleucodystrophy. Transverse section of cervical spinal cord, showing pallor of myelin staining due to loss of fibres in lateral corticospinal tracts and posterior columns.

Fig. 19.18 Electron micrograph of the cytoplasm of a macrophage in the white matter in a cerebral biopsy from a case of adrenoleucodystrophy. There are characteristic trilaminar inclusions (arrowed). Uranyl acetate and lead citrate, ×43000.

Fig. 19.19 Coronal T2W MR images (A–D: from back to front) of a 3-month infant with hypotonia, macrocephaly and seizures who was subsequently shown to have Canavan's disease. Diffuse symmetrical high signal is noted in the cerebral white matter bilaterally due to myelin spongy degeneration. The subcortical white matter is affected the worst with relative sparing of the internal capsule. (Alexander's disease is also associated with macrocephaly but myelin damage demonstrates a frontal predominance).

Spongiform leucodystrophy (Canavan's type of diffuse sclerosis)

This is a rare familial disease affecting infants or children, who develop enlargement of the head, mental retardation and spastic weakness. MRI shows diffuse high signal in the cerebral white matter (Fig. 19.19). The centrum semiovale is the most severely affected region, and it shows demyelination and a spongy state with vacuoles intersected by a meshwork of glial and axonal processes. The grey matter is relatively well preserved, but contains astrocytes with swollen, lobulated nuclei, similar to Alzheimer type 2 glia.

Cockayne's syndrome

This is an autosomal recessive disease commencing in late infancy, and characterized by dwarfism, cataracts, retinal pigmentation, optic atrophy, deafness, mental retardation, pyramidal and extrapyramidal motor disorders, ataxia

and peripheral neuropathy. The skull is abnormally thick, and the brain small and covered in thickened leptomeninges. On slicing the brain there is a gritty texture due to extensive calcification of blood vessels, particularly in the basal ganglia. Both grey and white matter are reduced in amount, and the ventricles dilated in compensation for this. Microscopically, apart from the vascular calcification, there is patchy demyelination of cerebral white matter, and a deficiency of Purkinje and granule cells in the cerebellum. The pathogenesis of the disease is unknown.

Cerebrotendinous xanthomatosis

This is an autosomal recessive disease presenting in late childhood with progressive dementia and cerebellar ataxia. There is a defect in the synthesis of bile acid, and over-production of cholesterol, which is converted to dihydrocholesterol, in which form it is deposited in tissues, including the brain. A pathological study reported softening and discoloration of the cerebellar white matter macro-

Fig. 19.20 Focus of cortical micro vacuolation and necrosis in a case of hepatic encephalopathy. H&E, ×200.

scopically, and clefts resulting from dissolved cholesterol crystals in white matter accompanied by a macrophage and foreign body giant-cell reaction microscopically.

Lipoprotein deficiencies

These are autosomal recessive conditions. Low-density lipoprotein deficiency (abetalipoproteinaemia, Bassen – Kornzweig syndrome) is characterized clinically by retinal degeneration, progressive neurological symptoms, acanthocytosis and fat malabsorption. Demyelination has been described in long tracts of the spinal cord and peripheral nerves, with some loss of neurons in the motor cortex and anterior horns of the spinal cord. In high-density lipoprotein deficiency (Tangier disease) there may be a severe peripheral neuropathy, with axonal degeneration and accumulation of lipid-containing macrophages in nerves.

Sporadic metabolic diseases chiefly affecting grey matter

Non-wilsonian hepatic encephalopathy

In some patients dying of chronic or acute-on-chronic liver disease there are no naked-eye abnormalities in the brain other than a variable degree of generalized swelling. However, there are frequently microscopic changes attributable to liver disease. Astrocytes are increased in number and contain enlarged, lobulated vesicular nuclei (Alzheimer type 2 glia) (Fig. 19.3). These altered astrocytes are most frequently seen in the deep layers of the cerebral cortex, subcortical white matter, basal ganglia, thalamus,

Fig. 19.21 Reye's syndrome. Low-power view of cortex and white matter, showing oedema of deep cortex and subcortical white matter, with some additional, patchy necrosis in more superficial layers of the cortex (arrowed). PTAH.

hypothalamus, and deep cerebellar grey and white matter. Some of these sites should be sampled for microscopy from cases of possible hepatic encephalopathy. There is also frequently a microcystic or spongy appearance in the deep cerebral cortex, with patchy necrosis and neuronal loss (Fig. 19.20), and widespread eosinophilic shrinkage of the cell bodies of some remaining neurons. This change may proceed to necrosis in cortical layers 5 and 6, and may also involve subcortical white matter. Experimental work in animals has shown that the histological changes of hepatic encephalopathy can be produced by raising the blood ammonia level.

In addition to the cerebral changes, a peripheral neuropathy of predominantly demyelinating type has been

Fig. 19.22 Cerebral calcification, with deposits of calcium in the cortex appearing as dark streaks.

described in hepatic failure. In practice, in an individual case of chronic liver disease due to alcoholism it is usually impossible to dissociate effects on peripheral nerves of thiamine deficiency from those due to liver disease.

Reye's syndrome

This is an acute disease of infants and children which should always be considered when performing a post mortem examination on a child who has died after a fulminating illness with epilepsy and coma. There is epidemiological evidence linking the disease to preceding acute viral infections, especially influenza or varicella, and with salicylate ingestion. In the course of the illness, liver function is abnormal and there is hyperammonaemia and hypoglycaemia. Post mortem there is panlobular, microvesicular fat deposited in liver hepatocytes, and a diffusely swollen brain, often with herniation. Microscopically the brain shows acute eosinophilic shrinkage of neurons in grey matter, sometimes affecting the cortex in a laminar distribution, and with associated oedema but no inflammation (Fig. 19.21). It is not clear whether the changes in the brain are wholly attributable to an acute derangement of liver function, hypoxia associated with swelling or hypoglycaemia, or whether there is also a primary metabolic brain abnormality. Mitochondrial structure has appeared abnormal in both neurons and hepatocytes in ultrastructural studies.

Hypoglycaemia

It is uncommon to find structural changes in the adult brain attributable to hypoglycaemia unless this has been profound and prolonged, as occurs after an overdose of insulin, or occasionally in patients with an insulin-producing islet cell tumour. Babies of low birth-weight may also suffer brain damage due to hypoglycaemia. In these circumstances the pathological changes in the brain are similar to those found in hypoxia (p.51). Neurons in the cerebral cortex, particularly in layers 3 and 5, are likely to show acute hypoxic change, or to have disappeared, depending how much time has elapsed between the episode of hypoglycaemia and death. The hippocampus and deep grey matter may be similarly affected. Damage in the cortex tends to be worst at the depths of sulci (Fig. 7.6), as in hypoxia. The cerebellar Purkinje cells are only slightly less susceptible to hypoglycaemia than to hypoxia.

Calcification of the basal ganglia

A mild degree of calcification in the walls of blood vessels in the basal ganglia is a common incidental finding in elderly brains. Occasionally it is much more severe, occurs more widely in the brain and is associated with clinical disturbances, chiefly extrapyramidal movement disorders. This is seen mainly in patients who are suffering from hypoparathyroidism, but it is also seen in those with mitochondrial cytopathies, Albright's hereditary osteodystrophy, or Cockayne's syndrome (see above), and in some patients without a demonstrable endocrine

Fig. 19.23 Very extensive calcification in the basal ganglia; small vessels are heavily affected. PTAH, ×100.

disorder. Calcification, in all these cases, occurs most heavily in the basal ganglia, internal capsules, lateral thalamic nuclei and dentate nuclei of the cerebellum (Figs 19.22–19.23). Also affected are the cerebral and cerebellar cortex. It is apparent on slicing the brain, as it imparts a gritty resistance to the knife. Calcium deposits occur in the walls of capillaries as tiny calcospherites and more diffusely in larger vessel walls. The surrounding nervous tissue is destroyed but there is little glial or inflammatory reaction.

Sporadic metabolic diseases chiefly affecting white matter

Alexander's disease

This is a rare, sporadic disease occurring in infants or children and presenting with progressive psychomotor retardation and epilepsy. At post mortem the brain tends to be larger than normal, and the cortical ribbon is relatively well preserved. The white matter is soft, almost jelly-like, and discoloured. Microscopically the white matter shows rarefaction with loss of myelin and of some of the axons. The brain stem is less severely affected. The distinctive feature is the presence of vast numbers of Rosenthal fibres (p.203), elongated, hyaline, eosinophilic structures, staining strongly with PTAH (Fig. 19.24). Many of these are oriented around blood vessels and pial and ependymal surfaces. The basic defect in this disease is not known.

Central pontine myelinolysis

This is a rare, sporadic disease affecting adults who are alcoholics or are suffering from a variety of other disorders such as carcinoma, severe malnutrition or chronic renal, pulmonary or hepatic disease. Symptoms and signs of a pontine lesion have usually been present for a few days before death. MRI shows an area of high signal in the pons (Fig. 19.25). The lesion consists of a circumscribed zone of of demyelination in the central part of the upper pons, involving the pontine nuclei and white matter of the base of the pons, but sparing the subpial and periventricular regions (Figs 19.25 and 19.26). In the affected area there is loss of myelin with preservation of axons and neuron cell bodies, an important distinction from pontine infarcts. Cases that have survived several days may show softening in the centre of the lesion, and macrophages containing neutral fat infiltrating the area. Oligodendrocytes are lost, but astrocytes survive, and appear reactive. A rapid rise in plasma sodium following treatment to correct an initially low level is thought to play a key role in the development of this lesion.

Fig. 19.24 Alexander's disease. Blood vessel in cerebral white matter, intensely rimmed with Rosenthal fibres. H&E, ×205.

Fig. 19.25 T2W axial MR image demonstrates an area of high signal due to myelin damage in the central part of the pons (arrow) with sparing of the subpial and periventricular regions. The MRI appearance of central pontine myelinolysis is however non-specific and may be confused with a glioma or with ischaemia and multiple sclerosis when multiple white matter lesions are present.

Table 20.1 summarizes the chief sites of damage in the various conditions considered in this chapter.

Many toxins produce their effects on cells by impairing their energy production. Neurons with very long axons are particularly dependent on a continuous supply of energy to maintain their very extensive cytoplasmic and surface membrane structure. It is frequently the structural integrity of these neurons that is most at risk from the effects of toxins. Because the blood–brain barrier often restricts entry of toxins to the CNS, large neurons here may be to some extent protected from their effects, so that it is the large peripheral sensory neurons (whose cell bodies in sensory ganglia are not protected by any vascular barrier) and motor axons that are most commonly affected by many toxins. Some of the toxins that solely affect the nervous system in this selective way are listed in Table 15.2, but most of these toxins are not further considered in the text. Some assistance when dealing with cases affected in this way may be obtained by consulting Chapter 22, and the section on nerve biopsies in Chapter 4. It should be noted that many toxins selectively affect *distal* peripheral nerves, and it is therefore essential that these are sampled if the pathology is to be identified. The rest of this chapter provides an alphabetical summary of other common toxins known to exert an adverse effect on the nervous system.

Alcohol

Effects of chronic excess alcohol on the nervous system are largely attributable to deficiencies, particularly thiamine (vitamin B₁) deficiency, to which alcoholics are peculiarly susceptible (see below). This gives rise to Wernicke's encephalopathy and possibly to the cerebellar degeneration found in some alcoholics. Alcoholic peripheral neuropathy is also due to nutritional deficiency. These deficiencies are due partly to an inadequate diet, partly to the increased need for thiamine that metabolism of alcohol demands, and possibly to a reduced absorption of thiamine from the gut in patients with gastritis. No specific neuropathological changes have been found in the cerebral cortex in alcoholics, although reversible 'atrophy' has been described in CT scans. Patients with cirrhosis of the liver may develop the clinical and pathological features of hepatic encephalopathy (p.345). Exceptionally, the changes of Marchiafava–Bignami disease (p.348) are found. Central pontine myelinolysis (p.347) is occasionally found in alcoholics but may have other causes. Amblyopia in smokers and alcoholics has been attributed to chronic cyanide intoxication (see below). Alcoholics are also at extra risk from head injuries (Chapter 5) and cerebrovascular accidents (Chapter 7).

In the *fetal alcohol syndrome*, from which infants exposed *in utero* may suffer, there is a characteristic facial appearance with short palpebral fissures, flattened nose and maxilla, and wide mouth. Various brain malformations (Chapter 16) are encountered in this syndrome. These include microencephaly, hydrocephalus, grey matter heterotopias, agenesis of the corpus callosum, schizencephaly and cerebellar malformations.

For the effects of methyl alcohol intoxication see p.359.

Aluminium

Encephalopathy with dementia occurs in some renal dialysis patients who are treated with dialysis water containing high levels of aluminium. No specific neuropathological changes occur in such cases, though non-specific features of neuronal shrinkage and reactive astrocytosis in white matter are described.

There is considerable interest in the possible involvement of aluminium in the pathogenesis of Alzheimer's disease (p.306). Aluminosilicates have been described in the cores of the argyrophilic plaques which develop in the cortex in that disease, and in neuronal nuclei, but it is not certain whether these deposits have a primary role in the disease or occur as a secondary consequence of the degenerative changes. Aluminium salts by direct injection have been experimentally shown to cause abnormal accumulation of neurofilaments in neuron cell bodies, but these do not have the ultrastructural characteristics of the neurofibrillary tangles of Alzheimer's disease.

Amphotericin B

This anti-fungal agent administered intravenously has been known to cause neurological disturbances including dementia and akinetic mutism. A diffuse cerebral encephalopathy can be seen in dogs administered the substance experimentally.

Arsenic

Chronic trivalent arsenic intoxication causes a peripheral sensory neuropathy with a minor motor component. Peripheral nerves show predominant wallerian degeneration, especially in the distal limb nerves. Pentavalent organic arsenic, used formerly to treat syphilis and still employed against trypanosomiasis, may cause an acute encephalopathy in which petechial haemorrhages and foci of haemorrhagic necrosis occur. In some cases the changes found were thought to be identical to those of acute haemorrhagic leucoencephalitis (p.179). Occasionally there is also a predominantly motor neuropathy resembling acute inflammatory polyneuropathy (Guillain–Barré syndrome) (p.382). These manifestations of toxicity are probably related to the development of an Arthus-type hypersensitivity response.

Bismuth

This is used medicinally for gastro-intestinal disorders. Excess ingestion can cause an encephalopathy with pyschiatric symptoms, gait disturbance and myoclonus. Pathological studies have shown necrosis in the hippocampus and loss of basal ganglia neurons and Purkinje cells.

Botulinum toxin

This exotoxin of *Clostridium botulinum* is occasionally ingested in contaminated food, and causes paralysis by blocking release of acetylcholine at neuromuscular junctions. Structural changes in motor end-plates in humans have not been described, perhaps because death occurs too rapidly for these to occur, but in experimental animals the toxin produces sprouting of terminal motor axons.

Carbon monoxide

Sources of carbon monoxide in the environment are numerous, and relate chiefly to the burning of fuel under conditions of insufficient ventilation and incomplete combustion. Poisoning is seen in subjects exposed to motor vehicle exhaust in a closed environment, improperly ventilated household heaters, and burning buildings and furniture. If acute carbon monoxide poisoning is suspected, a blood sample should be sent for analysis of the carboxyhaemoglobin content. In acute carbon monoxide poisoning, the brain, along with other viscera, muscle and skin are a deep pink–red colour and the leptomeninges are congested. Petechial or larger haemorrhages are common,

particularly in the cerebral white matter. There are characteristic alterations in the basal ganglia, which take at least 24 hours to become apparent, that take the form of well-circumscribed softenings, most commonly lying in the inner segment of the globus pallidus; they are usually bilateral (Fig. 20.1). Laminar cortical necrosis and acute hypoxic change (p.51) are frequently seen in the cerebral cortex, hippocampus and Purkinje cell layer of the cerebellum. White matter lesions are also common, and may accompany the grey matter changes or occur independently of them. They consist of microscopic foci of demyelination, mainly perivascular in distribution, or occurring as larger plaques or diffuse areas of myelin loss in cerebral white matter. Axons are relatively spared in some cases, and there is an associated astrocytic reaction. Old lesions are well demarcated from surrounding white matter.

Clioquinol

Used for treatment of 'travellers' diarrhoea', clioquinol has been found, when given in excessively large doses, to be responsible for a serious neurological disease with peripheral neuropathy, visual disturbances and an acute encephalopathy with prominent amnesia (subacute myelo-optico neuropathy, SMON). Pathological studies, chiefly from Japan, have shown grey matter oedema and white matter astrocytosis with, in the spinal cord, symmetrical posterior column fibre loss, some degeneration of spinocerebellar fibres and loss of distal corticospinal tract fibres (Fig. 20.2). In the peripheral nervous system there is degeneration of sensory and autonomic ganglion cells, secondary increase in satellite cells in ganglia, and axonal degeneration in posterior roots and peripheral nerves

Fig. 20.1 Coronal slice through the cerebrum from a case of acute carbon monoxide poisoning followed by prolonged survival of many years. Irregular areas of cystic necrosis are detectable in both segments of the globus pallidus (arrow heads). There is also severe white matter degeneration.

companying macrophages containing haemosiderin and some fibrillary gliosis. Neurons are relatively spared, though they may be shrunken. In the thalamus there may be neuronal shrinkage without the capillary changes described above. The dorsomedial thalamic nucleus is the one most commonly affected.

Thiamine deficiency also causes peripheral neuropathy, which is seen not only in alcoholics but also, in the form of beriberi, in victims of malnutrition and starvation. Peripheral nerves show a predominantly distal axonal degeneration with some sensory ganglion cell loss and degeneration of fibres in the posterior columns of the spinal cord.

In addition to the lesions of Wernicke's encephalopathy, thiamine deficiency is thought to be responsible for the cerebellar lesions often found in alcoholics. These consist of loss of Purkinje cells and to a lesser extent of granule cells from the cerebellar cortex, particularly in the superior vermis, at the crowns of the folia (Fig. 20.11). In severe cases most of the anterior parts of the anterior lobes of the hemispheres are also affected. Secondary loss of neurons caused by retrograde degeneration may also be seen in the inferior olives.

Pyridoxine deficiency

Deficiency of pyridoxal phosphate (vitamin B_6) in experiments in animals results in a peripheral neuropathy with axonal degeneration, but there has been no convincing demonstration that isolated deficiency of this vitamin causes a peripheral neuropathy in man.

Fig. 20.8 View of the mamillary bodies in Wernicke's encephalopathy. They show brown discoloration and atrophy (arrows).

Fig. 20.9 Wernicke's encephalopathy. Subacute lesion with capillary congestion, oedema and endothelial cell hypertrophy in the mamillary body. Note the survival of healthy-looking neurons. PAS, ×170.

Fig. 20.10 Wernicke's encephalopathy. Chronic lesion in mamillary body, with scarring and pericapillary fibrosis. Reticulin stain, ×22.

Nicotinic acid deficiency

Deficiency of this vitamin, one of the B group, or of its amino acid precursor tryptophan, causes pellagra. Most cases seen now are alcoholics or vegans. Morphological changes in the nervous system have been described in chronic deficiency, the most consistent being chromatolysis of neurons, particularly Betz cells in the motor cortex, pontine neurons in the brain stem and anterior horn cells. Degeneration is also described in peripheral nerves and long tracts in the spinal cord, principally in the posterior columns but also in the lateral columns.

Riboflavin deficiency

Deficiency of this member of the B group of vitamins causes a peripheral neuropathy with axonal degeneration, and skin lesions around the mouth.

Vitamin B₁₂ deficiency

Vitamin B_{12} deficiency causes pernicious anaemia and a myelopathy known as *subacute combined degeneration of the cord*. This is primarily a myelinopathy, but it is almost always accompanied by axonal loss in human cases if allowed to last long. The characteristic finding is of discontinuous foci of demyelination not conforming with anatomical or functional divisions, but situated mainly in lateral- and posterior-column white matter (Fig. 20.12). The thoracic level of the cord is usually the worst affected. The mildest lesions consist of patches of myelin sheath swelling and dissolution. In severe cases there is destruction of almost all the white matter around mid-thoracic cord level

Fig. 20.11 Low-power view of the cerebellar cortex from a chronic alcoholic. Purkinje cells are almost absent and granule cells reduced in number, and there is a proliferation of astrocytes in the molecular and Purkinje cell layers. H&E, ×100.

Table 21.6 Summary of intrauterine and congenital infections associated with cerebral pathology in infants.

Organism	Type of cerebral pathology	Extracerebral pathology	Diagnostic samples
Cytomegalovirus (exposure during pregnancy or birth)	Microencephaly, gyral malformations, foci of calcification, especially in periventricular regions, meningo-encephalitis with nuclear inclusion bodies	Hepatitis, chorioretinitis, cardio-vascular and skeletal malformations, purpura. Large inclusion-bearing cells in affected organs (often present in kidney); may be stillborn	Softened brain and kidney tissue for culture and IPX staining for viral antigen and PCR
Rubella virus (1st trimester infection)	Microencephaly, hydrocephalus, agenesis of corpus callosum, cerebral cysts and mild calcification. Very rarely progressive rubella syndrome	Cataracts, other ocular defects, deafness due to inner ear disease, cardiac abnormalities, liver disease, abnormalities of bone development, haematological abnormalities	Serum for IgM-specific antibody
HIV (AIDS) virus (exposure during pregnancy or birth)	Microencephaly, encephalitis, multinucleated giant cells, white matter degeneration and gliosis, vascular calcification	Thymic atrophy and lymphoid tissue depletion, disseminated infections with, e.g. atypical mycobacteria, CMV, fungi. Pneumocystitis in lungs	Serum for specific antibody, fresh brain samples for nucleic acid hybridization and PCR
Herpes simplex type II virus (exposure usually during birth)	Diffuse acute encephalitis. Inclusion bodies may be seen in glial and neuronal nuclei	Necrotic foci in lungs, liver and adrenal glands	Softened brain tissue for culture and IPX staining for herpes simplex antigen and PCR
Varicella virus (exposure in 1st trimester)	Microencephaly, meningoencephalitis or myelitis, occasionally cerebral mal-formations	Chorioretinitis, necrotic, scarred skin lesions and muscle atrophy in segmental distribution	Serum for specific antibody level
Treponema pallidum (2nd trimester onwards)	Leptomeningitis, hydrocephalus, vascular lesions associated with arteritis. Later in childhood there may be dementia due to loss of neurons in cerebral cortex and cerebellum with gliosis	Stillbirths, placental infiltration with spirochaetes which are also present in the liver, lungs, heart and bones	Serum and CSF for fluorescent treponemal antibody test; stain for spirochaetes in tissues
Toxoplasma gondii (especially end of 1st and during 2nd trimester)	Hydrocephalus, foci of calcification scattered throughout the brain, meningoencephalitis with necrotic foci. Free organisms and cysts in lesions	Chorioretinitis, hepatitis; may be stillborn; placenta infected also	Serum for IgM-specific antibody; detection of organisms or cysts in brain and placenta

AIDS, acquired, immune deficiency syndrome; CMV, cytomegalovirus; HIV, human immunodeficiency virus; IPX, immunoperoxidase; PCR, polymerase chain reaction.

virus causes a severe encephalitis with widespread macroscopic areas of softening, particularly in grey matter. If death occurs at the acute stage of the infection, viral antigen can be demonstrated in the brain in glial cells and neurons using immunohistological techniques on paraffin sections.

The AIDS virus, HIV, produces changes in the brain in congenitally infected infants. Brain weights are abnormally low, and an encephalopathy with white matter degeneration and gliosis has been described (Sharer *et al.* 1986). Variable inflammatory cell infiltrates, multinucleate giant cells and vascular calcification, particularly in the basal ganglia, are also found. Infection with opportunistic organisms may additionally be found in the brain and elsewhere.

Varicella infection *in utero* occasionally produces damage to the nervous system. This may take the form of necrosis in a segmental distribution in the spinal cord. Muscles and other tissues innervated by the destroyed neural segment(s) are atrophic, and the skin may be necrotic and scarred.

Toxoplasma gondii can cause a congenital meningoencephalitis which is usually manifest in the first few weeks of life. Lesions may be evident on inspection of the external

Fig. 21.14 Coronal slice through the cerebrum of an infant with congenital cytomegalovirus (CMV) infection. There are small foci of calcification (arrow heads), and areas of periventricular necrosis (arrowed).

Fig. 21.15 Intranclear inclusion bodies in the brain from an infant with congenital CMV infection (red). Immunoperoxidase for CMV counterstained with Mayer's haemalum, ×400.

Fig. 21.16 Low-power view of a section of periventricular area in an infant with congenital CMV infection. A periventricular focus of calcification (darkly stained) is present. H&E, ×150.

Fig. 23.12 Selective type 2 fibre atrophy. ATPase reaction at pH 9.4, ×110.

Fig. 23.13 Muscle fibre undergoing splitting (centre) from a case of limb girdle dystrophy. Trichrome, ×400.

disappear from the necrotic zone, and macrophages infiltrate and phagocytose the remnants (Fig. 23.14), following which regeneration is attempted. Focal necrosis of muscle fibres may occur non-specifically, for example in severe systemic infections.

Regeneration of muscle

The presence of regenerating fibres in muscle implies previous necrosis. Frequently a muscle will show evidence of both necrosis and regeneration. Satellite cells are the source of cells that proliferate and differentiate to produce muscle regeneration. These cells are not distinguishable by light microscopy, but can be seen lying outside the plasmalemma and inside the basal lamina of muscle fibres by EM (Fig. 23.16). Regenerating muscle fibres appear small, with basophilic cytoplasm and chains of prominent large, centrally placed, vesicular nuclei with clearly visible nucleoli (Fig. 23.11).

Alterations in muscle fibre architecture

Ring fibres (Ringbinden, spiral annulets) and sarcoplasmic masses. Ring fibres, *Ringbinden*, or spiral annulets, are myofibrils spirally wrapped around the inside of otherwise normally orientated, longitudinal muscle fibres (Fig. 23.17). Their striations can be seen in transverse sections of the fibre. Sarcoplasmic masses are accumulations of structureless material within the sarcolemma.

Vacuoles. Vacuoles of various types may occur in otherwise normal-looking muscle fibres. Some contain stainable material, most commonly glycogen. Others contain autophagic debris. Some contain fluid, and represent dilatations of the sarcoplasmic reticulum or T tubules.

Nemaline rods. These are short, rod-like structures, visible in a modified trichrome stain as red bodies, measuring up to 5 μm in length and 1.5 μm in width (Fig. 23.18). They consist of Z-band material.

Fig. 23.14 Muscle fibre undergoing segmental degeneration (centre). The sarcolemmal sheath is filled with phagocytes. H&E, ×300.

Fig. 23.15 Muscle fibres undergoing hyaline degeneration from a case of polymyositis. The affected fibres are swollen and their sarcoplasm structureless. H&E, ×200.

Fig. 23.16 Satellite cell lying between the basal lamina and plasmalemma of the adjacent muscle fibre. Uranyl acetate and lead citrate, ×16 430.

Whorled fibres. A disorderly swirling arrangement of myofibrils is sometimes seen in histochemical preparations. Neighbouring fibres may appear 'moth-eaten'.

Ragged red fibres. These are muscle fibres showing coarse intermyofibrillar granular material and irregular marginal zones which stain red with the modified Gomori trichrome stain. These regions consist of abnormal clumps of mitochondria, and they give an excessively strong reaction for oxidative enzymes (Fig. 23.19).

Fig. 23.17 Ring fibres, *Ringbinden*, or spiral annulets from a case of dystrophia myotonica. Transverse striations are seen in the spirally directed myofibrils situated at the margins of two transversely sectioned fibres (arrowed). PTAH, ×400.

Further architectural distortions of muscle fibres are detectable by EM, but are seldom visible by light microscopy. Details of altered ultrastructure are not described here but can be found in the textbooks of muscle disease listed at the end of the chapter.

Alterations in histochemical reactions and stored metabolites

Excessive storage material can be found in some diseases in otherwise normal muscle fibres. Glycogen or neutral fat can accumulate in this way in occasional fibres as a nonspecific abnormality in diseases unrelated to storage disorders. In the latter diseases there are usually many fibres containing abnormal amounts of the stored material. There are also usually alterations in enzyme activity relevant to the stored material, e.g. absence of myophosphorylase activity with excess glycogen deposition in McArdle's disease (type 5 glycogenosis).

Alteration in distribution and proportions of different histochemical fibre types

This change is common in muscle disease. In addition to type grouping, which occurs in denervating conditions, there may be predominance of one fibre type. In many myopathic disorders there is predominance of type 1 fibres, but in small biopsies this can be difficult to distinguish from type grouping, or from physiological alterations in fibre proportions which can to some extent be influenced by training and physical exercise. In isolation it is, therefore, not a reliable indication of a myopathy.

Fig. 23.18 Clusters of nemaline rods appearing as dark patches, many of them in a subsarcolemmal position close to myonuclei. Trichrome, ×200.

(a)

(b)

Fig. 23.19 (a) Abnormally heavy reaction product demonstrating succinic dehydrogenase activity in some muscle fibres throughout their fibre width, and in other fibres just beneath the sarcolemma, in a case of mitochondrial myopathy. (b) A 'ragged red' fibre from a case of mitochondrial myopathy. Trichrome, ×250.

Fig. 23.20 Polyarteritis nodosa. Intense inflammation in and around the walls of a small intramuscular artery. H&E, ×80.

Alterations in interstitial tissues

Abnormalities of interstitial structures may be of considerable diagnostic value when examining muscle. There may be an arteritis affecting intramuscular arteries, as in polyarteritis nodosa (Fig. 23.20), or reduced numbers of capillaries. Endomysial and perimysial fibrosis is very common in muscle disease, and as an early feature can have diagnostic value, particularly in the muscular dystrophies. Adipose tissue replacement of muscle is also a common late change occurring in many primary muscle or denervating diseases, but is particularly common and severe in muscular dystrophy. Amyloid is occasionally deposited in intramuscular connective tissue in systemic amyloidosis. Inflammatory cells are not normally found in muscle, and their presence in a focal or diffuse distribution is valuable evidence of muscle disease, particularly myositis.

Individual muscle diseases

Particular constellations of the changes outlined above are relatively, though seldom absolutely, specific for particular muscle diseases, as indicated alphabetically below. Table 23.4 summarizes some causes of the main types of pathological change.

Acute necrotizing myopathy

In this rare condition, which may cause massive myoglobinuria resulting in acute renal failure, there is extensive acute necrosis of many, often the majority of, muscle fibres in skeletal mucles. This necrosis is reflected in a high level of the creatine phosphokinase activity in the serum. Depending on the time that has elapsed since the onset, the muscle examined may contain macrophages infiltrating the dead muscle fibres, and there may be evidence of early regeneration. Inflammation is lacking. The causes are varied, but include damage secondary to viral infection (by a mechanism unknown), massive ischaemia of muscle (when it is limited to the ischaemic region), an acute episode of metabolic malfunction, a remote effect of carcinoma and the effect of certain toxins.

Arthrogryposis

The presence of limb joint deformities and associated contractures is referred to as arthrogryposis. This occurs in a number of neuromuscular diseases arising in early life and causing muscle weakness, such as Werdnig–Hoffmann disease, congenital muscular dystrophy, congenital myotonic dystrophy, central core disease and congenital fibre type disproportion. It is also sometimes found when there is a disease or malformation of the CNS which results in abnormal limb tone or movement. In some cases of arthrogryposis there may be no other abnormalities and in these cases microscopical examination of affected muscle usually reveals only non-specific abnormalities such as mild fibrosis or atrophy. This abnormality is thought to reflect abnormal positioning of the affected limb *in utero*.

Carcinomatous myopathy

The most common finding in weakness that is associated

with the presence of a carcinoma is selective atrophy of type 2 fibres. In patients with severe, acute or subacute weakness there may be myositis or acute necrotizing myopathy. Patients with malignant disease also commonly develop weakness due to peripheral nerve disease resulting from direct invasion of nerve roots by tumour, or from a remote effect of carcinoma on the nervous system (p.184).

Central core, multicore or minicore disease

These conditions produce weakness, usually mild and non-progressive, from childhood onward. Microscopy shows abnormal central regions in the type 1 muscle fibres, seen best in preparations for oxidative enzyme reactions (Fig. 23.21). These areas, or cores, extend the full length of the affected fibres in central core disease, but in multi- or minicore disease many small foci are seen in each affected fibre. EM studies show disruption of myofibrillar architecture in the region affected, with an absence of mitochondria (Fig. 23.22).

Centronuclear (myotubular) myopathy

There are several variants of this inherited myopathy which differ in age of onset, severity and pattern of inheritance. In the severe infantile form the extrafusal muscle fibres are small and most have centrally placed nuclei with myofibril-free sarcoplasm around the nuclei (Fig. 23.23). Milder forms show atrophy of type 1 fibres, type 1 fibre predominance and some central nuclei.

Fig. 23.21 Central core disease. Succinic dehydrogenase reaction on a transverse section of muscle, demonstrating an absence of reaction product in the centres of the fibres. ×270.

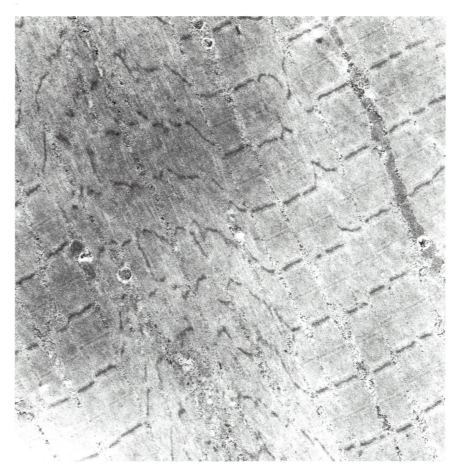

Fig. 23.22 Ultrastructure of a central core running from top left to bottom, midline. In the core region the sarcomeres are disorganized and mitochondria (seen top right between intact myofibrils) are absent. Uranyl acetate and lead citrate, ×10560.

Fig. 23.23 Longitudinal section of muscle from an infant with centronuclear myopathy. The nuclei are large, occupying much of the diameter of the fibres, and are often centrally situated. ×300.

Congenital fibre-type disproportion

This condition causes floppiness and delay in achieving motor milestones in infancy. In histochemical preparations of muscle it can be seen that the diameter of the type 1 fibres is unusually small, while the diameter of the type 2 fibres is normal or slightly increased (Fig. 23.24).

Cramps

In most subjects complaining of severe muscle cramps no morphological abnormalities are found in muscle. However, cramps may be a manifestation of muscle disease, particularly metabolic disease. A few cases have shown excess tubular aggregates on EM.

Distal myopathy

This is a rare autosomal dominant disease which causes a clinically fairly distinctive, slowly progressive weakness of the hands and feet in middle-age or later. Muscle biopsies show non-specific myopathic changes, including excess variation in fibre size, internal nuclei, occasional necrosis of

Fig. 23.24 Congenital fibre-type disproportion. ATPase reaction at pH 4.6 showing large type 2 fibres (pale) and abnormally small type 1 fibres (dark). ×280.

segments of muscle fibres and endomysial fibrosis. Autophagic vacuoles have been described with EM.

Drug-induced and toxic myopathies

Alcohol

There are acute and chronic forms of alcoholic myopathy. Acutely there may be a necrotizing myopathy or less widespread but similar features of scattered segmental necrosis, often with associated vacuolar change, phagocytosis and regeneration. In the chronic phase there are scattered atrophic fibres, internal nuclei and variable fibrosis.

Carbon monoxide poisoning

This may cause an acute necrotizing myopathy.

Chloroquine

High doses of chloroquine occasionally cause a severe myopathy with vacuolar necrosis particularly affecting the type 1 fibres. By EM the vacuoles can be seen to contain autophagic debris.

Clofibrate

High doses of this drug may cause a painful myopathy with segmental muscle fibre necrosis, phagocytosis and regeneration.

ε-aminocaproic acid (EACA)

This antifibrinolytic drug occasionally causes a myopathy with segmental necrosis of muscle fibres, phagocytosis and regeneration.

Penicillamine

This drug occasionally causes a myasthenic syndrome or a vasculitis which may involve intramuscular, among other, vessels.

Snake venom

Some snake venoms (e.g. Australian mulga snake, tiger snake and sea snake) cause an acute necrotizing myopathy.

Steroids

A painless proximal myopathy may complicate treatment with steroids or occur in subjects with Cushing's disease. Muscle microscopy shows selective atrophy of type 2 fibres.

Dystrophia myotonica

There are congenital and adult forms of this dominantly inherited disease which causes weakness and myotonia in varying proportions. Congenital myotonic dystrophy, in which weakness predominates, occurs in infants of affected mothers. There is smallness of muscle fibres, particularly the type 1 fibres, and internal nuclei (Fig. 23.25). Sarcoplasmic masses and ring fibres may also be seen. Ultrastructurally the muscle fibres contain a rim of peripheral sarcoplasm which lacks myofibrils. In adult cases type 1 fibres are usually small but type 2 fibres may be

Fig. 23.25 Congenital dystrophia myotonica. Section of muscle showing small muscle fibres with relatively large, central nuclei, in some fibres surrounded by a clear rim of sarcoplasm. H&E, ×400.

Fig. 23.26 Longitudinal section of muscle from a case of adult dystrophia myotonica. There are increased numbers of myonuclei, many of them arranged in chains. H&E, ×130.

hypertrophic. Nuclear clumps are frequently present. An increased number of internal nuclei is always found, and these characteristically form long chains (Fig. 23.26). Ring fibres and sarcoplasmic masses are also common (Fig. 23.17). There are occasional foci of necrosis and regeneration and endomysial collagen is increased. Adipose tissue replaces muscle at a late stage and muscle spindles tend to have increased numbers of intrafusal muscle fibres (Fig. 23.27).

Endocrine myopathies

Acromegaly

Proximal muscle weakness occurs in some acromegalic subjects. Muscle biopsies have shown non-specific changes of excess variation in fibre size and occasional segmental necrosis in such cases.

Cushing's disease

Selective type 2 fibre atrophy is the usual finding in cases of myopathy associated with Cushing's disease.

Hyperthyroidism

Thyrotoxic patients may have a proximal myopathy, but there are usually no structural changes found on muscle biopsy. Exophthalmos in thyrotoxicosis is due to severe oedema causing swelling of extraocular muscles and adjacent adipose tissue. There is also lymphocytic infiltration and segmental necrosis of extraocular muscle fibres.

Fig. 23.27 Muscle spindle from a case of adult dystrophia myotonica showing increased numbers of intrafusal muscle fibres (compare with Fig. 23.2). H&E, ×350.

Hypothyroidism

Mild type 2 atrophy and prominent collections of subsarcolemmal glycogen are described in hypothyroid patients with myopathy.

Eosinophilic fasciitis

In this condition inflammatory infiltrates are found in the deep fascia and immediately adjacent muscle fascicles. There may also be some segmental muscle fibre necrosis and regeneration. Eosinophils are sometimes prominent in the inflammatory infiltrates.

Fingerprint body myopathy

This is a rare congenital myopathy in which inclusions reminiscent of fingerprints are seen by EM of muscle.

Ischaemic myopathy

Ischaemic changes in muscle are seen commonly in lower limb muscles of subjects with severe atheroma or diabetes mellitus. They are also seen following acute interruption of the blood supply to a muscle, as can occur after trauma or as a result of prolonged, heavy pressure on a muscle, for example in deeply comatose subjects. Small muscle infarcts are also seen in muscle in polyarteritis nodosa. Microscopic appearances vary according to the age of the infarct. Initially there is acute necrosis affecting a sharply defined group of muscle fibres or fascicles, with loss of myonuclei. This is followed by phagocytosis and attempts at regeneration, but much of the healing in large infarcts is by scar formation.

Malignant hyperpyrexia

Occasionally apparently normal subjects react to certain anaesthetic agents, particularly succinyl choline or halothane, by developing a rise in temperature which may prove fatal. The tendency so to react is inherited in a dominant fashion. Muscle biopsy is occasionally undertaken to try to detect this tendency. Pharmacological and biochemical tests are much more useful for this purpose than is microscopy; so it is important that arrangements for these to be carried out are made before the biopsy is undertaken. There are no specific structural changes.

Metabolic myopathies

With glycogen storage

Acid maltase deficiency (type 2 glycogenosis). There is a severe infantile form and a milder adult form of this inherited disease. Affected infants have excessive deposits of glycogen in skeletal and cardiac muscle, and often die of cardiac failure. Cryostat sections of affected muscle show excess glycogen and acid phosphatase activity in the muscle fibres (Fig. 23.28). At the ultrastructural level some of this glycogen is seen to be membrane bound. Brain stem and spinal

Fig. 23.28 Infantile acid maltase deficiency (glycogenosis type 2, Pompe's disease). Transverse cryostat section of muscle showing vacuoles and excess, residual, dark-staining glycogen deposits in type 2 fibres. Type 1 fibres, though vacuolated, are better preserved. PAS, ×220.

Fig. 23.29 Adult acid maltase deficiency. Heavy glycogen deposition in scattered type 2 fibres. PAS, ×250.

cord neurons can be shown at post mortem also to contain excess glycogen. The deficiency of acid maltase activity can be demonstrated in muscle, liver, blood leucocytes and cultured fibroblasts. In the adult form of the disease some muscle fibres contain a few vacuoles filled with glycogen and reacting positively for acid phosphatase (Fig. 23.29).

Debranching enzyme deficiency (type 3 glycogenosis). In this rare disease there may be muscle weakness and wasting and exercise intolerance in childhood. Skeletal muscle fibres contain multiple glycogen-filled vacuoles and some fibres are atrophic. Subsarcolemmal glycogen particles are also increased. The enzyme deficiency can be demonstrated in liver, muscle or leucocytes.

Branching enzyme deficiency (type 4 glycogenosis). This rare inherited disease causes fatal liver disease commencing in infancy. Skeletal muscle is affected along with many other tissues. It shows circumscribed deposits of granular amylopectin stainable with PAS, colloidal iron and iodine. Enzyme assays for the enzyme should be performed on liver or leucocytes.

McArdle's disease (type 5 glycogenosis). Pain and fatigability of muscles on exercise clinically characterize this rare inherited disease. Another finding is failure of the blood lactate level to rise on ischaemic exercise of the forearm. Cryostat sections of muscle show excess subsarcolemmal deposits of glycogen and an absence of phosphorylase activity. The glycogen deposits are also evident on ultrastructural examination of muscle (Fig. 23.30).

Phosphofructokinase deficiency (type 7 glycogenosis). Muscle pain and exercise intolerance from childhood onward occur in this inherited disease, and as in McArdle's disease, there is a failure of the blood lactate level to rise after ischaemic exercise. Cryostat sections of muscle show excess subsarcolemmal deposits of glycogen, but phosphorylase activity is normal and phosphofructokinase deficiency can be demonstrated biochemically in muscle. Other rare enzyme deficiencies can give similar histochemical findings, details of which can be obtained from textbooks devoted to muscle disease.

With lipid storage

Metabolic disorders that influence oxidative metabolism are liable to give rise to excess storage of lipid which is a major source of energy in type 1 fibres. Carnitine deficiency produces increased storage of lipid droplets in muscle. Carnitine palmitoyl transferase deficiency may be, but is not always, associated with a slight increase in stored lipid; but it should be noted that there is a wide range of lipid stored in normal muscle. Disorders of mitochondrial metabolism can give rise to moderate storage of both fat and glycogen (Fig. 23.31). For the diagnosis of carnitine or carnitine palmitoyl transferase deficiency a sample of muscle should be deep-frozen and reserved for biochemical study.

With mitochondrial abnormalities

Mitochondrial myopathies are disorders in which symp-

Fig. 23.30 McArdle's disease (glycogenosis type 5). Subsarcolemmal, granular deposits of glycogen (above and left). Uranyl acetate and lead citrate, ×3890.

Fig. 23.31 Low-power electron micrograph showing excess fat droplets (pale) and glycogen (dark) in a transversely sectioned muscle fibre from an infant with a mitochondrial myopathy. Uranyl acetate and lead citrate, ×4490.

toms of myopathy, often very slight, are found associated with morphological changes in the fine structure of mitochondria and with an excess of oxidative enzyme activity detected histochemically (Fig. 23.19). Affected fibres appear as 'ragged red' fibres. Some cases have symptoms of CNS disease that are much more serious than the manifestations of muscle disease, as occurs in the Kearns–Sayre syndrome (p.425). Myoclonic epilepsy with 'ragged red fibres' (MERRF) and mitochondrial myopathy, encephalopathy, lactic-acidosis and stroke-like episodes (MELAS) are better termed *mitochondrial cytopathies*. Mitochondrial DNA has been found to be abnormal in a proportion of these cases and maternal transmission consistent with an inherited mitochondrial genetic defect is present in some cases. Clarification of the biochemical basis of a mitochondrial myopathy may entail specialized studies of freshly isolated mitochondria. If this is contemplated it may be desirable to confirm a tentative clinical diagnosis by performing light microscopy, histochemistry and EM on a needle biopsy sample of muscle before proceeding to an open biopsy which will be necessary for the removal of tissue for mitochondrial studies. Ultrastructural changes in the mitochondria are variable, some cases showing enlarged mitochondria and other abnormalities in the arrangement of the cristae, or paracrystalline intramitochondrial inclusions (Fig. 23.32). Not all mitochondria are affected, however, and several muscle fibres may need to be examined ultrastructurally before abnormal forms are found. The presence or absence of other myopathic features, the clinical presentation and biochemical findings all need to be taken into account when a diagnosis of mitochondrial myopathy is made, as some alteration in

mitochondrial numbers and structure can occur in other diseases, e.g. myositis.

Muscular dystrophy

Muscular dystrophies are genetically determined myopathies which share common structural abnormalities while differing in their age of onset and rate of progression. They all cause muscle weakness and, at some stage in the disease, an elevation in the serum level of creatine phosphokinase activity. This enzyme is present in high concentration in muscle, and is thought to leak out of muscle into the serum to produce the elevated levels seen in muscular dystrophy. Recently it has been demonstrated that muscle from patients with muscular dystrophy lacks, or contains abnormally low quantities of, a recently discovered protein, *dystrophin* (*Lancet* 1988). Pathologically the similarities of the muscular dystrophies outweigh their differences and most pathologists are rightly hesitant about classifying a case of muscular dystrophy solely on the basis of the histopathological features. Very late in the course of muscular dystrophy appearances of the muscle can be indistinguishable from long-standing denervation.

Fig. 23.32 Paracrystalline inclusions in abnormal mitochondria from a case of mitochondrial myopathy. Uranyl acetate and lead citrate, ×123 500.

The implied consequences for the patients and their families are so important that most clinicians rightly insist on obtaining pathological verification of the diagnosis of muscular dystrophy. Most of the pathological changes are detectable in routinely stained sections, and histochemistry adds no crucial information for the diagnosis of muscular dystrophy. The sections of muscle show excess variation in size of the fibres, with randomly scattered atrophic and hypertrophic fibres, an excess of internal nuclei, fibre splitting, foci of necrosis, generally sparse evidence of regeneration, and a marked excess of endoneurial collagen. In the late stages of the disease most muscle fibres disappear and are replaced to some extent by adipose tissue and collagen.

Pathological features that are relatively pronounced in the various types of muscular dystrophy are summarized below.

Duchenne dystrophy

Inheritance of this X-linked, recessive form affects boys in early childhood after a normal infancy. Death usually occurs in the late teens or early twenties, and cardiac failure supervenes in many cases. Necrosis of muscle fibres, with prominent hyaline change, is evident early in the course of the disease, as is endomysial fibrosis (Figs 23.33 and 23.34). Regenerating fibres are seen early on, but regeneration

Fig. 23.33 Duchenne muscular dystrophy. Transverse section of muscle showing variation in fibre diameters, with abnormally large (large arrow) and small (small arrow) fibres, and endomysial fibrosis. H & van Gieson, ×120.

Fig. 23.34 Duchenne muscular dystrophy. In this section many muscle fibres are abnormally rounded and swollen and there is perimysial fibrosis. Trichrome, ×120.

tends to fall off as the disease progresses. Histochemical differentiation of fibre types is usually rather difficult to confirm. In the late stage there is preservation of muscle spindles, intramuscular nerves and blood vessels, in sharp distinction from the virtually complete replacement of extrafusal muscle fibres by adipose tissue and collagen (Fig. 23.35). Ultrastructural studies have emphasized the frequent absence of stretches of the sarcolemma over regions of otherwise intact fibres, and reduplication of the basal lamina. Immunocytochemistry for dystrophia demonstrates a reduced or absent reaction.

Becker dystrophy

Pathological features resemble those of Duchenne dystrophy, but necrosis of muscle fibres tends to be less extensive, in keeping with the generally slower course of the disease.

Congenital muscular dystrophy

This form is less well defined than the other types of muscular dystrophy and is also unusual in showing little tendency to progress clinically. The main pathological features are excess variation in muscle fibre size, some necrosis and phagocytosis, and a marked excess of endomysial collagen.

Facio-scapulo-humeral dystrophy

Small angular-shaped fibres scattered singly or in small groups are a prominent feature in this very slowly progressive disease. Little necrosis is evident in biopsies, but 'moth-eaten' fibres are common.

Limb girdle dystrophy

This is a slowly progressive disease in which marked hypertrophy of muscle fibres and many internal myonuclei are prominent features. Atrophic fibres are also present, sometimes in small groups, and fibre splitting is also common. 'Moth-eaten' fibres may be seen, as in facio-scapulo-humeral dystrophy.

Oculopharyngeal dystrophy

Ophthalmoplegia, ptosis and dysphagia occur in this rare form of late-onset muscular dystrophy. Abnormalities in limb muscles are sparse and non-specific. A few 'ragged red' fibres may be present, together with mild atrophy and a few vacuolated fibres.

Myasthenia gravis

Routine microscopic examination of muscle is of little diagnostic value in myasthenia gravis and the various myasthenic syndromes. The diagnosis is usually made on the basis of the clinical features, backed up by a Tensilon test, electromyography and assay of serum for acetylcholine receptor antibody. That is not to say, however, that there are no features of interest in the microscopy and ultrastructure of myasthenic muscle. Examination of motor end-plates is of considerable interest, but requires that a motor point biopsy is taken to ensure that they are in-

Fig. 23.35 Appearance of muscle late in the course of muscular dystrophy. Most of the muscle is replaced by adipose tissue. A small cluster of muscle fibres remains (top right), with excess surrounding collagen. At this stage the appearances of muscular dystrophy are similar to those of late-stage denervation atrophy. H&E, ×80.

Fig. 23.36 Myasthenia gravis. Schofield-stained section showing a motor nerve terminal. The junctional area between terminal and muscle is expanded, abnormally branched and poorly formed. ×200.

cluded in the sample. They can be detected easily at the light microscope level with the non-specific esterase enzyme reaction on cryostat sections (Fig. 4.53) and with silver stains such as the Schofield stain in fixed samples. Intravitam methylene blue staining is another way by which they can be displayed. The end-plate region tends to be more spread out than in normal muscle, but the specialized terminations are ill-formed and the preterminal nerve is irregular in calibre (Fig. 23.36). EM shows widening of the synaptic clefts at the end-plates and loss of the secondary clefts in the postsynaptic membrane (Fig. 23.37). Elsewhere in the muscle small clusters of lymphocytes

(a)

(b)

Fig. 23.37 Low-power electron micrographs of a myasthenic motor end-plate (a) and normal end-plate (b). In myasthenia the secondary synaptic clefts (SS) are irregular, widened and shallow, and the presynaptic nerve ending is not closely applied to the postsynaptic muscle membrane. Uranyl acetate and lead citrate, (a) ×4800; (b) × 6860.

('lymphorrhages') may be found between muscle fibres and there may be occasional foci of segmental necrosis. Occasionally in long-standing myasthenia, denervation atrophy or selective type 2 atrophy may be seen. Denervation of the tongue can be particularly severe, and associated with fatty pseudohypertrophy and marked proliferation of terminal nerve fibres (Fig. 23.38). The thymus is almost always abnormal in myasthenia, showing either hyperplastic features or the presence of a thymoma.

Myasthenic syndromes, which also give rise to fatiguability of muscle, occur usually in association with carcinoma. They do not have any distinctive microscopic pathology.

Myositis

Inflammatory change in muscle is relatively commonly encountered by pathologists regularly examining muscle biopsies. It can occur to a mild extent as a non-specific feature in cases with a myopathy or muscular dystrophy. This can give rise to diagnostic confusion, particularly as some cases of primary myositis may also show only mild inflammation. Macrophages infiltrating necrotic muscle fibres do not constitute a myositis. Various forms of myositis occur, of which the idiopathic (probably auto-immune), forms are the commonest.

Dermatomyositis and polymyositis

These idiopathic forms differ mainly according to whether or not there is a skin rash associated with the muscle disease, whose chief manifestation is muscle weakness. There are associations with rheumatoid arthritis and other collagen diseases and, particularly for dermatomyositis, with malignancy. The key pathological features are a mononuclear inflammatory cell infiltrate in and around the muscle fascicles, scattered segmental necrosis of muscle fibres and the presence of regenerating fibres (Figs 23.11 and 23.39). The inflammatory cells consist chiefly of lymphocytes, many of them T-cells, macrophages and plasma cells. In childhood and some adult cases of dermatomyositis deposits of IgG and complement components C3 and C9 may be detectable in the muscle. In childhood myositis there is frequently atrophy of muscle fibres at the margins of the fascicles, thrombosis of vessels, loss of capillaries and relatively sparse inflammation. Scattered muscle fibre atrophy occurs in all forms of myositis, and there may be fibrosis of variable degree.

Granulomatous and giant cell myositis

Granulomas containing multinucleate giant cells, but without caseation, occur in muscle in some patients with sarcoidosis and others with a thymoma with or without accompanying myasthenia gravis. Occasionally extensive granulomatous myositis occurs as an isolated finding. In all these conditions the granulomas occur mainly in interstitial tissues between the muscle fibres, but occasionally they cause focal destruction of muscle fibres.

Inclusion body myositis

This rare condition is characterized pathologically by the presence of inclusion bodies visible by EM, which consist of collections of 15–18 nm filaments lying in muscle fibre cytoplasm or nucleus (Fig. 23.40). The muscle fibres may

Fig. 23.38 Myasthenia gravis. Proliferation of nerve fibres, with abnormal branching and formation of numerous lateral and terminal expansions in the tongue. Schofield, ×190.

Fig. 23.39 Polymyositis. There is a predominantly lymphocytic inflammatory cell infiltrate among the muscle fibres. H&E, ×170.

Fig. 23.40 Intranuclear filaments in a muscle fibre from a case of inclusion body myositis. Uranyl acetate and lead citrate, ×19 660.

also contain small vacuoles and show foci of segmental necrosis with mild inflammation.

Parasitic myositis

Trichinosis, due to the ingestion of insufficiently cooked meat infected with *Trichinella*, produces multifocal inflammation at sites in the muscles where larvae are deposited. At these sites there is focal segmental necrosis of muscle fibres with a mixed inflammatory cell infiltrate including lymphocytes, plasma cells, macrophages, neutrophils and eosinophils. Encysted larvae may also be present (Fig. 23.41). Other parasites may also invade muscle and cause a myositis. These include toxoplasma, sarcosporidium and cysticercus.

Pyogenic myositis

Myositis associated with gas gangrene due to *Clostridium welchii* infection may be seen complicating deep wounds. The infection produces extensive muscle necrosis and in-

Fig. 23.41 Longitudinal section of muscle from a case of parasitic myositis due to *Trichinella*, containing an encysted larva (arrow).

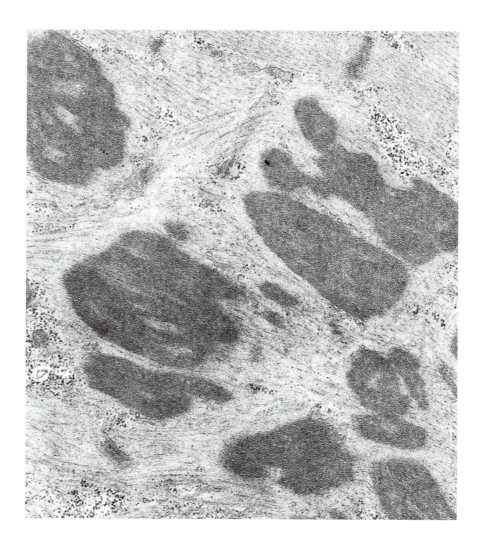

Fig. 23.42 Ultrastructural appearance of nemaline rods. Uranyl acetate and lead citrate, ×35 420.

tense infiltration with neutrophils and other inflammatory cells.

Muscle abscesses from which *Staphylococcus aureus* can usually be grown are quite common in the tropics. Intense inflammation and an abscess cavity develop. The pathogenesis of the condition is not clear.

Myositis associated with viral infection

Viruses have been implicated as a cause of occasional cases of acute localized myositis, usually in children. Biopsies of affected muscle show oedema and an inflammatory cell infiltrate of neutrophils and lymphocytes with segmental necrosis of some muscle fibres. In occasional cases virus has been demonstrated in muscle. A non-inflammatory acute necrotizing myopathy is another rare complication of systemic viral infection.

Fig. 23.43 Periodic paralysis. Vacuoles, and a few internal nuclei present in otherwise normal muscle fibres. H&E, ×340.

Myositis ossificans

Bone and cartilage are deposited in deep connective tissue in this condition. Muscle is only secondarily affected. In one familial form there are repeated episodes of ectopic bone formation from childhood, usually with congenital anomalies of the fingers or toes. There is also a localized sporadic form. For details, a textbook of muscle pathology should be consulted.

Myotonia congenita

Clinical manifestations of this rare disease are muscle hypertrophy and myotonia. Histologically the muscles show increased fibre diameters, especially of the type 2 fibres. Some internal nuclei and scattered atrophic fibres are also present.

Nemaline rod myopathy

This may present as a childhood disorder with hypotonia and weakness, or in adults with slowly progressive proximal muscle weakness. Clusters of nemaline rods are found in the type 1 muscle fibres. These are composed of material resembling Z-bands. Many muscle fibres are slightly atrophic and there tends to be a predominance of type 1 fibres. The rods are visible with a modified Gomori trichrome stain as red bodies up to 5 μm long and 1.5 μm wide. They are readily visible as electron-dense inclusions by EM (Figs 23.18 and 23.42).

Osteomalacia

Atrophy of type 2 muscle fibres has been described in muscle weakness associated with osteomalacia.

Fig. 23.44 Subsarcolemmal tubular aggregates (arrow heads) from a case of periodic paralysis in which many such aggregates were present. Uranyl acetate and lead citrate, ×8640.

Periodic paralysis

During attacks of paralysis there are vacuoles in the muscle fibres (Fig. 23.43). By EM these appear smooth walled and empty. They appear to communicate with the T tubules and there may also be proliferated T tubules or tubular aggregates present (Fig. 23.44). Between attacks of paralysis there are usually no abnormalities in muscle apart from occasional vacuoles.

Reducing body myopathy

This is a rare cause of severe muscle weakness commencing in childhood. Muscle fibres contain reducing bodies, so-called because they stain with a menadione nitro-blue tetrazolium stain. With H&E they appear reddish-pink and they show green autofluorescence. They have irregular margins, and large ones occupy the full diameter of the fibre.

Trauma to muscle

Mechanical trauma can itself directly damage muscle and it may interrupt the blood supply and thereby cause ad-

ditional ischaemic damage. Denervation of muscle may also occur if the nerve supply is damaged. Mechanical damage results in acute necrosis, phagocytosis and attempts at regeneration often with scar formation. A ruptured muscle may fail to reestablish continuity with its tendon and under these circumstances may show a variety of myopathic features.

Further reading and references

Dubowitz V. 1985. *Muscle Biopsy, a Practical Approach*, 2nd edn. Baillière Tindall, London.

Harriman DGF. 1992. Diseases of muscle. In Adams JH, Duchen LW (Eds) *Greenfield's Neuropathology*, 5th edn. Edward Arnold, London, pp.1026–96.

Hilton-Jones D, Squier MV, Taylor D, Matthews PM. 1995. *Metabolic Myopathies*. Sanders, London.

Lancet. 1988. Dystrophin Editorial **2**, 429–30.

Mastaglia FL, Walton J. 1992. *Skeletal Muscle Pathology*, 2nd edn. Churchill Livingstone, Edinburgh.

Walton JH, Karpati G, Hilton-Jones D. 1994. *Disorders of Voluntary Muscle*, 6th edn. Churchill Livingstone, Edinburgh.

24   Assorted Malfunctions

In this chapter we consider various signs and symptoms of disordered working of the nervous system, and suggest procedures for the post mortem examination of affected patients. The list is, of course, far from complete. It is in alphabetical order.

Acromegaly and gigantism

It may be assumed that the cause is an eosinophil adenoma of the pituitary, which may be either pure or mixed with chromophobe tumour. The mixed tumours, in particular, may reach a considerable size, and cause extra trouble by compressing the optic tracts, the nerves in the walls of the cavernous sinus, or the hypothalamic region of the forebrain. A block of the sphenoid bone should be removed at post mortem (see p.3); after fixation, coronal sections, including the upper cranial nerves and internal carotid arteries, may be examined histologically. If it is intended to carry out histochemical or immunohistological studies on the tumour (see p.243), samples of the tumour are taken at post mortem.

Ageusia (loss of taste)

This is most commonly due to trauma, involving either an olfactory tract or a chorda tympani. In acceleration injuries, one or both olfactory bulbs are avulsed from the cribriform plates, with rupture of fibres arising from the olfactory mucosa (see anosmia, below). Fractures of the petrous temporal bone may cause compression of the facial nerve, including the chorda tympani, within the facial canal, causing ageusia on one side of the tongue. If the pathologist fails to execute a thorough examination of these structures, they are unlikely to arouse fierce criticism from their colleagues.

Agnosias, various

The term *agnosia* implies a failure of perception, with inability to make sense of incoming sensory data. In general, the relevant lesions are found either in the parietal cortex or in subcortical white matter, where they are thought to disconnect the receiving areas (which remain more or less intact) from other areas of cortex where information is, as they say, processed. Auditory agnosia, for instance, is caused by *bilateral* lesions behind the auditory cortex (Heschl's gyri, in the buried upper surfaces of the temporal lobes; see Fig. 24.7). Visual agnosia, which may be one-sided, depends on disconnection of visual cortex from the temporal and parietal cortex of *both* sides. Loss of spatial orientation and failure to understand spatial relationships are commonly associated with lesions of the right parietal lobe. Agnosias involving the use of language tend to occur with lesions of the left parietotemporal region.

Akinetic mutism

Patients, not in true coma, who yet lie inert, not speaking or making 'voluntary' movements, may belong to one of three or more groups. In the first, there is widespread diffuse damage to the cerebral white matter, such as occurs in leucodystrophies and in severe cases of demyelinating disease. Strich (1956) described a series of cases in which the damage was caused by acceleration injuries to the brain. In her view, their state was one of profound and irreversible dementia. In another group there is an expanding lesion in the vicinity of the third ventricle and aqueduct. Cases of this type have been described in which the state of akinetic mutism could be almost instantaneously reversed by surgical relief of intracranial pressure. Similar states, without associated lesions, are said to occur in the course of mental illness, or the use of hypnotic drugs, or a combination of these. If a case of this kind comes to post mortem, even if no naked-eye lesions are found, it is reasonable to examine sections of the thalamus, hypothalamus and temporal lobe with the microscope.

Further reading and references

Strich SJ. 1956. Diffuse degeneration of the cerebral white matter in severe dementia following head injury. *J Neurol Neurosurg Psychiat* **19**, 163–85.

Amnesia

The neural mechanisms through which memories are formed, established, recalled at will, and lost, constitute one of the most fascinating areas of neuropsychological physiology, in which research is advancing rapidly. Disturbances of these mechanisms produce a variety of clinical disabilities, a few of which can be traced to lesions in some part of the so-called fornix system (hippocampus/fimbria/fornix/mamillary body/anterior nucleus of thalamus/cingulate cortex/hippocampus; see p.48. In the past, over-enthusiastic attempts to treat epilepsy by bilateral temporal lobectomy, with removal of large amounts of hippocampus, have resulted in loss of the ability to form new memories, although old memories were retained. In Korsakoff's syndrome, there is a similar inability to form new memories, combined with a failure to sort old memories into their proper temporal order. The syndrome is most often a feature of Wernicke's encephalopathy (see p.359), in which bilateral lesions occur in the mamillary bodies and elsewhere in the periventricular grey matter. Simple forgetfulness, beyond what is accepted as permissible in the elderly, is an early presenting feature of Alzheimer's disease (see pp.306–11).

Amusia

This term should perhaps be discarded. Several quite different activities are involved in the performance, memorizing, recognition, recall and composition of music; it is therefore not surprising if there is no recognized 'musical centre' in the brain. It is to be doubted, in fact, whether there is much consistency among different subjects in the 'localization' of an activity so recently acquired in primate history as music-making. Loss of various musical abilities is sometimes, but not always, associated with aphasia. The subject is discussed, with a review of the literature, by Benton (1977).

Further reading and references

Benton AL. 1977. The Amusias. In Critchley M., Henson RA (Eds) *Music and the Brain*. William Heinemann, London, Chapter 22.

Anosmia

This is usually a temporary inconvenience caused by the common cold. Lasting anosmia results when the olfactory bulbs are torn away from the cribriform plate. This may be due either to acceleration injury to the head, or to retraction of the frontal lobes in the course of a surgical operation. Traces of the injury may be found in the form of yellow staining of the bulbs and surrounding cortex.

One-sided anosmia is also a feature of tumours in the

floor of the anterior cranial fossa—in particular, olfactory groove meningiomas.

In Alzheimer's disease (pp.306–11) the sense of smell has recently been shown to be blunted early in the course of the illness. This may be related to the finding, in a number of cases of Alzheimer's disease, of numerous argyrophilic plaques and neurofibrillary tangles in the olfactory (periamygdaloid) cortex and in parts of the amygdaloid nucleus having intimate olfactory connections (corticomedial nuclei); also of neurofibrillary tangles and cell loss in the anterior olfactory nuclei.

Ataxia (see also Chapter 15, pp.275–81)

The term covers many manifestations of bad coordination of voluntary movements. Some of these have been given pleasing names such as dyssynergia and dysdiadochokinesis; for details, textbooks of neurology should be consulted. Most of them can be traced to lesions in the cerebellum and its connections; but in some cases the cerebellar network appears intact, and the relevant lesions are in some part of the sensory apparatus. The best-known example of a disease causing sensory ataxia is tabes dorsalis.

In examining a case of ataxia, if there is a suitably-placed lesion, apparent to the naked eye, such as a tumour, a haemorrhage or an infarct, there is little point in exploring the rest of the cerebellar and sensory systems. If, however, there is a history of progressive ataxia, and naked-eye inspection reveals nothing more than symmetrical shrinkage (associated, perhaps, with a palpable gliotic hardening), a system degeneration is the probable diagnosis; and multiple histological blocks are needed in order to determine the extent of the degeneration (see Chapter 15). When exploring the cerebellum, it should be borne in mind that lesions in a lateral lobe are associated with ataxia of the limbs on the same side of the body, whereas midline lesions are commonly associated with trunk ataxia.

Table 24.1 shows some sites where lesions bearing on ataxia may be found, along with the diseases in which such lesions are apt to occur. Anatomical relations are shown in Figs 2.27–2.29.

Autonomic failure

This term covers many functional disturbances, including anhidrosis (inability to sweat), retention of urine, impotence, orthostatic (or postural) hypotension, i.e. a tendency to faint in the upright posture, and other manifestations of defective vasomotor control. Four different types of morbid change have been implicated in autonomic failure.

1 Peripheral nerve diseases, of which by far the commonest is diabetic neuropathy (see p.382).

2 A group of rare genetic disorders, most of which involve

Table 24.1 Sites of lesions in diseases causing ataxia.

Sites of lesions	Diseases
Sensory ganglia and roots	Disc protrusions; toxic and inflammatory neuropathies; tabes dorsalis; FA; CMTD; AT; spinal radiculitis; carcinoma; chronic meningitis
Cord; posterior columns	As above; MS; spinal tumours
Dorsal (Clarke's) nuclei	FA; various spinocerebellar degenerations
Spinocerebellar tracts	FA; MS; various degenerations
Gracile and cuneate nuclei	'Chain' degeneration from posterior column lesions
Medial lemnisci	As above; MS
Accessory cuneate nuclei	FA
Inferior olives	Retrograde degeneration from cerebellar cortex; MSA; Leigh's disease
Inferior cerebellar peduncles	Degeneration of spino-, cuneo- and olivocerebellar tracts; lateral medullary syndrome; MS; MSA; FA
Cerebellar white matter	Degeneration of cerebellopetal fibres and Purkinje axons; MS; MSA; CCD; infarction
Cerebellar Purkinje cells	Hypoxia; epilepsy; toxins (including alcoholism); MSA; CCD; AT; old age
Cerebellar granule cells	Hypoxia; haemosiderosis; AT; CJD
Pontine nuclei	MSA; Leigh's disease
Middle cerebellar peduncles	MSA; MS
Dentate nuclei	FA; DRPLA; PSP
Superior cerebellar peduncles	FA; DRPLA; PSP; MS; trauma
Red nuclei	DRPLA; PSP

AT, ataxia–telangiectasia; CCD, cerebellar cortical degeneration; CJD, Creutzfeldt–Jakob disease; CMTD, Charcot–Marie–Tooth disease; DRPLA, dentato-rubro-pallido-luysian degeneration; FA, Friedreich's ataxia; MS, multiple sclerosis; MSA, multiple system atrophy; PSP, progressive supranuclear palsy.

both autonomic and sensory nerve fibres. Best known of these is familial dysautonomia (Riley–Day syndrome). For details, see Thomas *et al.* (1992). Most of the patients are children.

3 A group with destructive or expanding lesions in the region of the pituitary and hypothalamus.
4 In the most studied form of autonomic failure, the principal lesions are found in the CNS. The condition is progressive, affects middle-aged, and elderly people, and is often associated with degenerative lesions in many parts of the CNS. It is discussed in Chapter 15, p.275.

The clinical notes will usually indicate whether the main lesions should be looked for in the central or the peripheral nervous system. In any case, peripheral autonomic and sensory ganglia should be examined. If the vertebral column has been taken, the sympathetic chains will be available in the thoracolumbar region; and if a deep dissection of the neck has been carried out, there are cervical sympathetic ganglia and the (parasympathetic) inferior (nodose) ganglion of the vagus. The coeliac plexus provides a rich source of distal autonomic ganglia. This lies in the connective tissue around the origins of the coeliac, superior mesenteric and renal arteries.

Cases of progressive autonomic failure fall into two groups: in the first, there are Lewy inclusion bodies in pigmented cells of the substantia nigra and locus ceruleus; in the second, there is multiple system atrophy (see p.275) affecting the putamen and substantia nigra, and in many cases the pons, olives and cerebellar cortex. Cells of the intermediolateral columns, lying in the lateral horns of the thoracic cord, are depleted, sometimes devastated; but as their distribution is somewhat irregular, it is not safe to assess the degree of cell loss without examining five or more sections of thoracic cord and comparing these with sections of similar thickness from control material. Cell loss has recently been recorded from the intermediolateral columns of the sacral cord. These are the source of the sacral parasympathetic outflow. It has also been noted that cells are lost from the nucleus of Onufrowicz ('Onuf's nucleus'), a group of cells of somatic motor type, lying at the ventral edge of the anterior grey horn at level S2. These are believed to be the cells innervating the 'voluntary' sphincters of the anus and bladder neck. They are spared in motor neuron disease and in Werdnig–Hoffmann disease, even when the remaining sacral motor cells are devastated. For further discussion of the pathology of autonomic failure see Bannister & Mathias (1992).

The histological examination in any case of autonomic failure should include samples of both central and peripheral nervous systems. In a middle-aged or elderly subject with a progressive history, the two likely diseases are (i) multiple system atrophy of striatonigral type, and (ii) Parkinson's disease. Areas of the CNS at risk in these diseases are indicated in Table 15.1.

Further reading and references

Bannister R, Mathias C (Ed.). 1992. *Autonomic Failure*, 3rd edn. Oxford University Press, Oxford.

Thomas PK, Landon DN, King RHM. 1992. Diseases of the peripheral nerves. In Adams JH, Duchen LW (Eds) *Greenfield's Neuropathology*, 5th edn. Edward Arnold, London, Chapter 18.

Brown–Séquard syndrome

This is characterized by paralysis, of upper motor neuron type, of one lower limb, with loss of position and vibration sensibility on the same side, and loss of painful and thermal sensitivity on the opposite side. In its classical form it is due to hemisection of the spinal cord by a stab wound in the back. Other types of lesion may result in a more or less similar clinical picture. The neuropathologist's task is to identify the lesion, determine its segmental level, and observe, from sections taken a few centimetres above and below the lesion, the amount of upward and downward tract degeneration. In a 'classical' case, there will be a clear-cut myelin pallor and loss of axons in the pyramidal tract below the lesion, and in the gracile and spinocerebellar tracts above it. Upward degeneration of the so-called spinothalamic tract may be hard to appreciate, as the fibres in this group are mixed with others, many of them descending; but unless the lesion is very old, Marchi studies should reveal considerably more than can be seen by myelin staining. For cord tracts, see Fig. 2.29.

Cushing's disease

Cushing's disease, resulting from over-activity of the adrenal cortex, is sometimes due to excess production of ACTH by basophil cells in the anterior lobe of the pituitary. These may be scattered, or collected into a small discrete adenoma (for procedures, see pp.242–49). Rarer causes are adenomas and carcinomas of the adrenal cortex and oat-celled carcinomas of the lung, mischievously secreting ACTH or an analogous hormone. In all cases, the adrenals should be weighed, and studied histologically.

Diabetes insipidus

In a case of diabetes insipidus the structures needing detailed examination are the paraventricular and supra-optic nuclei of the hypothalamus (see Fig. 24.1), their efferent pathway in the infundibulum and pituitary stalk, and the posterior lobe of the pituitary itself. Some cases are 'primary', i.e. due to unknown causes. A few are familial. Among the rest, the causes include trauma, tumours and chronic inflammations. For details of anatomy and histopathology, see Treip (1992).

Further reading and references

Treip CS. 1992. The hypothalamus and pituitary gland. In Adams JH, Duchen LW (Eds) *Greenfield's Neuropathology*, 5th edn. Edward Arnold, London, Chapter 16.

poral bone should be removed with the vibrating saw at post mortem and fixed in formalin. The subsequent dissection can be planned and carried out after consultation between the clinician and the pathologist. Conditions in which such dissections may be informative include Ménière's disease, and a number of rare disorders in which sudden onset of deafness occurs, from unexplained causes.

Destructive lesions of an acoustic nerve will be reflected in myelin loss and, with time, gliosis, in the dorsal and ventral cochlear nuclei (see Fig. 15.8). The pathways from these to the inferior colliculi may be involved in vascular lesions or diffuse gliomas; but there are no well-defined clinical syndromes associated with particular lesions of the superior olives or trapezoid body. The input from each ear is relayed to both inferior colliculi (mainly to the contralateral one), and thence via the medial geniculate bodies to Heschl's gyri on the upper, buried surfaces of the temporal lobes. Lesions at these levels do not cause deafness unless they are bilateral.

In a case examined in this department there were bilateral temporal lobe infarcts, sparing a small amount of Heschl's gyrus on one side. The lesions were reflected in a severe retrograde loss of cells in the medial geniculate bodies. The patient was not deaf, but suffered from auditory agnosia, i.e. what he heard conveyed no meaning to him.

Hemiplegia

By far the commonest causes of hemiplegia are vascular accidents, occlusive or haemorrhagic, affecting the territory of a middle cerebral artery, with cerebral tumours in third place. Intracerebral haemorrhage is discussed in Chapter 6, infarction in Chapter 7, and tumours in Chapters 12 and 13. Causes of *hemiparesis* are varied: in addition to the above they include migraine, MS and trauma. In exploring the brain of a hemiplegic patient it is worth noting that the position of the corticospinal tract in the internal capsule is well behind the position commonly assigned to it in textbooks of anatomy. It occupies the middle third of the crus cerebri, and the entire medullary pyramid. The decussation is at the junction of medulla and cord; thus the tract degeneration is contralateral to the paralysis in the brain and ipsilateral in the cord (Figs 2.27 and 2.29).

Horner's syndrome

This consists in unilateral ptosis and enophthalmos, with pupillary constriction and relative flushing and dryness of the same side of the face. It is due to interruption of the sympathetic pathway which runs from the medulla via the lateral white column of the cervical cord to the intermediolateral cell column at the upper end of the thoracic cord. Here the upper sympathetic fibres end, and

the second-order sympathetic pathway begins. Its fibres run, via a white ramus communicans, to the sympathetic chain, ending in the superior cervical ganglion. The third-order fibres reach the face and eye by way of the carotid plexus, and thence via a multitude of little vessels and nerves. Clearly, interruption of the pathway may occur at many points. Here we will mention only a few such points. First, there is the lower medulla, where occlusion of the posterior inferior cerebellar artery may produce the lateral medullary (Wallenberg's) syndrome, which is discussed on p.424. In the cervical cord, a syrinx may destroy the upper sympathetic fibres. Injury to the lower cervical spine may sever an upper thoracic root; and a malignant tumour in the neck may destroy the upper stretches of the sympathetic chain.

Hypopituitarism

This term is generally taken to mean depression of anterior lobe functions—most conspicuously, sexual functions. The two best known causes are infarction and compression of the gland. The latter occurs with expanding lesions within or above the pituitary fossa, in particular chromophobe adenomas, craniopharyngiomas and meningiomas. With chromophobe adenomas, doubts have been expressed on whether in some cases depression of anterior lobe function is due more to excessive prolactin secretion than to mechanical compression. In *Sheehan's syndrome*, infarction is said to be due to massive blood loss, with resulting arterial hypotension, during the puerperium.

Hypopituitarism may also result from fracture of the base of the skull, or traumatic tearing of the pituitary stalk. Inflammatory processes within the sella include tuberculosis and sarcoidosis. Examination of the region is best carried out on a block of sphenoid bone removed as described on p.3.

Incontinence

In many cases, the causes of incontinence of urine and/or faeces are obvious to the clinicians, and there is no need for pathologists to strain their energies laying bare the structural changes responsible for it. In other cases, this is not so; for example, many an innocent prostate has been surgically assaulted in cases of progressive autonomic failure. Leaving aside the mechanical and psychiatric causes of incontinence, the post mortem examination should concentrate on the spinal cord. Plaques of MS are among the commoner causes of failure of sphincter control: but other parts of the CNS may be involved. In the heyday of prefrontal leucotomy, it was said that the operation seldom achieved its intended effect unless it rendered the patient incontinent for at least a few days.

Table 24.2 Some diseases associated with involuntary movements.

Type of movement	Diseases	Sites of lesions
Athetosis	Wilson's disease (p.335)	Striatum, etc; liver
	Perinatal hypoxia (pp.366–71)	
	Kernicterus (p.371)	Scattered in brain
	DRPLA (p.283)	Pallidum, etc.
Ballism	Vascular disease	Subthalamic nucleus
	DRPLA (p.283)	Subthalamic nucleus, etc.
Chorea	Sydenham's chorea (rheumatic fever)	? Basal ganglia
	Huntington's disease (p.281)	Striatum
	Wilson's disease (p.335)	Striatum, etc; liver
	DRPLA (p.283)	Pallidum, etc.
Myoclonus	Lafora body disease (p.326)	Scattered in brain
	Creutzfeldt–Jakob disease (pp.311–12)	Striatum, etc.
	SSPE (p.173)	Scattered in brain
Tremor	Paralysis agitans (p.273)	Substantia nigra; nucleus basalis
	'Senility'; multi-infarct dementia (p.315)	Thalamus; basal ganglia

DRPLA, dentato-rubro-pallido-luysian atrophy; SSPE, subacute sclerosing parencephalitis.

Involuntary movements

The commonly-used clinical terms, in alphabetical order are: *athetosis* (slow, writhing movements of head, trunk and limbs), *ballism* (or hemiballism: sudden wild flinging movements, commonly affecting one or two limbs on one side of the body), *chorea* (jerky movements, affecting many parts of the body), *clonus* and *myoclonus* (rhythmic or periodic contractions of a muscle or of a group of muscles), *tics* (irregular localized movements, to some extent under voluntary control), and *tremor*. Table 24.2 shows some of the CNS afflictions associated with abnormal movements, and sites where lesions may be found.

Irradiation

It sometimes happens, in the course of X-ray treatment of a tumour situated in the head, neck or back, that part of the CNS receives an intolerable dose of irradiation. When such a case comes to post mortem, the precise geometry of the area of radionecrosis and of its surroundings is (or should be) of intense interest to the radiotherapist, and the pathologist should be prepared to supply detailed information on this.

The lesions may take weeks, or months, or over a year to develop. Characteristically they consist of coagulative necrosis, with hyaline or fibrinoid necrosis of vessels (Fig. 24.2). According to one view, which we find plausible, the primary effect of the X-rays is exerted on vascular endothelium, which loses its ability to regenerate, and the parenchymal changes are attributable to ischaemia. The observation that white matter tends to be worse affected than grey matter may be related to the relatively poor blood supply of white matter (see Duchen 1992).

The effects of irradiation on the tumours themselves are discussed by Russell and Rubinstein (1989). A special case is the medulloblastoma, which is said to be one of the most radiosensitive of all malignant tumours. It has repeatedly been observed that 10 days or so after treatment the tumour is transformed into a highly pleomorphic tissue, with bizarre giant cells, indistinguishable from a giant-celled glioblastoma.

Occasionally, after a long delay, irradiation causes a tumour to develop at the irradiated site. Sarcomas have developed in the suprasellar region following irradiation of a benign pituitary adenoma, and in the meninges after irradiation of gliomas. In the past, irradiation of the scalp for tinea capitis has resulted in the late development of brain tumours, including both gliomas and meningiomas.

Further reading and references

Duchen LW. 1992. Effects of irradiation on the nervous system. In Adams JH, Duchen LW (Eds) *Greenfield's Neuropathology*, 5th edn. Edward Arnold, London, pp. 42–5.

Fig. 24.2 Cluster of abnormal blood vessels in a necrotic left temporal lobe biopsy from a patient with progressive dysplasia developing 2 years after radiation to the left upper neck for an aggressive parotid gland tumour. H&E, ×200.

Russell DS, Rubinstein LJ. 1989. *Pathology of Tumours of the Nervous System*, 5th edn. Edward Arnold, London.

Lateral medullary (Wallenberg's) syndrome

This syndrome, well loved by teachers of neuro-anatomy, is caused by an infarct in the territory of the PICA, which includes a variable amount of cerebellum and an area in the dorsolateral quadrant of the lower medulla (see Fig. 7.14). The syndrome consists of cerebellar ataxia, palatal palsy, Horner's syndrome and loss of pain and temperature sense over the face, all on the side of the lesion, and loss of pain and temperature sense on the other side of the body. The accompanying diagram is intended to show how this combination of disturbances is produced (Fig. 24.3).

After identifying and mapping the infarct, it remains to discover its cause. In some cases there is an occlusive thrombus in the vertebral artery, blocking the origin of the PICA; in others, the same effect is produced by atheroma, without thrombosis. In a few cases the vertebral artery is patent, but the PICA itself is thrombosed. A rare cause, which we have encountered, is a mechanical buckling of a loop of the PICA as it passes between the medulla and cerebellum. The course, size and territory of the artery are all variable, and the clinical syndrome varies accordingly.

'Locked-in' syndrome

Patients who, though alert, are unable to carry out any voluntary movements except of the eyes and eyelids are said to suffer from the 'locked-in' syndrome. The lesion responsible is one that interrupts descending tracts in the pons, or occasionally in the midbrain. This is usually due to infarction associated with occlusion of the basilar artery; but a few cases are due to the effects of trauma, tumour, or demyelination.

Mental defect

This is distinguished from dementia in being (in most cases, at least) congenital and non-progressive. Examination of the cerebral hemispheres of severe mental defectives usually reveals naked-eye abnormalities. When none are found, and the histology appears normal, the pathologist may well conclude that the subject simply lay at the left-hand end of the normal distribution curve for intelligence, or was autistic.

Most of the recognized lesions responsible for mental defect fall into one of three categories: (i) *developmental anomalies*, which are discussed in Chapter 16; (ii) *perinatal vascular mishaps*, discussed in Chapter 21; and (iii) *metabolic disorders*, discussed in Chapter 19. Examples of these are (i) tuberous sclerosis, (ii) cerebral palsy, and (iii) lipidosis. More rarely, the defect is traceable to intrauterine or perinatal infections, for instance, by cytomegalovirus, *Treponema pallidum* or *Toxoplasma* (Chapters 9 and 10). Some metabolic disorders, e.g. phenylketonuria, are identifiable biochemically, but have no recognized histopathology. For the most part they cause progressive dementia rather than congenital mental defect. Milder

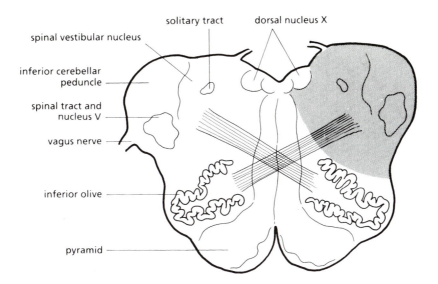

solitary tract   dorsal nucleus X

spinal vestibular nucleus

inferior cerebellar peduncle

spinal tract and nucleus V

vagus nerve

inferior olive

pyramid

Fig. 24.3 Area of the medulla commonly supplied by the posterior inferior cerebellar artery (stippled). Structures involved in the lateral medullary syndrome include: the inferior cerebellar peduncle, containing the dorsal spinocerebellar tract and olivocerebellar fibres from the opposite side; the spinal (descending) vestibular tract and nucleus; emerging and entering fibres of the vagus nerve; the spinal (descending) trigeminal tract and nucleus; and a mixture of ascending and descending pathways, continuous with the anterolateral columns of the cervical cord, including the spinothalamic and spinoreticular (sensory) pathways and the upper sympathetic fibres running from the hypothalamus to the intermediolateral columns of the spinal cord.

forms of mental retardation are associated with genetic defects e.g. fragile X syndrome, but they have as yet no recognized neuropathology.

Nystagmus

The physiology of the various types of nystagmus is discussed in considerable detail by Brodal (1981). In general, the lesions associated with it are to be found in the labyrinth, in the vestibular nerves and the nuclei in the lower brain stem to which they project, or in the connections between the vestibular nuclei and (i) the cerebellum, and (ii) the nuclei of the third, fourth and sixth cranial nerves, including the medial longitudinal fasciculus (see Fig. 2.27). Diseases in which such lesions occur include acute labyrinthitis, Ménière's disease, posterior fossa tumours (in particular acoustic schwannomas), occlusion of a posterior inferior cerebellar artery, brain stem gliomas and MS.

Further reading and references

Brodal P. 1992. *The Central Nervous System*, 3rd edn. Oxford University Press, Oxford.

Ophthalmoplegia

Unilateral oculomotor palsy may be caused by: intra-orbital tumours, pseudotumours and granulomas; trauma, including difficult birth; or by an expanding lesion—tumour or internal carotid aneurysm—in or near the cavernous sinus. Isolated nerve palsies occur in both acute and chronic forms of meningitis, meningeal carcinomatosis and sarcoidosis, and may also be a feature of diphtheritic neuropathy.

Bilateral ocular palsy may be due to a variety of myopathies and neuropathies. The myopathies, discussed by Harriman (1992), include the Kearns–Sayre syndrome ('ophthalmoplegia plus'), a slowly progressive disease of childhood, in which ocular palsy is associated with retinitis pigmentosa, mental defect, and deafness. The characteristic finding is of 'ragged red' fibres, containing abnormal mitochondria (see p.406).

In cases labelled *progressive external ophthalmoplegia*, the clinical diagnosis between myopathy and neuropathy is often difficult and dependent upon finding evidence of one or the other condition elsewhere in the body. The histological diagnosis from a tiny, often damaged, biopsy specimen is likewise difficult. In the post mortem examination it is important to be aware of the differences between normal external ocular muscle and skeletal muscle elsewhere in the body. Silver preparations of normal eye muscles show a wide scatter of fibre calibres, including groups of small fibres, and a bewildering tangle of irregular branching nerve fibres.

In system degenerations of the CNS causing denervation of muscle elsewhere in the body, the oculomotor (III,

IV and VI) nuclei are very rarely involved. An exception is *progressive supranuclear palsy*, which is discussed on p.282.

In the condition *exophthalmic ophthalmoplegia*, met with in some cases of thyrotoxicosis, the ocular palsy appears to be due largely to mechanical factors.

Further reading and references

Harriman DGF. 1992. Disease of muscle. In Adams JH, Duchen LW (Eds) *Greenfield's Neuropathology*, 5th edn. Edward Arnold, London, Chapter 21.

Pain syndromes

Cases of severe persistent or episodic pain (other than headache) which call for post mortem examination by a neuropathologist tend to belong to one of four categories: (i) 'central' pain (see Pagni 1984), including the *thalamic syndrome*; (ii) cases that have undergone *surgery* on the CNS for the relief of pain; (iii) cases of *tic douloureux* (trigeminal neuralgia); and (iv) cases of *post-herpetic neuralgia*.

1 *Thalamic syndrome.* In its classical presentation, the lesion is an infarct or haemorrhage involving the posterolateral area of the thalamus, which results in a condition of *hyperpathia* or *hyperalgesia* on the opposite side of the body. Thresholds for common sensation are raised, and normal stimuli evoke a spreading, slowly subsiding, discomfort which the patient may describe as 'agonizing'. In all such cases the thalamus should be examined in multiple sections, and the damaged area mapped. If no lesion is found in the thalamus, the search should include the sensory pathways from the brain stem to the parietal white matter and cortex.

2 The commonest surgical procedures for the relief of pain include *anterolateral chordotomy* and *posterior rhizotomy*. The post mortem examination has two aims: first, to give the surgeon accurate information on the extent of the lesion; and, second, to trace the resulting tract degeneration in the CNS. Even if it is decided not to pursue the second aim, the material should be kept for the benefit of colleagues with neuro-anatomical interests.

3 In cases of *trigeminal neuralgia*, whether or not they have undergone surgical attack on the affected nerve root or its ganglion, these should be preserved and carefully dissected after fixation (see p.3 and Fig. 1.3 for details of removal at post mortem). There are published reports of apparently successful operations for this condition in which abnormal relations of the nerve with the surrounding dura have been observed. Trigeminal neuralgia is said to be unduly frequent in patients with MS; and small plaques have repeatedly been seen in the trigeminal root entry zone (Fig. 2.27, level E) in such cases (see Loeser 1984).

4 In cases of *post-herpetic neuralgia*, the suspected dorsal root ganglion (or trigeminal ganglion) should be examined histologically; likewise one or two spinal ganglia above and below the suspected one. It has been suggested (Noordenbos 1959) that pain ensues when there is selective destruction of large myelinated nerve fibres. To prove this point, many controlled fibre counts would be necessary. If such counts are contemplated, portions of ribs may be taken at post mortem, and intercostal nerves dissected out after fixation. The fifth intercostal nerve, for instance, is found in the costal groove on the under-surface of the fifth rib.

The pathology of *causalgia* is discussed by Schott (1986).

Further reading and references

Boivie J. 1994. Central pain. In Wall PD, Melzack R (Eds) *Textbook of Pain*, 3rd edn. Churchill Livingstone, Edinburgh, pp. 871–902.
Loeser JD. 1994. Tic douloureux and atypical facial pain. In Wall PD, Melzack R (Eds) *Textbook of Pain*, 3rd edn. Churchill Livingstone, Edinburgh, pp. 699–710.
Noordenbos W. 1959. *Pain: Problems Pertaining to the Transmission of Nerve Impulses which give rise to Pain*. Elsevier, Amsterdam.
Schott GD. 1986. Mechanisms of causalgia and related conditions. *Brain* **109**, 717–38.

Paraplegia and paraparesis

Paralysis of both lower limbs is usually due to a transverse lesion of the spinal cord; less often, to compression of the roots of the cauda equina. In the former (except perhaps for a few days following a back injury) the paralysis is of spastic type, with pathologically brisk tendon reflexes; in the latter it is flaccid, with loss of reflexes, and eventually with wasting of muscles. For obvious reasons it is desirable, where possible, to remove the vertebral column at post mortem in cases of paraplegia.

Some of the causes of paraplegia are listed below.

1 MS.

2 Expanding lesions in the spinal canal.

3 Spinal deformity causing compression of the cord.

4 Spinal trauma.

5 Infarction of a length of spinal cord, which may in turn be due to:

    (a) atheroma of the abdominal aorta;

    (b) malignant infiltration of, or accidental damage to, a major radicular artery;

    (c) arteriovenous malformation ('angioma of the spinal cord'; see p.35).

The term *transverse myelitis* is freely used by clinicians to denote any acute ailment causing blockage of conduction in the long tracts of the spinal cord with a definite sensory level. It does not refer to any specific pathological process. In most of the cases thus labelled the cause is either a vascular disorder or an acute demyelinating process.

Whatever the cause of the paraplegia, the blood supply of the affected stretch of cord should be examined. The lesion itself is of interest; the amount of glial and fibrous scarring, and the extent of invasion of the necrotic tissue by sprouting of peripheral fibres from the central processes of sensory ganglion cells, are all worth looking at; and sections should be taken from above and below the lesion, to determine whether *any* nerve fibres, ascending or descending, were getting through. In cases of cauda equina compression, the lumbosacral cord should be examined for central chromatolysis in motor cells and wallerian degeneration in the posterior columns. When the lesion is recent, Marchi preparations may be more informative than myelin stains.

Parkinsonism

Patients who have responded well to L-dopa are almost certainly cases of *Parkinson's disease*, which is discussed on p.273. Where this is not the case, especially if there were also cerebellar or autonomic disturbances, one may suspect the striatonigral variety of *multiple system atrophy* (p.275). Rigid muscles are a feature of *progressive supranuclear palsy* (p.282). Tremor and bradykinesia are common in elderly patients, and may be related to scattered rarefactions in the thalamus and lentiform nuclei, which are generally attributable to atheroma of the basal arteries. This, we feel, is probably the pathological basis of the *'arteriosclerotic parkinsonism'* spoken of in textbooks of neurology. The other parkinsonian syndrome discussed in the textbooks—the *post-encephalitic* type—is becoming increasingly rare, as survivors from the 1920s outbreak of encephalitis lethargica die off. The lesions to be looked for consist in massive loss of pigmented cells in the substantia nigra, which to the naked eye may be totally depigmented; and scattered gliotic foci, shown up in Holzer or PTA preparations, throughout the basal grey matter (hypothalamus, subthalamic area and tegmentum); and neurofibrillary tangles in nerve cells in a similar distribution. Whether this picture can be produced by other virus infections is at present unknown. These tangles, unlike those seen in Alzheimer's disease, are not particularly well displayed in silver impregnations, but show up well enough in H&E and van Gieson preparations. Cases are occasionally met with having the histological stigmata of post-encephalitic parkinsonism but no history of encephalitis.

After Parkinson's disease, the commonest type of parkinsonism is probably an effect of *phenothiazine drugs*. Clear evidence on the pathology of this condition is still lacking. Another toxic state which sometimes gives rise to a parkinsonian syndrome is *carbon monoxide poisoning*. The principal lesion here is usually bilateral necrosis of the globus pallidus. This involves not merely the cells of the pallidum but also most of the outflow from the putamen.

Precocious puberty

This has repeatedly been found associated with gliomas or hamartomas involving the hypothalamus. It affects boys more often than girls (Fig. 24.4); but the patient in Fig. 24.5 was a woman.

Pseudobulbar palsy

This is a term used by clinicians when bilateral weakness of muscles supplied by cranial nerves is attributed to vascular lesions in the cerebral hemispheres. The affected muscles do not undergo atrophy. Post mortem, the diagnosis is confirmed by finding lesions in the hemispheres and none in the brain stem. Plaques of MS should be looked for, if infarcts are not present; and progressive supranuclear palsy (p.282) should be borne in mind as a possible diagnosis.

Psychosis

Psychotic behaviour, sometimes closely resembling schizophrenia, may occur in a number of organic brain diseases—frontal gliomas, for instance, and Huntington's chorea—in the absence of positive neurological signs. Transient psychosis due to various drugs is exceedingly common. Psychosis is also not infrequently an early presenting feature of inherited metabolic diseases (Chapter 19). We have seen two cases of adult leucodystrophy—one metachromatic, the other adrenoleukodystrophy—in men who suffered from apparently typical schizophrenia for many years before they developed additional progressive neurological disease. An association of psychosis with temporal lobe epilepsy has long been recognized (Trimble 1984). In these cases the local pathology (p.326) is usually on the left side. Outbursts of *maniacal behaviour* may occur in hypoglycaemic attacks due either to an overdose of insulin or to a secreting islet-cell adenoma. In a case examined in this department, a middle-aged man, in good health, suddenly went mad. After about two hours of maniacal behaviour he lapsed into coma and stayed there, undiagnosed, for six months. At post mortem he was found to have multiple necrotic foci in the brain, and diffuse hyperplasia of islet cells in the pancreas. Serious mental disturbances associated with excessive consumption of alcohol include *Korsakoff's psychosis*, most commonly associated with Wernicke's encephalopathy (p.359), and the *Marchiafava–Bignami syndrome*, discussed on p.348.

Infections causing madness are dealt with in Chapters 9 and 10. The best documented of these is *chronic syphilitic encephalitis* (also known as general paralysis of the insane;

Fig. 24.4 T1W coronal MR image demonstrates a hamartoma of the hypothalamus (white arrow) in a 6-year-old boy with precocious puberty. The lesion is typically a non-progressive, non-enhancing, sessile or pedunculated mass attached to the tuber cinereum, isointense with grey matter.

Fig. 24.5 Hamartoma of hypothalamus in a woman of 24, with epilepsy since the age of 4 and precocious puberty since the age of 8. There is a normal mamillary body on the right. The left hypothalamus is expanded by a mass of ectopic grey matter, with no evidence of neoplasia.

see p.316). Since the introduction of penicillin, the full-blown pathology described in the older literature is very rarely seen, but it is still worth looking for in suspect cases. In general, the cruder and more easily recognizable brain diseases are apt to cause dementia rather than madness.

In a typical case of *schizophrenia*, with onset after puberty, the disease is idiopathic, i.e. utterly mysterious. There are now generally agreed changes in medial temporal lobe structure with atrophy of the parahippocampal gyrus and compensatory enlargement of the inferior horns of the lateral ventricles. These changes have been described in post mortem brains (Brown *et al.* 1986) and with MRI scans on living patients. There is no general agreement about the various fine histological changes which have been reported from time to time. The subject is reviewed by Bogerts (1993). The fact that the manifestations of the disease can be modified by drugs suggests that the basic disorder may be a biochemical one; and a public-spirited pathologist will preserve the brains of schizophrenic patients and hand them over to colleagues in centres where the neurochemistry and neuropharmacology of madness are studied. The same applies for cases of 'idiopathic' manic-depressive psychosis. Some addresses are given in Appendix B.

Further reading and references

Bogerts B. 1993. Recent advances in the neuropathology of schizophrenia. *Schiz Bull* **49**, 431–45.

Brown R, Colter N, Corsellis JAN *et al.* 1986. Post mortem evidence of structural brain changes in schizophrenia: differences in brain weight, temporal horn area and parahippocampal gyrus compared with affective disorder. *Arch Gen Psychiat* **43**, 36–42.

Kovelman JA, Scheibel AB. 1986. Biological substrates of schizophrenia. *Acta Neurol Scand* **73**, 1–32.

Trimble MR. 1984. Interictal Psychosis of epilepsy. *Acta Psychiat Scand* (suppl) **313**, 9–20.

Rigidity

The commonest form of muscular rigor is *cramp*, of the type that afflicts many elderly people, most commonly in the legs and feet. The physiological disorder in this condition is unknown. In *miner's cramp* and *tetany*, on the other hand, electrolyte imbalance is given the blame. The second commonest is the rigidity of hemiplegic limbs following a stroke. Since pure lesions of the corticospinal tracts do not cause rigidity, this is presumably due to interruption of extrapyramidal pathways which inhibit reflex muscular contractions. The same principle may apply to so-called *decerebrate rigidity*, and to the 'cog-wheel' and 'lead pipe' rigidity of parkinsonism. There have been reports of intense, painful muscular rigidity in which the responsible lesion appears to have isolated groups of motor neurons from descending inhibitory influences; and we have encountered a case of rigid hemiplegia in a patient with selective infarction of the striatum, with intact corticospinal tracts.

Sensory loss

From the pathologist's point of view, the simplest cases are those with peripheral nerve lesions. When there is a localized area of anaesthesia, reference to a textbook of anatomy will usually indicate where to look for the lesion, and the clinical notes should make it plain whether the cause of the lesion is leprosy, a slipped disc, a glass splinter or a horse's hoof. More generalized disturbances call for procedures outlined in Chapter 22, to determine whether the neuropathy is of toxic, metabolic or inflammatory origin. To these three categories one may add a fourth, namely 'idiopathic', i.e. 'having no apparent cause'. Some would add a fifth: neurotic.

Dulling of sensation in the limbs is a regular feature of some diseases of the CNS—in particular, MS. In this condition, numbness is commonly associated with *paraesthesiae*, among them *Lhermitte's sign*—a sensation like an electric shock running down the back when the neck is flexed. When this is known to have occurred, the cervical cord should be carefully examined. MS is the commonest but not the only disorder causing this symptom.

Cases of *congenital indifference to pain* have been found to show a deficiency of sensory ganglion cells. We have no experience of such cases. They are discussed by Thomas, Landon & King (1992).

Cases of *dissociated sensory loss* (the dissociation being between 'posterior column' and 'spinothalamic' sensibility) usually offer a good ratio of reward to effort. In most cases the lesion lies in the spinal cord; less often in the brain stem; rarely elsewhere, e.g. in the thalamus. Interruption of a sensory tract will produce a sensory *level*, with sensation normal above, and impaired below. An exception to this rule occurs in some cases of syringomyelia, in which the decussation of the 'spinothalamic' pathway is destroyed over a few segments. Thermal and noxious stimuli are ignored over the relevant segments, but felt normally above and below.

Further reading and references

Thomas PK, Landon DN, King RHM. 1992. Diseases of the peripheral nerves. In Adams JH, Duchen LW (Eds) *Greenfield's Neuropathology*, 5th edn. Edward Arnold, London, Chapter 18.

Sleep disturbances

Most disorders of sleep patterns occur as part of the rough-and-tumble of life—anxiety, pain, air travel, intoxication, banal feverish illnesses and so forth. In such cases it is generally assumed that the disturbances are caused by variations in the discharge of impulses in the *brain stem reticular formation*—a convenient term used to cover numerous scattered small groups of nerve cells whose connections are difficult to trace, but which exert profound influence upon our normal physical and mental functions, including waking and sleeping. Indeed, sleep disturbances are among the common features of cases of MS and brain stem glioma. They also occur with lesions of the hypothalamus. Von Economo (1931) observed that in fatal cases of 'sleeping sickness' lesions affecting the posterior hypothalamus and upper midbrain were usually associated with excessive sleep, while lesions in the anterior hypothalamus often resulted in insomnia; and the examination of the hypothalamus and its immediate surroundings remains the first requirement when a sleep disturbance figures large in the clinical history. The anatomy and physiology of the subject are reviewed by Moruzzi (1963) and Brodal (1992).

In fatal cases of *sleeping sickness* due to infection by *Trypanosoma gambiense*, a diffuse meningoencephalitis is described. Since much of the hypothalamus lies exposed at the base of the brain, the disturbance of sleep may be due to its involvement in the inflammatory process. In a recently reported remarkable Italian family in which some members developed an inability to go to sleep, the pathology was described as that of a transmissible spongiform encephalopathy (p.311) (Lugaresi *et al.* 1986).

Further reading and references

Brodal P. 1992. *The Central Nervous System*. Oxford University Press, Oxford.

von Economo C. 1931. *Encephalitis Lethargica. Its Sequelae and Treatment*. Oxford University Press, Oxford.

Lugaresi E, Medori R, Montagna P *et al.* 1986. Fatal familial insomnia and dysautonomia with selective degeneration of thalamic nuclei. *New Engl J Med* **315**, 997–1003.

Moruzzi G. 1963. Active processes in the brain stem during sleep. *Harvey Lectures*, Academic Press, New York, **58**, 233–97.

Spasticity

We understand this term to denote increased muscular tone, resistance to passive stretch, and enhanced tendon reflexes. Spastic paralysis is conventionally attributed to lesions of 'upper motor neurons' (UMNs). If UMNs are taken to include non-pyramidal descending pathways and their cells of origin, this is probably correct; if it refers only to the corticospinal (pyramidal) tracts, it is not. The clearest evidence on this is the report by Bucy *et al.* (1964) on a case of incapacitating hemiballismus, treated by transection of the outer two-thirds of one crus cerebri. The resulting hemiplegia, without ballismus, delighted the patient. A few months later, power returned to the affected limbs, along with control of fine finger movements. The Babinski sign was positive, and reflexes were slightly brisker. Tone was normal. The patient died of a malignant lymphoma. Post mortem showed almost total degeneration of the medullary pyramid on the side of the operation.

Spasticity is usually associated with weakness or paralysis of the affected limbs, whether the lesion lies in a cerebral hemisphere or in the brain stem or spinal cord. In the cerebrum, vascular accidents and tumours are the commonest lesions; in the brain stem, MS; and in the spinal cord, MS and compressing lesions. In none of these conditions is the corticospinal tract affected in isolation from other descending pathways.

Obviously, the corticospinal tracts should be examined in cases of spastic paralysis; and if the pathologist's interests lie elsewhere, he need do little more than that. Our justification for introducing unsolved problems in motor physiology into a practical treatise is that a careful examination may provide useful general information, if it is not hampered by traditional myths, repeated through successive editions of medical textbooks.

Further reading and references

Bucy PC, Keplinger JE, Siqueira EB. 1964. Destruction of the pyramidal tract in man. *J Neurosurg* **21**, 385–98.

Speech and language disorders

Two areas of cerebral cortex are concerned with speech functions. The better known, and less important, of these is *Broca's area*—a small patch at the hind-end of the left inferior frontal convolution. The main 'speech centre' is *Wernicke's area*, which includes the posterior third of the left superior temporal convolution, and a certain amount (there is disagreement about how much) of neighbouring temporal and parietal cortex (Fig. 24.6). Regarding this disagreement, it has been pointed out (Bogen & Bogen 1976) that whereas Broca's area is clearly defined anatomically while its function remains uncertain, Wernicke's area is *defined* as the main centre for the organization of language functions, but there is no agreement about its *extent*. Regarding function, it is a suggestive fact that Broca's area is very close to the motor area for the face, while the 'speech area' of the temporal lobe lies immediately behind the auditory receiving area in the transverse (Heschl's) gyri (Fig. 24.7). In conformity with this, clinicians sometimes speak of 'Broca's dysphasia' in cases with a predominantly motor, or expressive, disability, and of 'Wernicke's dysphasia' for the rest of the dysphasic syndromes—word deafness, word blindness, dyslexia, dysgraphia, and so forth.

Human language is a recently evolved faculty; it is therefore not surprising that it has no hard-and-fast, genetically determined, cerebral localization. In some people, dysphasic disorders result from lesions in the right hemisphere. Children with congenital or acquired lesions of the left hemisphere nevertheless learn to talk, read and write. The area in the right hemisphere responsible for the takeover in such cases is not known.

Language 'centres', if they are to be of any use, must be adequately connected with other 'centres'—for hearing vision, thought, memory, and so on. Geschwind (1965, 1972) drew attention to various *'disconnection' syndromes*, in which the important lesion lies not in this or that area of cortex, but in the white matter connecting these. From what has been said, it follows that the examination of the brain from a case of aphasia or dysphasia may involve more than the inspection of the 'speech centres' of the left hemisphere.

By definition, *dysphasia* implies a defect in the use of language, either on the receptive side, in the understanding of spoken or written words, or on the expressive side, in the choice of words and phrases. *Dysarthria*, on the other hand, implies defective utterance. Lesions responsible for dysphasia are assumed to lie in the cerebrum—most commonly in the left hemisphere. *Dysarthria* may be due to lesions in many places, including motor cortex (strokes, tumours, etc.), basal ganglia (as in Huntington's and Parkinson's diseases), pathways in the brain stem (commonly affected in MS), motor nuclei (motor neuron disease, bulbar polio), the cerebellum and its connections; not to mention the effects, which may be transitory, of various neuropathies and myopathies. Dysarthria is also an effect of congenital deafness. Careful reading of the clinical notes, plus appropriate histology, will usually elucidate the cause of dysarthria; of dysphasia, not so often.

Further reading and references

Bogen JE, Bogen GM. 1976. Wernicke's region—where is it? *Ann NY Acad Sci* **280**, 834–43.
Brain WR. 1965. *Speech Disorders*. Butterworth, London.
Geschwind N. 1965. Disconnexion syndromes in animals and man. *Brain* **88**, 237–94, 585–644.
Geschwind N. 1972. Language and the brain. *Sci Am* **226**, 76–83.
Luria AR. 1970. *Traumatic Aphasia: its Syndromes, Psychology and Treatment*. Mouton & Co, New York.

Tremor

A mild tremor, occurring at rest, with a frequency around 10 per second, and unassociated with known lesions in the brain, is commonly referred to as physiological tremor. A somewhat coarser tremor, seen particularly in elderly people with atheroma, has been attributed to multiple rarefactions in the lentiform nuclei and thalamus. In Parkinson's disease and striatonigral degeneration coarse

Fig. 24.6 'Speech areas' (see text, p.430). Disagreement persists on the precise extent of Wernicke's area (stippled). (Redrawn, after Geschwind 1972.)

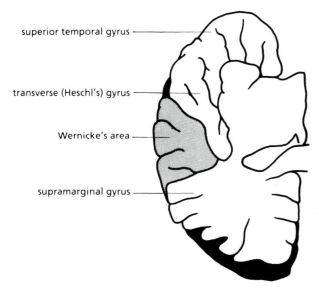

Fig. 24.7 Drawing to show the upper surface of the left temporal lobe. The Sylvian fissure has been opened up, and the frontal lobe removed. Wernicke's area (stippled) lies immediately behind the transverse (Heschl's) gyrus, which is the auditory area, receiving its main input from the medial geniculate body. (Redrawn, after Geschwind 1972.)

resting tremor of the limbs may become a fairly violent flapping movement. This is still sometimes relieved by stereotactic operations aimed at the ventrolateral nucleus of the thalamus (less often, the globus pallidus) on one side or both. In the post mortem examination, it is worth mapping the precise extent of the resulting lesion, if only to reassure the surgeon as to the accuracy of his technique.

Intention tremor—that is, tremor not present at rest, but coming into play in the course of voluntary movements, especially of the hands—is generally associated with disease involving the cerebellum and its connections. It is commonly seen in cases of MS.

Unconsciousness

Neuropathologists are seldom asked to explain why a particular patient was unconscious at the time of his death. They may, however, be moved by curiosity as to why, of two patients with similar lesions, one was conscious and the other not. This question arose in the course of looking for microscopic lesions in the brain following head injury. One of the patients was a man of 66 who was knocked down by a motor scooter and suffered multiple rib fractures. He was concussed, but was fully conscious 20 minutes later. He died of a chest infection 13 days later. The brain, which was macroscopically normal, was found to contain microglial clusters, characteristic of acceleration injury, in all areas, including the brain stem. The other case was of a 19-year-old girl who drove a car into a telegraph pole, and was deeply unconscious, responding to painful stimulation with 'decerebrate' movements, until her death 5 days later. There were naked-eye lesions in the cerebral hemispheres, but no tentorial hernia, and the brain stem looked normal apart from some bruising around the aqueduct. Sections of the brain stem resembled those in the previous case, except for a concentration of microscopic lesions in the peri-aqueductal grey matter.

Descartes placed the soul in the pineal body, apparently because this lies at the geometrical centre of the brain. It may seem equally childish to imagine that the 'centre' for consciousness lies about a centimetre below the site of Descartes' soul, but it is scarcely less childish to speak of 'centres' for sleep a centimetre in front of this. It may be recalled that one of the cardinal signs that the upper brain stem is being compressed by a transtentorial hernia is a progressive lowering of the level of consciousness.

When death has been preceded by a period of *coma*, the cause of the coma is usually made fairly clear by the clinical history, signs and investigations. The commoner causes of progressive clouding of consciousness include *cerebral hypoxia* (which in very many instances results from impaired lung function, as in pneumonia), *toxic and metabolic disorders*, and *space-occupying lesions* causing transtentorial herniation (see Chapters 7, 11, 19 and 20). Regarding toxic states, it hardly needs stressing that if there is the least suspicion of coma and death being due to drugs, self-administered or otherwise, the coroner will be displeased if the pathologist has not taken the stomach contents and samples of blood. Similarly, in a case of acute encephalopathy of unknown nature, the possibility of an infection should be kept in mind, and appropriate specimens taken for bacteriological and virological examination. It should also be remembered that two factors may be working together to produce coma; for instance, a diabetic may lapse into ketosis when assailed by pneumonia or meningitis; and either the infection or the ketosis may have been missed in the ward. Again, hypoglycaemic coma due to an overdose of insulin in a fasting diabetic will usually be spotted; but when it is due to a sudden release of insulin from an islet-cell tumour, it may be missed.

Prolonged coma following a head injury is sometimes attributable to brain stem damage. It may also result from a combination of cerebral trauma and cerebral hypoxia—due, for example, to aspiration of vomit during a period of concussion (see Table 5.1). There is also a state referred to as *vigil coma* or *persistent vegetative state*, in which the patient remains inert and unresponsive for months or even years; yet appears, from movements of the eyes, to have periods of alternating sleep and waking. Some such cases, following cardio respiratory arrest, show neuronal loss particulary affecting the thalamus.

Vertigo

True vertigo, as opposed to dizziness due to circulatory disturbances, is attributed to lesions in the vestibular system. These may be peripheral, as in Ménière's disease and acute labyrinthitis, or due to nerve damage by, for instance, an acoustic schwannoma, or central, involving the vestibular nuclei and their connections in the brain stem and cerebellum, as in the lateral medullary syndrome. Vertigo is nearly always associated with *nystagmus* (see above).

Visual disturbances

The common disorders of vision which may call for investigation by a neuropathologist include: loss of acuity in one eye or both, up to the point of total blindness; loss of vision in a particular visual field in one eye or both; loss of stereoscopic vision; double vision; and loss of the ability to interpret what one sees (visual agnosia), which is sometimes confined to loss of reading ability.

For a crude map of the visual pathways see Fig. 2.31, and p.47. The retina, which is developmentally a part of the brain, lies outside the usual scope of neuropathology. Not so the optic nerves, which should be taken in all cases of optic atrophy, from whatever cause, and in all cases with a history of optic neuritis or in which the diagnosis of MS has been suggested. In cases of double vision not attributable to congenital squints, the cause may be found to be an orbital tumour displacing the eyeball, or interfering with the third, fourth or sixth cranial nerves, or more proximally in the nuclei of these nerves (see Fig. 2.27), or in their intracranial course. The commonest site for such interference is probably in the side walls of the pituitary fossa, where they are at risk from tumours and from aneurysms of the internal carotid arteries. The optic nerves themselves are likewise at risk in this area, which is best explored by dissection, after fixation, of a block of the sphenoid bone, removed as described on p.3. Figure 24.8 and Fig. 3.32 show two uncommon causes of blindness from trouble in this region.

Causes of *bitemporal field loss* are to be looked for just in front of, or just behind, the optic chiasm. They are nearly always neoplastic. Causes of *homonymous field loss* are found on the side opposite the field defect, anywhere between the chiasm and the visual cortex. Causes of the various forms of *visual agnosia* are commonly due to vascular or neoplastic lesions in the white matter connecting the visual cortex with other parts, in particular the cortex of the parietal and temporal lobes (for a discussion of 'disconnection syndromes' see Geschwind 1965).

The raw material, so to speak, of vision is processed and re-processed in the retinae, in the lateral geniculate bodies, and in the striate cortex. Physiological research has revealed a certain amount about the further stages involved in *seeing*—that is, making sense of the visual input; but at present there is no more than a vague hope that neuropathology can contribute to the understanding of such disorders as colour anomia and visual agnosia. All we can suggest is that material which might in future be used to throw light on these subjects should be carefully preserved. For the anatomy of the visual system see Polyak (1957).

Further reading and references

Geschwind N. 1965. Disconnexion syndromes in animals and man. *Brain* **88**, 237–94, 585–644.
Polyak S. 1957. *The Vertebrate Visual System*. University of Chicago, Chicago.

Weakness

Weakness of limbs, trunk and cranially-innervated muscles is a common affliction in neurological practice. In searching for the pathological cause of weakness it is helpful to discover from the clinical notes whether it is general-

Fig. 24.8 An uncommon cause of blindness, in a hypertensive woman aged 83, with severe calcifying atheroma of the cerebral arteries. Both optic nerves (arrowed) are compressed by calcified internal carotid arteries.

ized or restricted to one side of the body or to one limb; and whether it is accompanied by spasticity and hyper-reflexia, or by flaccidity and reduced or absent reflexes. Spastic weakness and involvement of one side of the body usually point to damage to motor pathways in the CNS, while if weakness is flaccid and generalized there is usually damage in the periphery, in nerves or in the muscles themselves. Flaccid weakness is often accompanied by wasting of muscles. In motor neuron disease (p.271) both upper and lower motor neurons are affected, and the relative severity of damage to each will determine whether weakness is predominantly spastic (upper motor neuron damage) or flaccid (lower motor neuron damage), but both need to be examined at post mortem together with samples of muscles. In other cases of spastic weakness the causes are varied, and can be found anywhere from the cerebrum to the spinal cord. If a lesion such as a cerebral infarct is found that will account for the weakness experienced during life, there is no indication to examine peripheral nerves and muscles. Cases in which there is generalized flaccid weakness are likely to have suffered from one of the diseases discussed in Chapters 22 and 23, and require examination of spinal cord and samples of peripheral nerves and muscles. If eye muscles were clinically affected, these and their innervating nerves should be taken for histological examination (see also ophthalmoplegia, above).

25   Other Matters

Neuropathologists run little risk of developing *folie de gran-deur*. They need only to remind themselves that, whereas their clinical colleagues can manage quite nicely without their help, they are lost without theirs. Clinicians, of course, need someone to examine their patients' blood, pus, urine and CSF; but in many—perhaps most—centres these tasks are carried out by other kinds of pathologist. On the whole, clinicians assisted by radiologists, can judge for themselves what kind of tumour they are dealing with, whether the patient is losing his motor neurons, and what he finally dies of. Diagnostic neuropathologists, on the other hand, cannot function without raw materials, which are either supplied directly, as biopsy specimens, or steered in their direction after the patient's death, by clinicians. Their pronouncements are generally not treated as oracles, but taken into consideration in conjunction with the rest of the available evidence.

Relations with clinicians

Ideally, the relation between pathologist and clinician is a kind of symbiosis, or, using another analogy, a mystical brotherhood, reinforced by periodical 'love-feasts' in the form of slide-showing sessions and brain cuttings. These ceremonies are supposed to enable the clinicians to compare their previous guesses with the truths revealed by the microscope. In practice, they have a slightly different function—that of allowing the clinicians to recollect their patients in tranquillity, and to discuss with one another the merits of different lines of treatment. Pathologists may grow impatient with these debates, and may wish to recall attention to their carefully assembled slices and slides; but it is unwise to show this too openly. It is a still greater mistake to stress the point in cases where the clinician has got the diagnosis wrong. Pathologists who appear to exult in their superior cleverness are not quickly forgiven.

'Brain cuttings'

'Brain cuttings' is a term in general use for demonstrations of post mortem material. These are of two types. In the first, the pathologist, robed in a protective apron and armed with a long knife, listens to the clinical history, and the general discussion of possible diagnoses, before displaying the fixed brain and/or spinal cord and proceeding with the dissection and slicing of the specimens. Sometimes the diagnosis, previously in doubt, becomes clear at this point. At other times, it does not. Somebody says 'It will be interesting to see what the histology shows', and the discussion turns to the next case. In the second type, the brain and cord are cut up in the laboratory; blocks are taken, sections are stained, mounted, photographed, and reported on. Six months or more after the post mortem the case is demonstrated. The proceedings tend to begin with the query, 'Does anybody remember this case?'

Avoidance of delay

Delays of this magnitude can generally be avoided. The irreducible minimum is about three weeks—the time taken for fixation of the brain. In an interesting and complicated case, multiple blocks, and multiple stains, may be needed before the case can be adequately reported on; but for the simple purpose of making a diagnosis, a few may suffice. These few may be hurried through along with the current surgical specimens. Histological details may be demonstrated either with the aid of a projector—still better, if it can be afforded, by a closed-circuit television unit—or in the form of colour transparencies. Delays greater than about two months between post mortem and demonstration are rarely necessary.

A situation in which delay should be kept to a minimum is when the patient is a child with an undiagnosed progressive encephalopathy. A number of such patients turn out to have been suffering from a genetically determined disease—Leigh's encephalopathy, for instance, or a lipidosis, or a leucodystrophy. The author has more than once suffered remorse, having let some months elapse between making the diagnosis and issuing a report, only to learn that by the time the news reached the family doctor the child's mother was already pregnant again.

Reporting

In a letter to the General Assembly of the Church of Scotland in the year 1650, Oliver Cromwell is said to have written: 'I beseech you, in the bowels of Christ, think it possible you may be mistaken'. This admonition is as applicable to diagnostic pathology as it is to politics and religion. From time to time the pathologist receives a polite letter referring to one of his previous reports, giving details of the patient's subsequent progress, and enquiring whether, in the light of these, the pathologist would care to modify his earlier opinion. The response to such an enquiry should not be distorted by personal vanity. A rather more delicate situation arises when the pathologist is asked to review another pathologist's report. Here again the response should not be coloured either by loyalty or by malice. In any case, the author of the previous report should be told what the response has been.

Regarding biopsy reports, it is important that the pathologist should know what are the questions which the clinician wants answered. For instance, most surgeons will not be very interested in whether a particular meningioma is of syncytial or transitional type, but would like to know whether the tumour shows signs of transgressing its capsule and invading the brain.

Relations with other pathologists

In centres where neuropathologists and general pathologists work in close proximity, the importance of maintaining friendly relations between the two need hardly be stressed. If pathologists are aware of the research interests of each of their colleagues, exchanges of pathological material bring both scientific and social rewards. Often the question of shared post mortems arises, and it is important to avoid demarcation disputes by having agreed conventions about these. Situations where coroners' fees may be involved – in post mortems on cases of fatal head injury, for example – may call for some diplomatic delicacy.

It is also important to maintain good communications with pathologists in neighbouring areas. In the Oxford region, for example, there are a dozen or so hospitals with pathology departments, but only one teaching hospital with a department of neuropathology, associated with departments of clinical neurology, neurosurgery, neuroradiology, neurophysiology, and the rest. Clinicians from the centre pay regular visits to other hospitals in the region; patients are transferred to the centre for investigation and treatment, and subsequently returned to the regional hospital. If a patient dies, the clinicians in both places are likely to be interested in the outcome of the post

mortem. This may be arranged in various ways: for instance, the body may be transported to the centre, where the neuropathologist carries out the post mortem, and the body is returned; or the neuropathologist drives out to the regional hospital, where the post mortem is shared with the local pathologist; or the local pathologist does the post mortem, and keeps the relevant material, fixed in formalin, for the neuropathologist to deal with. This last is a good arrangement, but very dependent on good communication; in particular, on the local pathologist's knowledge of the neuropathologist's requirements in a particular type of case, and readiness to satisfy them. In a case diagnosed clinically as Friendreich's ataxia or motor neuron disease, the brain, unaccompanied by the spinal cord, is not really adequate. In return, neuropathologists must be ready to display their findings in a form which evokes the interest of the pathologist and their clinical colleagues. Failing this, a detailed histological report should be sent out with the least possible delay.

In this context, it is worth stressing the advantages of the practice of taking the spinal cord within the vertebral column, as described on p.4. Not only does this give access to spinal ganglia, roots, and sympathetic chain, it also preserves the cord from the hazards of unskillful dissection, and the further hazards of storage and transit. Besides, it involves the pathologist in less expense of time and effort than would the careful removal of the cord at post mortem.

It is hardly necessary to stress the importance to research of close communications between neuropathologists in their own and in other countries, and of awareness of what lines of research are being pursued at many different centres. One hears growls of criticism directed against the self-advertising antics observed at international congresses, but the value of the conversations over cups of inferior coffee in the intervals between sessions should not be underestimated.

Relations with laboratory staff

Pathologists should never forget how much their own success depends on good rapport with the laboratory staff. This involves being aware of the factors which may diminish that rapport. Perhaps the most important of these is the temptation to take their work for granted. The production of consistently good histological preparations requires not merely the application of an acquired technique, but the willingness to try again, with modifications of the technique, if it does not work well the first time. This willingness cannot be taken for granted; it has to be earned. In other words, pathologists must show that they really care about the result, and share the technician's delight when the result is good. Conversely, they must not let it be thought that they ask for sections to be cut, stained and mounted which they do not require, and which they do not trouble to examine. In practice, some skilled technicians are concerned about the aesthetic merits of their work rather than about the information derived from it, while others are keenly interested in pathological interpretations. Appreciation in the first case, and explanation in the second, will not be wasted. Finally, and most important, technicians' worries about health hazards must be taken very seriously. These may arise, for instance, over the handling of material from suspected cases of Creutzfeldt–Jakob disease, or about the toxic effects of exposure to aniline (used in the Holzer technique) or xylol (xylene), which is widely used as a clearing agent.

Behaviour in court

At this point we feel that for the sake of completeness we ought to make some recommendations to pathologists on how to behave in a court of law, including the coroner's court. As witnesses, we are enjoined, on oath, to tell the truth, the whole truth, and nothing but the truth; but this injunction cannot be taken literally. In general, the truth is an elusive thing, and what we are being asked for is our opinions. If we set out to tell the whole truth, we should only succeed in being tedious, irrelevant, and in most cases unintelligible to our audience. We do not favour telling downright untruths—for instance, that the cause of death in a case of closed head injury was a fractured skull; on the other hand, giving 'foraminal herniation' as a cause of death is not likely to enlighten a coroner's jury. We can only advocate the use of common sense, and of extreme wariness in answering a barrister's questions.

Indexing

A word is needed about the tedious but necessary business of indexing. We do not know how many different systems are in use, and are not in a position to recommend one rather than another. We are, however, in no doubt about what the system should achieve: in a word, accessibility. For our own convenience, we need an indexing system which gives each case a departmental (as opposed to hospital) number, assigned as soon as the material is received, which from then on will lead us to the jar in which the material is stored, the case notes and/or diagnostic report, the stored histological preparations, the black-and-white negatives and prints and colour transparencies of the case, and any correspondence relating to it. For dealing with enquiries from outside the department, we need an index of patients' names, with initials, ages and dates, with hospital and departmental numbers. Computerized databases run on stand-alone personal computers can be readily put to use by neuropathology departments and have more

than adequate storage capacity for the numbers of specimens they handle. Fax machines offer a rapid means of communicating biopsy results to surgeons that side-steps the delays of most hospital postal systems.

For research based on series of cases of particular conditions, a diagnostic index, though not essential, is extremely useful, and saves time in the long run. For this purpose many laboratories have adopted the classification of disease compiled by the American Medical Association (SNOMED: systematized nomenclature of medicine) as a basis. This index can be maintained either by the pathologists themselves, or by the departmental secretary. In the past we have tried it both ways, and are in no doubt that it is far better if the pathologists do the work themselves. This is particularly so for half-remembered, peculiar 'one-off' findings in old cases. The same applies to the indexing of photographs; one needs to know where to look for pictures illustrating particular points; and having found a suitable print, where to find the negative. Last and not least, there is the job of instructing each new departmental secretary in the intricacies of the filing system, and imparting a general understanding of what it is all about. Rapport with the secretary is hardly less important than rapport with the technicians.

The neuropathologist's role

The last few years have seen health services in all parts of the world rightly emphasizing the importance of obtaining value-for-money from those who deliver medical care, and concentrating their resources on proven diagnostic and treatment procedures. Post mortem examinations are not a top priority. Histopathologists concentrate on coping with ever larger surgical work loads while non-invasive imaging techniques seem to provide many of the answers that clinicians might previously have sought from pathologists. Is there a future, therefore, for neuropathologists in health services of the future? The answer is surely 'yes' while so many of the major diseases afflicting humans of all ages, from neonates to the elderly, have their basis in nervous system dysfunction. Until we understand a great deal more about these diseases neuropathologists will be needed to recognize and classify them and work with others to understand them better. They will perhaps need to organize and coordinate their work better than in the past, working in teams with clinicians to enable the details of clinico-pathological correlations to be worked out and to allow autopsy work to be focused where it can yield the greatest value. They will need to apply new techniques eagerly and grasp opportunities to extend the range of their investigations in response to clinicians' needs, and they will need to look critically at what they do and how they do it. But provided they do all these things neuropathologists will continue to have a role that extends from the local reporting of individual biopsies and teaching of medical students to national and international collaborations aimed at understanding neurological and psychiatric disease. And they also have a part to play in understanding normal human behaviour.

In our undoubtedly biased opinion, biology is the most interesting province of natural science. We think that animals are more interesting than plants, and that the most interesting thing about animals is their behaviour, and the complex of mechanisms giving rise to their behaviour. Doubtless, because we are ourselves human, we think that man is the most interesting animal of all. As matters stand, neurology and psychology are separate fields, and those who cultivate these two fields use different conceptual models and different terminologies. Yet both groups know that animal behaviour, including thinking and talking, depends on the functioning of a nervous system. They know that in theory their fields overlap, although in the present state of ignorance, the overlap—that is, the area sometimes referred to as neuropsychology—is pathetically small. At the same time it constitutes what we regard as one of the most enthralling parts of biological science. Working in

collaboration with practitioners in the clinical parts of these fields, there is now something worthwhile that the neuropathologist can do to enlarge the area of overlap. We hope that in future there will be more and better facilities for cooperative work involving psychologists, anatomists, physiologists, radiologists, chemists, pharmacologists and molecular biologists, with clinicians and pathologists playing their part.

The pleasures of problem-solving

The world will have to wait for answers to the really big questions in biology; in the meantime, there are thousands of little questions, a few of which lie within the power of neuropathologists to answer. For most of us, solving puzzles is fun. And the fun is enhanced if the solution—unlike the solution of a crossword puzzle—leads one on to further puzzles, calling for further solutions. Furthermore, there is the chance that the solution of little puzzles may in time contribute to the solution of bigger, and yet bigger, puzzles. We end, therefore, by wishing our readers fun, in the form of successful problem-solving.

Appendix A
Neurohistological Staining Methods

Most of the staining methods referred to in this book are described in the following commonly used textbooks of histopathological techniques.

1 Drury RAB, Wallington EA. 1980. *Carleton's Histological Technique*, 5th edn. Oxford University Press, Oxford.

2 Culling CFA. 1985. *Handbook of Histopathological Techniques*, 4th edn. Butterworth, London.

3 Bancroft JD, Stevens A. 1982. *Theory and Practice of Histological Techniques*, 2nd edn. Churchill Livingstone, Edinburgh.

4 Ráliš HM, Beesley RA, Ráliš ZA. 1973. *Techniques in Neurohistology*. Butterworth, London. (A useful neuro-histological textbook, unfortunately out of print at the time of writing.)

In what follows, details are given of a number of neurohistological techniques which are in common use in our laboratory. When a technique is already well known in general pathology, it is referred to with numbers (1, 2, 3 or 4) indicating which of the textbooks listed above contain details of the method. For some methods which have not yet reached the standard textbooks, references are given for published articles in journals.

Amyloid

Method
Congo Red.

Fixation
Not critical; formalin is satisfactory.

Sections
Paraffin or frozen, 10 μm.

Technique
1 Take sections down to 70% alcohol.
2 Stain in Congo Red in 0.2% potassium hydroxide in 80% alcohol for 25 minutes.
3 Wash in tap water.
4 Counterstain lightly with haematoxylin.
5 Blue.
6 Dehydrate, clear and mount.

Results
| Amyloid | pink |
| Nuclei | blue |

Astrocytes

Methods
Cajal's gold sublimate (1, 2, 3, 4).
Holzer (1, 2, 3, 4).
Mallory's phosphotungstic acid/haematoxylin (PTAH) (1, 2, 3, 4).
When using the PTAH method with surgical specimens we get better results by pre-mordanting in a solution of equal parts of potassium dichromate and acetic acid, as shown.

Fixation
Usually formalin.

Sections
Paraffin, 5–10 μm.

Technique
1 Take sections down to water.
2 Incubate in a 60°C oven for 60 minutes in a solution of equal parts of 5% acetic acid and 5% potassium dichromate.
3 Wash well in tap water to remove residual chromate.
4 Oxidize with 0.5% potassium permanganate for 3 minutes. *NB* This time must not be exceeded.
5 Remove potassium permanganate with 2% oxalic acid.
6 Wash well in tap water.
7 Stain for 5–6 hours in PTAH or overnight if PTAH is not fresh.

Results
| Glial fibres, myelin and astrocytes | slaty blue |
| Nerve cell bodies | pink |

Axons

Methods
Palmgren (1, 3, 4).
Schofield (1, 4).
Holmes (1, 2, 3, 4).
Marsland, Glees and Erikson (1, 2, 3, 4).
Palmgren, Holmes, and Marsland, Glees and Erikson methods are suitable for demonstrating axons in both CNS and PNS material. Schofield's is the method of choice for the demonstration of axons and nerve endings in muscle and other peripheral tissues.

Fat

The technique preferred in our laboratory is shown below.

Technique
1 Cut frozen formalin-fixed sections at 10 μm.
2 Mount on gelatinized slides or free-float.
3 Stain in 0.5% Oil red O in 60% triethyl phosphate for 15 minutes.
4 Wash in tap water.
5 Lightly counterstain with haematoxylin.
6 Blue.
7 Mount in glycerin jelly.

Results
Fat   red
Nuclei   blue
Myelin   pale pink

Fungi

Methods
Periodic-acid–Schiff reaction (PAS) (1, 2, 3).
Grocott (1, 3).

Glial fibres

Methods
Holzer (1, 3, 4).
PTAH (1, 2, 3, 4).
NOTE: in the Holzer method a frequent problem is the deposition on the section of granules of dark blue stain. If during differentiation under the microscope such deposits become visible, allow the section to dry completely. When it is dry, flood the section with pure aniline. The deposits are dissolved by the aniline, and can be seen to disperse. This step may be repeated if necessary. Differentiation is then continued as before.

NB Because of the use of aniline and chloroform, this technique should be performed only in a fume cupboard. Aniline is toxic in contact with skin, and gives off a poisonous vapour. (Threshold limiting volume (TLV) 5 p.p.m.). Inhalation or absorption causes headache, drowsiness and other troubles.

Inclusion bodies in Parkinson's disease

Method
Lendrum's phloxine tartrazine (1, 2, 3, 4).

Melanin

Method
Masson–Fontana (1, 2, 3, 4).

Muscle biopsy

The muscle biopsy should be received in the laboratory as soon as possible after removal from the patient, to prevent the loss of labile enzymes. We find that we can still attain good results after 30 minutes. For best results, ideally the specimen should measure about 3 × 1 × 1 cm with muscle fascicles running in the long axis. We cut the muscle, where possible, into segments, as shown in the figure. The shaded area (2) is reserved for EM. This area should have escaped surgical damage. Portions (1) and (4) are placed on a stiff card for about 10 minutes. The muscle will dry onto the card, and so avoid distortion. The card with the muscle attached is placed in formalin to fix. Portion (3) is placed on a cork disc in a small amount of Tissue Tek and then orientated, using a dissecting microscope if required, so that the fibres may be sectioned transversely. The cork disc is then placed on a freezing microtome chuck with a blob of Tissue Tek to hold it in place. The whole is then held by forceps in iso-pentane, which has been cooled with liquid nitrogen until it is viscous. This will prevent the formation of ice-crystal artefact, which sometimes occurs if muscle is placed directly into liquid nitrogen, owing to the production of an insulating pocket of nitrogen gas. Ten–fifteen seconds immersion should be sufficient: too short a period will allow ice-crystal artefact to form; too long may cause cracking. Sections are then cut in a cryostat at not more than 10 μm. If ice crystals have formed, they can be removed by allowing the tissue to come up to room temperature and then refreezing in chilled iso-pentane. The disadvantage of thawing and refreezing is that the muscle fibres swell and become more rounded. They do, however, keep their relative proportions and are easily identifiable. The histochemistry also appears to be unaltered.

Methods
Haematoxylin and eosin.
Fat — see above.
PAS.
PAS with glycogen digestion. } 0.25% celloidinized slides.
ATP pH 9.4.
NADH.
Gomori one-step trichrome pH 3.4 (1, 4).
Acid phosphatase (Gomori lead acetate method) — see below.

from which airborne particles are retained on a filter. Such a cabinet is best housed in a separate containment room, level 3, on the door of which is posted a biological hazard warning notice (Health and Safety Executive, 1991 (HMSO 1990a)). Blocks from brain slices for histological processing should be placed in formic acid for at least one hour following which they may be processed normally. Formic acid treatment has been found effectively to inactivate the CJD agent whilst retaining normal morphology of the tissue (Brown *et al.* 1990). Potentially HIV-infected material can be dealt with wearing gloves at containment level 2 (HMSO 1990b, 1991), at a designated, secluded and easily cleaned work bench which is always disinfected after use. All infected waste material must be autoclaved or disposed of by incineration. To destroy prions autoclaving needs to take place at 134°C for at least 18 minutes. After fixation blocks for paraffin embedding should be immersed in formic acid for five minutes.

With appropriate safety precautions established and regularly followed staff in a neuropathology laboratory can be reassured that there is negligible risk to health from their work. It is important to discourage unnecessary fear and anxiety. Most difficulty in our experience is encountered in pathology departments that have little or no exposure to infective cases. Under these conditions some personnel may, through ignorance, exaggerate the risks involved and cause unnecessary anxiety.

Further reading and references

Bell JE, Ironside JW. 1993. How to tackle a possible Creutzfeldt–Jakob disease necropsy. *J Clin Pathol* **46**, 193–7.

Brown P, Wolff A, Gajdusek DC. 1990. A simple and effective method for inactivating virus infectivity from formalin-fixed tissue samples from patients with Creutzfeldt–Jakob disease. *Neurol* **40**, 887–90.

Centers for Diseases Control. 1982. National Infections Study Report. US Department of Health and Human Services, Atlanta.

Committee on Health Care Issues of the American Neurological Association 1986.

Department of Health and Social Security. 1984. Report of the advisory group on the management of patients with spongiform encephalopathy (Creutzfeldt–Jakob disease (CJD)), Circular DA (84) 16 DHSS, London.

Department of Health, Scottish Home and Health Department, Department of Health and Social Services Northern Ireland and Welsh Office. 1991. Code of Practice for the prevention of infection in clinical laboratories and post mortem rooms, 2nd edn. HMSO, London.

HMSO. 1988. Control of substances hazardous to health regulations. HMSO, London.

HMSO. 1989. Monitoring strategies for toxic substances–Guidance. HMSO, London.

HMSO. 1990a. Advisory Committee on Dangerous Pathogens–Categorisation of pathogens according to hazard and categories of containment, 2nd edn. HMSO, London.

HMSO. 1990b. Advisory Committee on Dangerous Pathogens–HIV, the causative agent of AIDS and related conditions. HMSO, London.

HMSO. 1991. Safe working and the prevention of infection in clinical laboratories. HMSO, London.

HMSO. 1994. Health Services Advisory Committee. Precautions for work with human and animal transmissible spongiform encephalopathies. HMSO, London.

Index